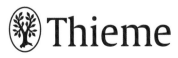

Flow Diversion of Cerebral Aneurysms

Min S. Park, MD
Director of the Endovascular Neurosurgery Fellowship and Associate Residency Program Director
Department of Neurosurgery
University of Utah Health
Salt Lake City, Utah

Philipp Taussky, MD
Section Chief of Neurovascular Surgery
Associate Professor
Chief Value Officer
Department of Neurosurgery
University of Utah Health
Salt Lake City, Utah

Felipe C. Albuquerque, MD
Director of the Endovascular Neurosurgery Fellowship and Associate Residency Program Director
Department of Neurosurgery
Barrow Neurological Institute
St. Joseph's Hospital and Medical Center
Phoenix, Arizona

Cameron G. McDougall, MD, FRCSC
Medical Director
Cerebrovascular Neurosurgery
Swedish Neuroscience Institute
Seattle, Washington

104 illustrations

Thieme
New York • Stuttgart • Delhi • Rio de Janeiro

Executive Editor: Timothy Hiscock
Managing Editor: Sarah Landis
Director, Editorial Services: Mary Jo Casey
Editorial Assistant: Nikole Connors
Production Editor: Naamah Schwartz
International Production Director: Andreas Schabert
Editorial Director: Sue Hodgson
Vice President, Editorial and E-Product Development: Vera Spillner
International Marketing Director: Fiona Henderson
International Sales Director: Louisa Turrell
Director of Sales, North America: Mike Roseman
Senior Vice President and Chief Operating Officer: Sarah Vanderbilt
President: Brian D. Scanlan

Library of Congress Cataloging-in-Publication Data

Names: Park, Min S. (Min Sik), 1975- editor. | Taussky, Philipp, editor. | Albuquerque, Felipe C., editor. | McDougall, Cameron G., editor.
Title: Flow diversion of cerebral aneurysms / [edited by] Min S. Park, Philipp Taussky, Felipe C. Albuquerque, Cameron G. McDougall.
Description: New York : Thieme, [2018] | Includes bibliographical references.
Identifiers: LCCN 2017022626| ISBN 9781626233867 (print) | ISBN 9781626233874 (e-ISBN)
Subjects: | MESH: Intracranial Aneurysm–therapy | Endovascular Procedures–methods | Neurosurgical Procedures–methods
Classification: LCC RC693 | NLM WL 355 | DDC 616.1/33–dc23 LC record available at https://lccn.loc.gov/2017022626

Thieme Publishers New York
333 Seventh Avenue, New York, NY 10001 USA
+1 800 782 3488, customerservice@thieme.com

Thieme Publishers Stuttgart
Rüdigerstrasse 14, 70469 Stuttgart, Germany
+49 [0]711 8931 421, customerservice@thieme.de

Thieme Publishers Delhi
A-12, Second Floor, Sector-2, Noida-201301
Uttar Pradesh, India
+91 120 45 566 00, customerservice@thieme.in

Thieme Publishers Rio de Janeiro, Thieme Publicações Ltda.
Edifício Rodolpho de Paoli, 25º andar
Av. Nilo Peçanha, 50 – Sala 2508
Rio de Janeiro 20020-906 Brasil
+55 21 3172-2297 / +55 21 3172-1896

Cover design: Thieme Publishing Group
Typesetting by DiTech Process Solutions

Printed in China by Everbest Printing Co.   5 4 3 2 1

ISBN 978-1-62623-777-3

Also available as an e-book:
eISBN 978-1-62623-387-4

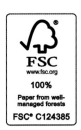

Important note: Medicine is an ever-changing science undergoing continual development. Research and clinical experience are continually expanding our knowledge, in particular our knowledge of proper treatment and drug therapy. Insofar as this book mentions any dosage or application, readers may rest assured that the authors, editors, and publishers have made every effort to ensure that such references are in accordance with **the state of knowledge at the time of production of the book.**

Nevertheless, this does not involve, imply, or express any guarantee or responsibility on the part of the publishers in respect to any dosage instructions and forms of applications stated in the book. **Every user is requested to examine carefully** the manufacturers' leaflets accompanying each drug and to check, if necessary in consultation with a physician or specialist, whether the dosage schedules mentioned therein or the contraindications stated by the manufacturers differ from the statements made in the present book. Such examination is particularly important with drugs that are either rarely used or have been newly released on the market. Every dosage schedule or every form of application used is entirely at the user's own risk and responsibility. The authors and publishers request every user to report to the publishers any discrepancies or inaccuracies noticed. If errors in this work are found after publication, errata will be posted at www.thieme.com on the product description page.

Some of the product names, patents, and registered designs referred to in this book are in fact registered trademarks or proprietary names even though specific reference to this fact is not always made in the text. Therefore, the appearance of a name without designation as proprietary is not to be construed as a representation by the publisher that it is in the public domain.

Contents

Foreword

The field of endovascular surgical neuroradiology is rapidly changing and advancing with new technology, innovations, and devices. The advent of flow diversion, however, represents a true paradigm shift in the treatment of cerebral aneurysms. Before flow diversion, our endovascular treatment of cerebral aneurysms could best be characterized as intrasaccular embolization, most notably utilizing coils. Additionally, other agents such as liquid embolics have been used. Advances in our field focused on the development of adjunctive devices and techniques (i.e., balloon microcatheters, stents) to enable intrasaccular embolization of wide-necked or other complex aneurysms.

Flow diversion, however, has shifted the paradigm from intrasaccular embolization to true luminal reconstruction. The parent artery is remodeled to resemble the native, undiseased vessel. Elegant computational flow dynamic studies followed by animal studies have demonstrated that flow diversion devices disrupt the pathologic flow into the aneurysm resulting in stasis, thrombosis, and the eventual occlusion of the aneurysm. The results from our collective experience are exciting and further advances in the future are promising. However, as with any innovation, questions and challenges remain.

What do you do when there is persistent aneurysm after flow diversion? The luminal reconstruction with the tight mesh design limits other options for treatment of a cerebral aneurysm; conventional intrasaccular embolization is no longer an option because the aneurysm orifice is now jailed by the flow diversion device. There is a broad spectrum of practices and very little evidence to support a treatment algorithm in this situation. Possible options include reducing dual antiplatelet treatment to monoplatelet treatment (usually stopping clopidogrel and continuing aspirin), placing additional flow diversion device(s), or proceeding to an open surgical procedure.

The optimal number of flow diversion devices remains in question. Should we place just one device at the initial treatment or use multiple devices until convincing intrasaccular contrast stasis is demonstrated? My practice has evolved from using multiple devices to now typically placing a single device when possible—reserving multiple devices generally for longer constructs.

The rate of delayed in-device stenosis or occlusion seems to be lower than what was seen in initial experiences, but still remains a concern. Additionally, the pathophysiology behind in-device stenosis is not completely understood.

The interval, frequency, and modality for re-imaging are varied among practices. Should one re-image at 6 months after flow diversion? 12 months? 3 months? Should we use digital subtraction angiography? Computed tomographic angiography (CTA)? Magnetic resonance angiography (MRA)?

While initial animal studies demonstrated the preserved patency of branch vessels jailed by flow diversion devices, there are multiples examples in the collective experience and in the literature of branch vessel occlusion on follow-up imaging. In certain instances (i.e., ophthalmic artery) the occlusion may be asymptomatic, but when devices cover other vessels (i.e., the posterior communicating artery or anterior choroidal artery) occlusion can result in neurologic deficit.

The need for dual antiplatelets presents a challenge particularly in the setting of subarachnoid hemorrhage or other instances when platelet inhibition is undesirable. Additionally, the use of flow diversion devices following aneurysmal subarachnoid hemorrhage is also limited by the delayed aneurysm occlusion that occurs with flow diversion. The risk of acute re-bleeding is a significant concern when using a device that does not immediately secure the bleeding source. As a result, I use flow diversion devices sparingly in acute subarachnoid hemorrhage.

This also raises the question as to the proper levels of platelet inhibition. Although we believe that dual antiplatelet therapy is necessary, this has not been definitively proven. Additionally, how long is it necessary? My practice is to continue dual antiplatelets for 6 months after placement of a flow diversion device, and then aspirin indefinitely. However, I am the first to admit that this approach has not been proven by a high level of evidence.

For those of us who use platelet inhibition assays to help guide dual antiplatelet therapy, there have been publications that supported specific target ranges of P2Y12 reaction units (PRU). However, we certainly do not have prospective randomized data to support these practices. But what if a therapeutic PRU cannot be achieved with aspirin and clopidogrel, the most commonly used dual antiplatelet combination? Practices vary widely and include increasing the dose of clopidogrel, or switching to other agents such as prasugrel or ticagrelor–but again, there is no consensus on the right strategy.

At the time of this writing, the Pipeline Embolization Device (PED, Medtronic) is currently the only FDA-approved flow diversion device in the United States and is only approved for large aneurysms in specific locations. Therefore, the on-label indications are limited. There is growing experience with the use of flow diversion devices in off-label locations such as the posterior circulation. While early experience in this location demonstrated intolerably high rates of complications with poor outcomes, we have seen improvements in morbidity and mortality with added experience. Thus, we are hopeful that the indications for use will be expanded in the future.

In its current form, flow diversion devices are not ideal to address bifurcation aneurysms, which are still some of the most common cerebral aneurysms encountered. While successful treatment of middle cerebral artery bifurcation aneurysms has been reported, I still have a great deal of trepidation jailing one limb of the MCA when treating aneurysms in this location.

The cost of flow diversion devices is also a nontrivial matter. Cost comparison analysis has demonstrated that flow diversion is more cost effective than primary coiling for larger aneurysm sizes, whereas smaller aneurysms are still more cost-effectively treated with coiling. We often require a large inventory of devices to account for the wide variety in size, shape, and location of aneurysms. Keeping this large of an inventory on hand can be financially prohibitive for some institutions.

There is a continued need to improve the navigability and ease-of-use of flow diversion devices. The second generation devices are certainly a welcome advance, but larger sizes are still stiff and can be challenging to navigate in tortuous anatomy. Additionally, deploying the flow diversion device from the advancer wire can still be quite finicky.

Editors Min S. Park, Philipp Taussky, Felipe C. Albuquerque, and Cameron G. McDougall and the contributors should be congratulated on assembling this insightful and comprehensive compendium on what is currently known and understood about flow diversion. The topic is timely and valuable to all of us practitioners. As with any innovation in our field, I am excited for what the future brings.

Brian L. Hoh, MD
James and Brigitte Marino Family Professor and Associate Chair
Chief, Division of Cerebrovascular Surgery
Lillian S. Wells Department of Neurosurgery at the
University of Florida
Gainesville, Florida

Preface

Practitioners of neurointerventional techniques have been fortunate to work in an era of rapid and exciting advances. From detachable balloons, to GDC coils, and most recently to the advent of flow diversion, those of us who practice in this sphere can experience multiple paradigm shifts over the course of a career. But despite its recent introduction, flow diversions has, rather quickly, become an accepted and required component to all of our practices and the raison d'etre for the existence of this book

While the first commercially available flow diverter in the United States was originally approved for only a small subset of cerebral aneurysms, recent experience has demonstrated its utility in treating a wider complement of aneurysms safely and efficaciously. The design of these devices, however, requires a rather significant departure from the techniques used in the deployment of other, non-braided stents. Additionally, the complications that we have all witnessed, firsthand or otherwise, can also be unique to these devices.

We have attempted to create an all-inclusive text on all things flow diversion for the neurointerventionalist learning to deploy a flow diverter for the first time to the seasoned veteran. Specific chapters are dedicated to the early history and design, illustrative cases, detailed deployment instructions of the most common devices, pre- and post-procedural management, and areas of current and future research and development. We harnessed the combined experience and knowledge from dedicated experts and leaders in the field in order to provide the reader with the best information currently available. We hope that you will perceive this as a worthwhile endeavor and find some piece of information in this textbook which helps you provide better and safer care for your patients.

Min S. Park
Philipp Taussky
Felipe C. Albuquerque
Cameron G. McDougall

Contributors

Peter Abraham, BA
Medical Student and Pre-Doctoral Clinical Researcher
Department of Neurosurgery
University of California, San Diego
San Diego, California

Amin Nima Aghaebrahim, MD
Interventional Neurologist
Department of Neurology
Baptist Health
Jacksonville, Florida

Pedro Aguilar-Salinas, MD
Research Associate
Lyerly Neurosurgery
Baptist Health
Jacksonville, Florida

Felipe C. Albuquerque, MD
Director of the Endovascular Neurosurgery Fellowship
   and Associate Residency Program
Director
Department of Neurosurgery
Barrow Neurological Institute
St. Joseph's Hospital and Medical Center
Phoenix, Arizona

Yaaqov Amsalem, MD
Director
Interventional Neuroradiology Unit
Rambam Health Care Center
Haifa, Israel

Adam S. Arthur, MD, MPH, FAANS, FACS, FAHA
Professor
Department of Neurosurgery
University of Tennessee Health Sciences Center and
   Semmes-Murphey Clinic
Memphis, Tennessee

Brandon Burnsed, MD
Cerebrovascular Fellow
Department of Neurosurgery
Semmes Murphy Clinic
University of Tennessee Health Science Center
Memphis, Tennessee

Or Cohen-Inbar, MD, PhD
Attending Physician and Neurosurgeon
Department of Neurological Surgery
University of Virginia
Charlottesville, Virginia
Department of Neurological Surgery
Rambam Health Care Center
Haifa, Israel

R. Webster Crowley, MD
Assistant Professor
Department of Neurosurgery and Radiology
Rush University Medical Center
Chicago, Illinois

Jason M. Davies, MD, PhD
Assistant Professor
Department of Neurosurgery
Jacobs School of Medicine and Biomedical Sciences
University at Buffalo, State University of New York
Department of Neurosurgery
Gates Vascular Institute/Kaleida Health System
Buffalo, New York

Andrew F. Ducruet, MD
Endovascular Neurosurgeon
Department of Neurosurgery
Barrow Neurological Institute
St. Joseph's Hospital and Medical Center
Phoenix, Arizona

David Fiorella, MD, PhD
Professor
Departments of Neurosurgery and Radiology
SUNY Stony Brook University Medical Center
Stony Brook, New York

Paul M. Foreman, MD
Resident
Department of Neurosurgery
University of Alabama at Birmingham
Birmingham, Alabama

W. Christopher Fox, MD
Associate Professor
Department of Neurosurgery
University of Florida
Gainesville, Florida

David Frakes, BSEE, MSME, MSEE, PhD BioE
Associate Professor
Department of Biological and Health Systems Engineering
Arizona State University
Tempe, Arizona

Douglas Gonsales, MD
Fellow
Department of Neurosurgery
Baptist Medical Center
Jacksonville, Florida

L. Fernando Gonzalez, MD
Assistant Professor
Department of Neurosurgery
Duke University
Durham, North Carolina

Bradley A. Gross, MD
Assistant Professor
Department of Neurological Surgery
University of Pittsburgh
Pittsburgh, Pennsylvania

Ricardo A. Hanel, MD, PHD
Neurosurgeon
Lyerly Neurosurgery
Baptist Health
Jacksonville, Florida

Mark R. Harrigan, MD
Professor
Department of Neurosurgery
University of Alabama at Birmingham
Birmingham, Alabama

Ryan Hebert, MD
Assistant Professor
Department of Neurosurgery
Yale University School of Medicine
New Haven, Connecticut

Pascal Jabbour, MD
Associate Professor
Department of Neurosurgery
Director
Division of Neurovascular Surgery and Endovascular
  Neurosurgery
Thomas Jefferson University Hospital
Philadelphia, Pennsylvania

M. Yashar S. Kalani, MD, PhD
Assistant Professor
Departments of Neurosurgery and Radiology
University of Utah School of Medicine
Salt Lake City, Utah

Alexander Khalessi, MD, FAANS
Director of Neurovascular Surgery
Acting Clinical Chief of Neurosurgery
Associate Professor of Surgery and Neurosciences
University of California, San Diego
San Diego, California

Louis J. Kim, MD
Professor
Department of Neurological Surgery
University of Washington School of Medicine
Seattle, Washington

Michael J. Lang, MD
Resident
Department of Neurosurgery
Thomas Jefferson University Hospital
Philadelphia, Pennsylvania

Avra Laarakker, MS
Ruth and Bruce Rappaport Faculty of Medicine
Technion-Israel Institute of Technology
Haifa, Israel

Elad I. Levy, MD, MBA, FACS, FAHA
Professor
Departments of Neurosurgery and Radiology
Jacobs School of Medicine and Biomedical Sciences
University at Buffalo, State University of New York
Department of Neurosurgery
Gates Vascular Institute/Kaleida Health System
Toshiba Stroke and Vascular Research Center
University at Buffalo, State University of New York
Buffalo, New York

Baruch B. Lieber, PhD
Professor
Department of Neurological Surgery
Cerebrovascular Center
State University of New York at Stony Brook
Stony Brook, New York

Marcus Mazur, MD
Resident
Department of Neurosurgery
Clinical Neurosciences Center
University of Utah
Salt Lake City, Utah

Cameron G. McDougall, MD, FRCSC
Medical Director
Cerebrovascular Neurosurgery
Swedish Neuroscience Institute
Seattle, Washington

Lynn B. McGrath Jr., MD
Resident
Department of Neurological Surgery
University of Washington
Seattle, Washington

Scott McNally, MD
Assistant Professor
Department of Neuroradiology
University of Utah Hospitals and Clinics
Salt Lake City, Utah

Bartley Mitchell, MD, PhD
Medical Director
Department of Endovascular Surgery
Moody Brain and Spine Institute
Methodist Dallas Medical Center
Dallas, Texas

Karam Moon, MD
Resident
Department of Neurosurgery
Barrow Neurological Institute
St. Joseph's Hospital and Medical Center
Phoenix, Arizona

Christopher J. Moran, MD
Professor
Department of Radiology
Division of Diagnostic Radiology
Neuroradiology Section
Department of Neurological Surgery
Washington University School of Medicine
St. Louis, Missouri

Priya Nair, PhD
Postdoctoral Research Assistant
Image Processing Applications Laboratory
Arizona State University
Tempe, Arizona

John D. Nerva, MD
Resident
Department of Neurological Surgery
University of Washington
Seattle, Washington

Christopher Nickele, MD
Assistant Professor
Department of Neurosurgery
Semmes Murphy Clinic
University of Tennessee Health Science Center
Memphis, Tennessee

J. Scott Pannell, MD
Assistant Professor
Department of Neurosurgery
University of California, San Diego
San Diego, California

Min S. Park, MD
Director of the Endovascular Neurosurgery Fellowship and
  Associate Residency Program
Director
Department of Neurosurgery
University of Utah Health
Salt Lake City, Utah

Shervin Rahimpour, MD
Resident
Department of Neurosurgery
Duke University
Durham, North Carolina

John Reavy-Cantwell, MD
Reynolds Associate Professor
Department of Neurosurgery
Director
Department of Endovascular/Interventional Neurosurgery
Virginia Commonwealth University
Richmond, Virginia

Dennis J. Rivet II, MD, FACS
Associate Professor
Department of Neurosurgery
Virginia Commonwealth University
Richmond, Virginia

Robert H. Rosenwasser, MD, MBA, FACS, FAHA
The Jewell Osterholm Professor and Chairman
Department of Neurological Surgery
President/CEO Vickie and Jack Farber Institute for
  Neuroscience
Jefferson Hospital for Neuroscience
Thomas Jefferson University
Philadelphia, Pennsylvania

Eric Sauvageau, MD
Neurosurgeon
Lyerly Neurosurgery
Baptist Health
Jacksonville, Florida

Philip G. R. Schmalz, MD
Resident
Department of Neurosurgery
University of Alabama at Birmingham
Birmingham, Alabama

Robert M. Starke, MD, MSc
Assistant Professor
Department of Neurosurgery and Radiology
University of Miami
Miami, Florida

Jeffrey A. Steinberg, MD
Resident
Department of Neurosurgery
University of California at San Diego
San Diego, California

William R. Stetler Jr., MD
Assistant Professor
Department of Neurosurgery
University of Alabama at Birmingham
Birmingham, Alabama

Michael F. Stiefel, MD, PhD, FAANS
Director, Capital Institute for Neurosciences
Director, Stroke & Cerebrovascular Center
Chief, Division of Neurosurgery
Capital Health System
Trenton, New Jersey

Philipp Taussky, MD
Section Chief of Neurovascular Surgery
Associate Professor
Chief Value Officer
Department of Neurosurgery
University of Utah Health
Salt Lake City, Utah

Stavrapola I. Tjoumakaris, MD
Associate Professor of Neurosurgery
Associate Residency Program Director
Fellowship Director of Endovascular Surgery & Cerebrovas-
  cular Neurosurgery
Director of Neurosurgery Clerkship
Thomas Jefferson University Hospital
Philadelphia, Pennsylvania

Edison P. Valle-Giler, MD
Vascular Neurosurgeon
Ochsner Healthcare System
New Orleans, Louisiana

Ajay K. Wakhloo, MD, PhD, FAHA
Professor
Departments of Radiology, Neurology, and Neurosurgery
University of Massachusetts Medical School
Division Neuroimaging and Intervention
New England Center for Stroke Research.
Worcester, Massachusetts

Arthur Wang, MD
Resident
Department of Neurosurgery
New York Medical College, Westchester Medical Center
Westchester, New York

1 THE BEGINNINGS OF FLOW DIVERSION: A HISTORICAL REVIEW

AJAY K. WAKHLOO and BARUCH B. LIEBER

Abstract

This chapter is a historical review of flow diverter (FD) development from its inception to clinical application. The journey spans two decades of in vivo and in vitro research in hemodynamics and engineering prior to the introduction of a reliable and safe technology in the endovascular treatment (EVT) of cerebral aneurysms. Encouraged by impressive results from early clinical studies on treatment for complex and non-treatable aneurysms, multiple medical device manufacturers have created FDs that currently are at various stages of clinical evaluation and approval. Experimental studies demonstrate that the device design influences the time required and location of endothelialization on the FDs and that circulating CD34 + progenitor cells participate in the endothelialization of the implant. FD treatment represents a significant paradigm shift in cerebral aneurysm treatment with the ability to remodel the diseased vessel segment and exclude the aneurysm from the circulation.

Keywords: aneurysm-parent-artery flow dynamics, cerebral aneurysms, Computational Fluid Dynamics (CFD), endovascular scaffold for endothelial growth, endovascular treatment (EVT), flow diverter porosity and pore density, laser-induced fluorescence (LIF), stents—flow diverters (FD), particle imaging velocimetery (PIV)

1.1 Introduction

The past nearly three decades of endovascular treatment (EVT) of intracranial aneurysms (IA) have demonstrated coiling to be superior to standard surgical treatment for ruptured and unruptured IA.[1,2,3] Thus globally, EVT is progressively replacing the latter. However, EVT occlusion rates remain highly dependent on aneurysm morphology and location, the coils used, and the operators' experience and skill.[2,3,4,5] Subsets of large, giant, and wide-neck aneurysms, fusiform and blister aneurysms, as well as aneurysms associated with segmental artery disease remain difficult to treat because of the significant risk of coil herniation from the aneurysm into the parent artery. Using EVT, a subtotal aneurysm occlusion, aneurysm regrowth, and/or recanalization remain a challenge in 20 to 80% of cases due to coil compaction and migration of coils into the aneurysm thrombus.[4,6,7] Previous *Computational Fluid Dynamics* (CFD) studies show that complex interaction between parent artery and aneurysm hydrodynamics induces significant forces on the coil mass.[8,9] These calculations demonstrate that a higher coil packing density and a lower permeability of the coil mass at a given packing density could promote faster intra-aneurysmal thrombosis due to increased blood residence time and potentially create a more stable and durable occlusion.

Adjunctive techniques, such as balloon-assisted EVT and intracranial stents, were introduced into the clinical realm to enable embolization of giant and wide-neck aneurysm and reduce recanalization with coils alone.[7,10,11,12,13,14,15,16,17] However, recanalization requiring retreatment remained a challenge in this subset of IA.[18,19,20] In addition, some aneurysms were amenable neither to EVT nor to a safe surgical repair.

To address these challenges in the early days of aneurysm embolization, research was conducted on a new treatment paradigm for IA that later became known as *flow diversion*. This chapter is a historical review of the development of *flow diverters* (FDs) from their inception to mature clinical products. The journey spanned nearly two decades of research and development prior to the introduction of a reliable and safe technology in one of the most challenging systems of the human body, the cerebrovasculature.

1.2 In Vivo Observations

Disappointing results with detachable latex and silicone balloons in the 1970s and the early generation of pushable coils in the late 1980s led several researchers to devise other solutions to circumvent existing challenges. Initially, Fedor Serbinenko[21] introduced detachable balloons for IA with preservation of the parent artery in 1974. His success and vast experience attracted the interventional neuroradiologist Gerard Debrun to visit and bring Dr. Serbinenko's techniques to Paris, France.[22,23,24,25] Other centers in Europe soon followed in his footsteps.

In the late 1970s, Grant Hieshima at the University of California Los Angeles (UCLA) developed silicone balloons. Later, his first fellow and colleague Randy Higashida at University of California San Francisco published their large series of IA successfully treated with detachable balloons.[25,26,27,28] Moret et al developed refinements in the technique to optimize position of the balloon in the aneurysm to achieve a more stable occlusion.[29,30] Unfortunately, these results were infrequently hampered by parent artery occlusion due to balloon rupture or migration resulting in thromboembolic ischemic events, as well as leak or rupture of the aneurysm due to a ball-valve mechanism created by movement of the balloon inside the aneurysm.

The next evolution in EVT of IA began more than a decade later. In the late 1980s, Fernando Vinuela at UCLA invited Guido Gugliemli from Italy to work in California. Joined later by Ivan Sepetka, these early pioneers developed the electrically detachable coil system from the bench to the bedside. Their work, however, relied on the development of a microcatheter that could be safely introduced into the cerebrovasculature and shapable tip microwire by Erik Engelson, a bioengineer at Target Therapeutics. This culminated in the first successful reported use of the Tracker microcatheter by Alex Berenstein and In Sup Choi at New York University in 1986.[31]

Target Therapeutics then began work on the first prototypes of Guglielimi's coils. In 1990, the first patient with a ruptured superior hypophyseal artery aneurysm was treated with this new technology under compassionate use at UCLA. Based on their experience, the Food and Drug Administration (FDA) approved the commercial sale of the Guglielmi detachable coils (GDCs) in 1995.

Simultaneously in 1989, Ajay Wakhloo was recruited by Martin Schumacher, department chief, to join as a junior attending physician in the Department of Neuroradiology at the University of Freiburg, Germany. It was there that Wakhloo was introduced to Hans Peter Strecker, a body interventional radiologist (IR) and inventor who was working in Karlsruhe, Germany, on a knitted tantalum stent for athero-occlusive disease of the peripheral circulation. Schumacher encouraged Wakhloo and his research team to further develop the stent technology for use in the cerebrovasculature. The tantalum stent, which was manufactured at the time by Boston Scientific Corporation (Watertown, MA) was a knitted tubular-shaped stent.[32,33] Owing to reports of increased intimal hyperplasia and frequent restenosis, tantalum was replaced by nitinol (▶ Fig. 1.1).[34]

In 1990, Wakhloo introduced the stent technology for stent-assisted EVT of IA with coils or balloons. His early observations were presented in 1992 at the 18th Congress of The European Society of Neuroradiology in Stockholm, Sweden (▶ Fig. 1.2).[36] Further experimental work was conducted in a canine model using bare and venous graft-covered tantalum and nitinol stents for occlusion of carotid aneurysms and arteriovenous fistulas, respectively. To assess the feasibility of the technology, venous pouch side-wall aneurysms were created in the canine common carotid arteries by Joost de Vries, as described previously by Varsos et al.[37] After a maturation period of 2 weeks, the balloon-expandable tantalum stents and self-expanding nitinol stents were placed through a transfemoral approach into the common carotid artery covering the aneurysm. The stent provided a scaffold through which a Tracker microcatheter could be advanced allowing for the deployment of the pushable coils. Due to lack of sophisticated delivery systems, the stents were mounted on a percutaneous transarterial (PTA) balloon (Schneider, Lausanne, Switzerland) for delivery. A crochet technique with nylon threads was used to anchor and deploy the stents.

The balloon-expandable tantalum stents were deployed in the carotid artery at an inflation pressure of 3 to 4 atmospheres and, in most cases, immediate postdeployment angiograms had no evidence of residual aneurysms (▶ Fig. 1.3). Follow-up angiograms demonstrated a complete and stable aneurysm

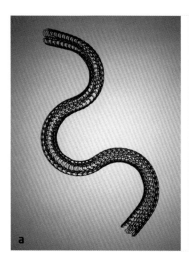
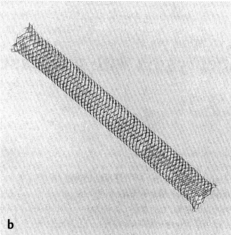

Fig. 1.1 (a) Fully expanded, 5 mm in diameter, self-expanding, nitinol-knitted Strecker stent (Boston Scientific Corporation, Watertown, MA) and (b) cobalt alloy Wallstent (Schneider, Minneapolis, MN, with permission from Geremia et al[35]) from 1992. The filaments have a diameter of 100 μm.

5 COATED AND NON-COATED STENTS FOR VESSEL RECONSTRUCTION AND TREATMENT OF ANEURYSMS AND AV-FISTULAS: AN EXPERIMENTAL STUDY

A.K. Wakhloo, MD, F. Shellhammer, J. de Vries, MD, J. Schumacher, MD, Departments of Neuroradiology and Neurosurgery, University of Freiburg, D-7800 Freiburg, Germany

Purpose of this study was to assess the efficacy of coated and non-coated endovascular prosthesis (stent) for reconstruction of carotid vessels.

Material and methods: 16 balloon-expandable and 10 self-expandable stents were placed in 12 labrador dogs with experimentally constructed carotid aneurysms and AV-fistulas. Non-coated tantalum and nitinol stents were introduced through a transfemoral approach for closure of 11 carotid aneurysms. For treatment of carotid-external jugular fistulas coated stents were used. The coating material consisted of fresh harvested autologous vein graft which covered the inside of the stent. The vein was fixed to the stent with 10-0 prolene sutures. In two cases the vein was attached with cyanoacrylate. In 8 cases lyophilized human vein graft covered the prosthesis. Control angiograms were obtained after 1 and 3 weeks and after 3, 6 and 9 months.

For histologic investigations the vascular prosthesis were explanted after 3 and 9 months.

Results: Except in 2 cases placement of non-coated stents lead to complete occlusion of aneurysms with patency of the carotid artery. The histopathologic examination revealed a thin layer of intimal fibrocellular proliferative tissue which covered the stent. The placement of coated stents showed an immediate closure of the AV-fistulas with patency of carotid artery. Histopathologic investigations showed no necrobiotic changes of the sutured autologous vein graft which seems to be nourished through capillaries arising from the adjacent arterial wall. Between the vein and the arterial intimal wall the stent was encased in fibrocellular tissue without significant narrowing of the vessel lumen. Lyophilized sutured vein graft and autologous vein attached with cyanoacrylate lead to an early and complete thrombosis of the endoprosthesis one week after the implantation due to immunologic rejection and distinct foreign-body reaction, respectively.

Conclusion: Non-coated stents may be promising in vessel reconstruction, e.g. in skull-base surgery and treatment of large carotid aneurysms. Stents inside coated with autologous vein graft showing a good biocompatibility may be excellent for vessel reconstruction as well as for treatment of fusiform aneurysms and large AV-fistulas.

Fig. 1.2 First published observation on bare stents for the treatment of aneurysm in a canine carotid side-wall aneurysm model.[36]

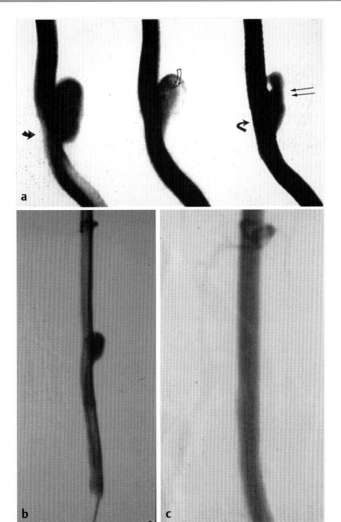

Fig. 1.3 Placement of a woven, knitted nitinol stent across a canine venous pouch side-wall aneurysm model. **(a)** Common carotid artery (CCA) angiogram shows a wide-neck aneurysm with associated narrowing of the CCA due to surrounding scar tissue (*arrow*). A typical flow pattern is seen within the aneurysm pouch (*open arrow*). Follow-up angiogram after deployment of a stent across the aneurysm neck (*curved arrow*) shows an incomplete aneurysm filling and change of inflow pattern and delayed contrast material washout (*double arrow*); a reduction of previously seen narrowing is noted due to radial force of the stent. **(b)** CCA angiogram before stent placement. **(c)** 6-month follow-up angiogram after stent placement shows lack of aneurysm filling (*continued*).

occlusion up to 9 months after the stent implantation. Over time, the stents became covered by a "thin layer of intimal fibrocellular proliferative tissue" on histologic specimens.[36] Macroscopic inspection also demonstrated aneurysm scarring and shrinkage (▶ Fig. 1.3). However, Turjman et al, in a porcine side-wall aneurysm model, described instances of incomplete aneurysm obliteration following deployment of the knitted stents, as well as instances of complete parent vessel occlusion.[38] Thus in 1994, Turjman et al recommended the combined use of coils and knitted stents.[39]

In 1994, Wakhloo et al proposed that the number of pores of a stent (higher number of pores = smaller pore

size) may determine the occlusion rates based on up to 9 months of follow-up studies in a canine aneurysm model, a finding that would become the basis to flow diversion.[34] Nitinol stents with a higher number of pores as compared with knitted tantalum Strecker stents (62.4 pores/cm^2 and 34.7 pores/cm^2 at 5 mm diameter, respectively) had less intimal buildup within the implant, but also increased the aneurysm obliteration rate at follow-up. A stent-induced regional flow alteration was suggested as a mechanism for the aneurysm thrombosis which was documented on high-frame rate digital subtraction angiography (DSA) at 4 to 6 frames/sec. DSA also showed that stent placement within the parent artery led to the redirection of contrast material toward the distal part of the artery, with decreased inflow into the aneurysm pouch and delayed contrast material washout due to *increased circulation time*.[34] These findings were described as *blood diversion or channeling effect* (▶ Fig. 1.4).

To prevent carotid thrombosis, the research specimens were treated with periprocedural heparin along with aspirin (80 mg/daily) in their diet for the duration of the study. In addition to *pore density*, the choice of the *stent alloy* was thought to be important to minimize in-stent intimal buildup.[34] In 1994, Geremia et al published their experience with self-expanding Wallstents (Schneider, Minneapolis, MN) in a canine carotid side-wall aneurysm model (▶ Fig. 1.1).[35] The cobalt alloy Wallstent, which was designed for use in peripheral athero-occlusive disease, was available premounted on a 7F delivery system. Unlike Turjman et al, the investigators found high aneurysm occlusion rates on follow-up angiography up to 2 months after stent implantation without any in-stent stenosis.[35] Hematoxylin and eosin staining revealed the presence of dense fibrous tissue within the aneurysm pouch (▶ Fig. 1.4). Immediately after stent placement, not only was delayed filling of the aneurysm observed but a *gradual puddling* of contrast medium was also noted. Vortex flow patterns as calculated previously by Perktold et al[40] in 1984 and observed by Steiger et al in 1987 in aneurysm models[41] and by Graves et al in a canine side-wall aneurysm model[42] was disrupted by placement of the stent. In this study, the carotid arteries remained patent despite lack of anticoagulation most likely due to the high fibrinolytic activity of the canine clotting system.

Besides the initial lack of availability of sophisticated stent delivery systems for the tortuous neurovascular circulation, another major challenge for the clinical use of stents to treat IAs was the preservation of critical perforators or side branches that are often intimately related to the aneurysm. Subsequently, the fate of those small vessels when covered by stents was studied using small muscle branches originating from the vertebral artery in a canine model.[43] Fortunately, no branch occlusions were observed angiographically during an observation period of 9 months after the stent implantation. Nearly a decade later, Kallmes et al and Sadasivan et al used the rabbit lumbar and vertebral arteries, respectively, as substitutes for perforators and side branches to assess mature FDs with high mesh densities in a preclinical setting (▶ Fig. 1.5).[44,45] The investigators did not report any branch occlusions, even in cases where several overlapping FDs were deployed.

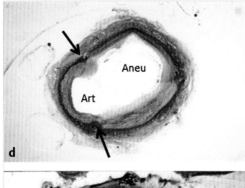
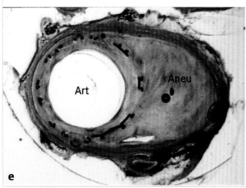
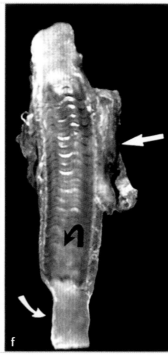

Fig. 1.3 (*continued*) **(d)** Cross-section of venous pouch side-wall aneurysm without a device. Note surgical sutures between artery and vein (*arrows*). **(e)** Cross-section through an aneurysm 6 months following a stent placement shows complete aneurysm thrombosis, circular remodeling of the artery, and endothelial coverage of the stent of various thickness. **(f)** Longitudinal section through the stented artery of a treated aneurysm shows endothelial coverage of the implant (*curved arrow*), scarring, and size reduction of aneurysm (*arrow*) (with permission from Wakhloo et al[34]).

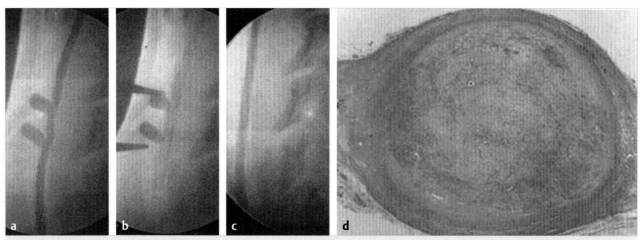

Fig. 1.4 Common carotid artery angiograms 2 weeks after surgical construction of venous pouch side-wall aneurysms in a canine model. **(a)** Two aneurysms are seen next to each other with a widely patent carotid artery. **(b)** Placement of a Wallstent covering both aneurysms with delayed washout of contrast medium. **(c)** Eight weeks after placement of the stent, both aneurysms are obliterated with patency of the carotid artery. **(d)** Cross-section through the bases of the aneurysms reveals dense fibrous tissue within aneurysm pouch (hematoxylin and eosin stain; with permission from Geremia et al[35]).

1.3 Principle of Flow Diversion: In Vitro and In Vivo Findings

Encouraged by these early amorphous, but compelling findings, Wakhloo and Lieber drove the development of endoluminal scaffolds for vascular reconstruction and coined them as *flow diverters* (▶ Fig. 1.6).[45,46,47] While stents were developed to support percutaneous transluminal angioplasty (PTA) in athero-occlusive disease and prevent arterial recoil, the FD was designed to serve a different objective: to create a stable aneurysm occlusion and

repair the diseased vessel segment. In the mid-1990s and early 2000s, a series of preclinical studies were performed to determine the optimum materials for device composition, to refine the device design to ensure consistent and complete vessel wall apposition, as well as to address the challenges of navigating through the tortuous neurovascular system. In addition, studies were designed to ensure optimization of the flow diversion effect and the device's long-term biomechanical stability.

CFD, as well as semiquantitative *laser-induced fluorescence* (LIF) followed by quantitative *particle imaging velocimetry* (PIV) methods, was utilized to refine and optimize the properties of

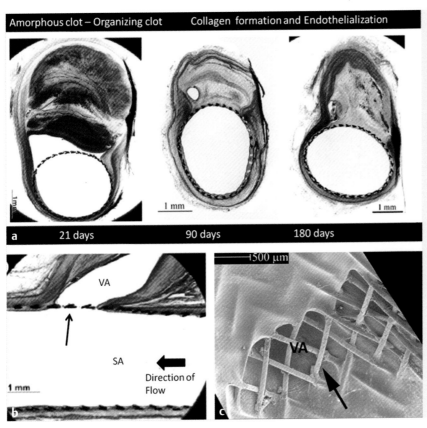

Fig. 1.5 Histology of rabbit elastase aneurysms after treatment with flow diverters (FDs) at various time points. **(a)** Amorphous clot is found initially within the aneurysm pouch. Progressive replacement of clot by collagen starting at the aneurysm perimeter toward the neck and endothelialization of the FD. **(b)** Patency of the vertebral artery (VA) that is covered by FD (*arrow*) and serves as surrogate for side branches. (Note: SA = Subclavian Artery) **(c)** SEM shows patency of the VA origin (*arrow*) and no endothelial coverage (with permission from Lieber and Sadasivan[46]).

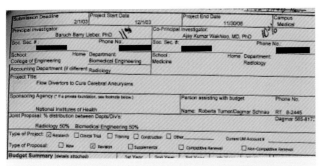

Fig. 1.6 National Institute of Health (NIH) project on "FD to cure aneurysms" and creation of the terminology *flow diverter* (2003).

the FD to ensure obliteration of the aneurysm with the preservation of critical perforators (▶ Fig. 1.7, ▶ Fig. 1.8, ▶ Fig. 1.9).[48,49,50] Two major parameters were found to be important for FDs to be hydrodynamically effective: (1) *porosity* and (2) *pore or mesh density* of the implant (▶ Fig. 1.10). The *in vivo* and *in vitro* hemodynamic studies indicated that fine tuning was required to balance the *porosity* (metal free/metal area) and *pore or mesh density* (number of pores/mm²) of the FD to optimize the effect on flow reduction within the aneurysm sac while keeping perforators and side branches patent.[46,51]

Flow diverters create a resistance to flow at the aneurysm neck and subsequently decrease the hydrodynamic circulation and the peak and mean kinetic energy transfer from the parent artery into the aneurysm with each pulse cycle. They also modify the predominantly convective flow to a more diffusive form.[53,54] As calculations demonstrate after FD placement, there is a reduction in shear rates at the aneurysm neck without a pressure increase within the aneurysm pouch (▶ Fig. 1.7).[49]

Experimental studies in 2009 showed that hydrodynamically optimized FDs placed in a rabbit elastase aneurysm model led to progressive aneurysm thrombosis, scarring, and finally endothelialization of the FD across the aneurysm neck.[46] Similar findings were reported by Kallmes et al with the pipeline embolization device (PED).[44] Importantly, Sadasivan et al discovered that to maintain consistent effect of FDs on reducing the momentum transfer between the parent artery and the aneurysm with each pulse cycle, the increased blood flow in larger arteries had to be taken into consideration.[45] Thus, to maintain a nearly consistent mesh density in various parent vessel diameters and to keep *mesh density* consistent over various implant sizes, the number of wires had to be increased.

Furthermore, the braid angle of the implant had to be designed to withstand any major deformation to maintain consistent mesh density across the neck, that is, minimize "herniation" of the construct into the aneurysm which would alter the device structure and change the effect on flow diversion, as recently shown by Raymond et al.[55] This eliminated the potential risk for areas of larger openings between struts or areas with higher metal density when deployed around tight bends. This may necessitate the use of multiple FDs to mitigate unwanted high impingement zones within the aneurysm pouch to minimize the risk for rupture.

In vivo evaluation in a rabbit elastase aneurysm model demonstrated that a progressive thrombosis of the aneurysm pouch occurs within the first 3 weeks with gradual transformation of

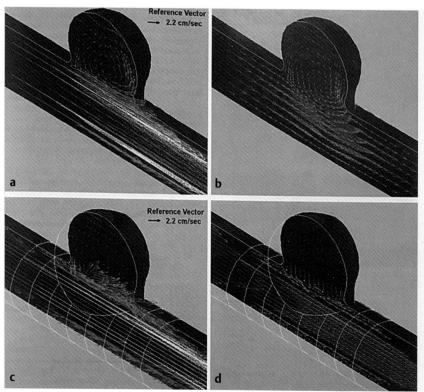

Fig. 1.7 Computational fluid dynamics (CFD) simulation in a straight stented and nonstented side-wall aneurysm model. Velocity profiles of nonstented and stented aneurysm models under pulsatile flow conditions at maximum (**a** and **c**) and minimum flow rates (**b** and **d**).

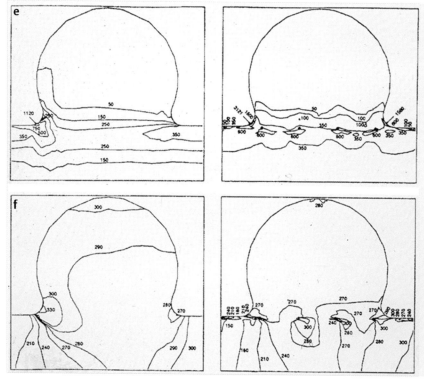

Fig. 1.7 (*continued*) (**e**) Shear rate distribution (dyne/cm^2) and (**f**) pressure distribution at the aneurysm neck during peak flow rate for nonstented (left) and stented (right) models (with permission from Aenis et al[49]).

the stable aneurysmal clot to collagen as the FD serves as a scaffold for endothelial growth (▶ Fig. 1.11).[46,55] This earlier thrombus formation enables the exclusion of the aneurysm sac from the circulation while remodeling of the parent artery occurs around the implant. Animal model testing of vertebral arteries or lumbar arteries that were covered by the implant and served as surrogate for intracranial side branches remained patent (▶ Fig. 1.12).[44,45,56]

A recently published study in a rabbit aneurysm model demonstrated that the device design influences the time required

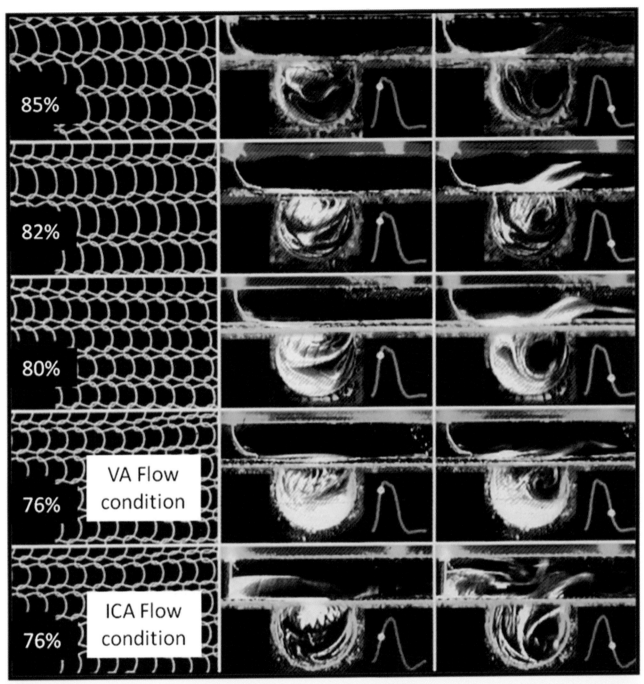

Fig. 1.8 Laser-induced fluorescence (LIF) study in a simplified side-wall aneurysm model. Knitted nitinol stents with various porosities (76–85% metal free/metal area, left panels) have been placed across the aneurysm. The flow condition is similar to that found in the vertebral artery (VA, upper four rows) and the internal carotid artery (ICA, lower row). A decrease in stent porosity (from top row to bottom row) leads to increased accumulation of laser dye inside the aneurysm during systole (center column) and diastole (right column). However, at same stent porosity (76%, lower panel), flow resumes within the aneurysm pouch under ICA as compared to VA flow conditions, indicating less effectiveness of the stent in higher flow environment (with permission from Lieber et al[50]).

and location of endothelialization on the FD. The investigators reported that circulating CD34 + progenitor cells participate in the endothelialization of the implant.[57] In recent years, additional modifications of FDs were tested in experimental models, including a low porosity PTFE patch on a self-expanding microstent and a thin film, high-mesh density nitinol FD. These modifications generally need a "carrier stent" as a base with the mesh attached to them. Because of the possibility of compromised vessel wall apposition, an endoleak of a hybrid system may be of potential concern.[58,59]

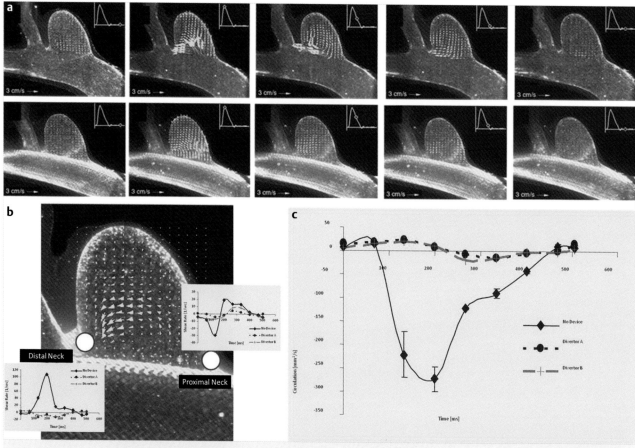

Fig. 1.9 Particle imaging velocimetry (PIV) in a silicone replica of a rabbit elastase aneurysm model. **(a)** Upper panel shows direction and magnitude of flow in the aneurysm during the entire pulse cycle before (upper panel) and after placement of a flow diverter (lower panel). Note change in flow magnitude and pattern. **(b)** Change in shear rate at distal and proximal aneurysm neck during the pulse cycle before and after placement of two different flow diverters (FDs). **(c)** Temporal evolution of intra-aneurysmal circulation before and after placement of two different FDs (with permission from Lieber et al[52]).

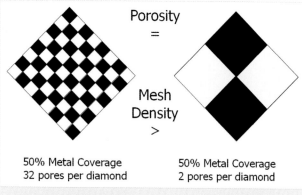

Fig. 1.10 Illustration shows equal porosities in both cases (50%, ratio of black and white) but different pore densities (×16 on the left as compared to the right; with permission from Lieber and Sadasivan[46]).

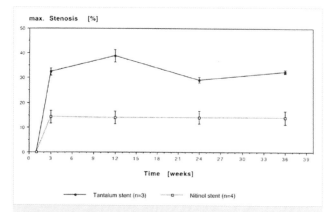

Fig. 1.11 Angiographic follow-up of stented common carotid artery aneurysms in a canine model. Higher intimal buildup and narrowing of the artery is seen with tantalum stent at 3 months with improvement on 6-month follow-up angiography as compared with nitinol self-expanding stent. Maximal narrowing of the vessel is seen at week 3 without any further progression (with permission from Wakhloo et al[34]).

1.4 Human Use of Flow Diverters

Encouraged by this research, early attempts were made to use coronary stents in conjunction with coils for IA.[60,61,62,63,64] However, owing to the lack of a sophisticated stent delivery system and access products for the tortuous neurovascular anatomy, as well as the absence of a dedicated neurovascular stent, nearly a decade passed before the first laser-cut stent from Smart

Therapeutics Inc. (San Leandro, CA) became available for intracranial use (▶ Fig. 1.13).[65]

Based on previous experimental studies, various companies embarked on the development and manufacturing of FDs for

clinical applications. As mentioned previously, the initial experience with stents in the cerebrovascular circulation was hampered by access to the tortuous cerebrovasculature with the existing technology.[44,66] However, improvements in plastics, catheter coating materials, laser etching and cutting, as well as in fine wire braiding enabled a more aggressive approach to the brain. The *Pipeline Embolization Device* (PED; Chestnut Medical Technologies, Menlo Park, CA), the first commercially available FD, received CE mark in June 2008 and entered the U.S. market after receiving an FDA approval on April 6, 2011.[67] Chestnut Medical was incorporated in 2000 by Aaron L. Berez, a neuroradiologist, to work on the Alligator, a foreign body–retrieval device. Berez joined Smart Therapeutics Inc. (San Leandro, CA), a startup company founded by Arani Bose, an interventional neurologist, that later was acquired by Boston Scientific Corporation (Natick, MA).

Later in 2003, Peter Kim Nelson joined Berez and Quang Tran, a biomedical engineer. After a few iterations, Alec Piplani (lead engineer at Smart Therapeutics Inc.) and Quang develop a 32-strand braided implant, which was later revised to a 48-strand implant.[56] The first patient treated with this device was in December 2005. Further improvements were made to the implant, as well as to the delivery system through 2007. The Marksman microcatheter was also specifically developed for delivery of the PED and used for the initial clinical trials. On June 2, 2009, ev3 Inc. (Plymouth, MN) announced a definitive agreement to acquire Chestnut Medical Technologies.

Surpass Medical Ltd. was founded in April 2005 by Ygael Grad, Barry B. Lieber, and Ajay K. Wakhloo and based in Tel Aviv, Israel, with manufacturing, research, and development located in Miramar, Florida. The company's focus was to develop the next generation of FD technology using cobalt chrome braided tubular mesh premounted on an over-the-wire delivery system. The *Surpass NeuroEndoGraft (NEG)* system was designed to treat large or giant wide-neck or fusiform IAs that are not amenable to surgical or current standard EVT due to location, morphology, or other risks factors. The NEG family of FDs with a nominal diameter of 2.5 to 5.3 mm and 48 to 96 cobalt chrome wires was tailored to the local flow environment. When placed in the parent artery, this FD redirects blood flow in a consistent and predictable fashion. The first patient was treated with Surpass in 2009 at the University of Heidelberg, Germany. Evaluated both preclinically and clinically, Surpass FD received a CE mark in the European Union in 2010.[68,69] The results of these evaluations demonstrated overall product safety and efficacy. In 2012, Stryker (Kalamazoo, MI) acquired Surpass Medical Ltd. A pivotal investigational device exemption (IDE) clinical study was conducted in the United States and in 2016, the SCENT study (The Surpass IntraCranial Aneurysm EmbolizatioN System Pivotal Trial to Treat Large or Giant Wide

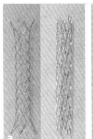

Fig. 1.12 (a,b) Placement of two overlapping flow diverters (FDs) with each 72-wire braid chromium cobalt in the rabbit aorta. (c) Both renal arteries and lumbar arteries are covered by FDs as seen on cone beam CT. (d) Three-month follow-up angiogram shows patency of lumbar and renal arteries without any flow compromise. (e,f) SEM of a lumbar artery covered by an FD.

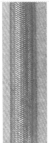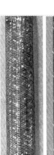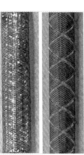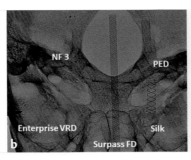

Fig. 1.13 (a) Examples of stents and flow diverters for clinical use. (b) Corresponding radiographs of selected implants. NF, Neuroform EZ; PED, Pipeline Embolization Device.

Neck Aneurysms) was completed. At the time of this writing, U.S. FDA approval was pending.

Encouraged by impressive results from the PITA and PUFS study on PED treatment for complex and nontreatable aneurysms, other medical device manufacturers in the neurovascular realm embarked on the development of their own FDs.[67,70] The *Silk* stent (Balt Extrusion, Montmorency, France) is made of 48-braided nickel-titanium (nitinol) strands with two radiopaque platinum markers of 35 μm. The device is a braided mesh cylinder with flared ends and provides a 35 to 55% metal coverage of the target vessels with a pore size of 110 to 250 μm at nominal diameter. The Silk stent system includes a self-expanding FD, a delivery system, and a reinforced catheter for its placement. The delivery procedure is similar to other self-expanding FDs and has the ability to resheath with up to 90% of the FDs deployed. The first patients were treated in 2009.[71,72,73] Silk subsequently received a CE mark in Europe, but currently does not hold an approval for commercial use in the United States.

The Flow-Redirection Endoluminal Device (FRED, MicroVention, Tustin, California) is a newer entry into FDs. FRED is composed of a dual-layer design consisting of a low-porosity inner mesh and a high-porosity outer stent and is placed through a microcatheter.[74] The first reported patient was treated in 2012.[75] Currently, a pivotal IDE clinical study is under way.

The *p64* (Phenox, Bochum, Germany) is a braided tubular implant consisting of 64 nitinol wires. Visibility under X-ray fluoroscopy is provided by two platinum wires wrapped around in a helix on the braided shaft. The 64 wires of the implant are grouped into 8 bundles proximally, each consisting of 8 individual wires. The ends of each bundle carry a radiopaque marker with a 0.5-mm length. The eight bundles are mounted onto a slotted crown on the distal end of a stainless steel delivery wire.[76]

The DERIVO FD (Acandis, Pforzheim, Germany) is made of nitinol composite wires with a platinum core for improved radiopacity. The device allows for the treatment of vessels with diameters ranging from 2.5 to 6.0 mm. The broad range of available FD sizes includes diameters from 3.5 to 6.0 mm and lengths from 15 to 50 mm (Acandis GmbH & Co. KG, Pforzheim, Germany).[77]

The Tubridge FD (MicroPort Medical Company, Shanghai, China) is a braided, self-expanding tubular implant similar to Silk and is available in various diameters (2.5–6.5 mm) and lengths (12–45 mm). The larger Tubridge is a braid of 62 nickel-titanium microfilaments and 2 platinum-iridium radiopaque microfilaments, while the small Tubridge (3.5 mm) is composed of 46 nitinol and 2 platinum-iridium microfilaments.[78]

The BRAVO FD (Codman Neurovascular, Raynham, MA) is a variable count, braided implant made of nitinol wires for optimized wall apposition, with platinum wires for radiopacity. The implant also has laser-cut nitinol expansion rings at each end for instant opening and accurate placement.[79] Currently, clinical information is not available.

1.5 Summary

Initial experimental observations and descriptions of the effect of stents on aneurysm flow in the early 1990s lead to the refinement of the tubular implants using innovative in vitro and in vivo experimental hydrodynamic studies leading to the development of flow diversion (FD). Since 2005, multiple medical device manufacturers have developed FDs that are currently at various stages of clinical evaluation and approval. Multicenter data continue to demonstrate an acceptable safety profile married with a high efficacy in the treatment of large, wide-necked IAs. Although the reported durability and high rate of progressive occlusion and ultimate obliteration of aneurysms are promising, longer-term follow-up studies are still needed. FD treatment represents a significant paradigm shift in brain aneurysm treatment with the ability to remodel the diseased vessel segment and exclude the aneurysm from the circulation.

References

[1] Molyneux A, Kerr R, Stratton I, et al. International Subarachnoid Aneurysm Trial (ISAT) Collaborative Group. International Subarachnoid Aneurysm Trial (ISAT) of neurosurgical clipping versus endovascular coiling in 2143 patients with ruptured intracranial aneurysms: a randomised trial. Lancet. 2002; 360 (9342):1267–1274

[2] Sluzewski M, van Rooij WJ, Slob MJ, Bescós JO, Slump CH, Wijnalda D. Relation between aneurysm volume, packing, and compaction in 145 cerebral aneurysms treated with coils. Radiology. 2004; 231(3):653–658

[3] Alshekhlee A, Mehta S, Edgell RC, et al. Hospital mortality and complications of electively clipped or coiled unruptured intracranial aneurysm. Stroke. 2010; 41(7):1471–1476

[4] Gallas S, Pasco A, Cottier J-P, et al. A multicenter study of 705 ruptured intracranial aneurysms treated with Guglielmi detachable coils. AJNR Am J Neuroradiol. 2005; 26(7):1723–1731

[5] Murayama Y, Nien YL, Duckwiler G, et al. Guglielmi detachable coil embolization of cerebral aneurysms: 11 years' experience. J Neurosurg. 2003; 98 (5):959–966

[6] Wakhloo AK, Gounis MJ, Sandhu JS, Akkawi N, Schenck AE, Linfante I. Complex-shaped platinum coils for brain aneurysms: higher packing density, improved biomechanical stability, and midterm angiographic outcome. AJNR Am J Neuroradiol. 2007; 28(7):1395–1400

[7] Raymond J, Guilbert F, Weill A, et al. Long-term angiographic recurrences after selective endovascular treatment of aneurysms with detachable coils. Stroke. 2003; 34(6):1398–1403

[8] Cha KS, Balaras E, Lieber BB, Sadasivan C, Wakhloo AK. Modeling the interaction of coils with the local blood flow after coil embolization of intracranial aneurysms. J Biomech Eng. 2007; 129(6):873–879

[9] Pierot L, Wakhloo AK. Endovascular treatment of intracranial aneurysms: current status. Stroke. 2013; 44(7):2046–2054

[10] Bendok BR, Parkinson RJ, Hage ZA, Adel JG, Gounis MJ. The effect of vascular reconstruction device-assisted coiling on packing density, effective neck coverage, and angiographic outcome: an in vitro study. Neurosurgery. 2007; 61 (4):835–840, discussion 840–841

[11] Moret J, Cognard C, Weill A, Castaings L, Rey A. Reconstruction technic in the treatment of wide-neck intracranial aneurysms. Long-term angiographic and clinical results. Apropos of 56 cases [in French]. J Neuroradiol. 1997; 24 (1):30–44

[12] Pierot L, Spelle L, Leclerc X, Cognard C, Bonafé A, Moret J. Endovascular treatment of unruptured intracranial aneurysms: comparison of safety of remodeling technique and standard treatment with coils. Radiology. 2009; 251 (3):846–855

[13] Pierot L, Cognard C, Anxionnat R, Ricolfi F, CLARITY Investigators. Remodeling technique for endovascular treatment of ruptured intracranial aneurysms had a higher rate of adequate postoperative occlusion than did conventional coil embolization with comparable safety. Radiology. 2011; 258(2):546–553

[14] Sluzewski M, van Rooij WJ, Beute GN, Nijssen PC. Balloon-assisted coil embolization of intracranial aneurysms: incidence, complications, and angiography results. J Neurosurg. 2006; 105(3):396–399

[15] Shapiro M, Babb J, Becske T, Nelson PK. Safety and efficacy of adjunctive balloon remodeling during endovascular treatment of intracranial aneurysms: a literature review. AJNR Am J Neuroradiol. 2008; 29(9):1777–1781

[16] Akpek S, Arat A, Morsi H, Klucznick RP, Strother CM, Mawad ME. Self-expandable stent-assisted coiling of wide-necked intracranial aneurysms: a single-center experience. AJNR Am J Neuroradiol. 2005; 26(5):1223–1231

[17] Biondi A, Janardhan V, Katz JM, Salvaggio K, Riina HA, Gobin YP. Neuroform stent-assisted coil embolization of wide-neck intracranial aneurysms: strategies in stent deployment and midterm follow-up. Neurosurgery. 2007; 61 (3):460–468, discussion 468–469

[18] Fiorella D, Albuquerque FC, Deshmukh VR, McDougall CG. Usefulness of the Neuroform stent for the treatment of cerebral aneurysms: results at initial (3–6-mo) follow-up. Neurosurgery. 2005; 56(6):1191–1201, discussion 1201–1202

[19] Mocco J, Snyder KV, Albuquerque FC, et al. Treatment of intracranial aneurysms with the Enterprise stent: a multicenter registry. J Neurosurg. 2009; 110(1):35–39

[20] Piotin M, Blanc R, Spelle L, et al. Stent-assisted coiling of intracranial aneurysms: clinical and angiographic results in 216 consecutive aneurysms. Stroke. 2010; 41(1):110–115

[21] Serbinenko FA. Balloon catheterization and occlusion of major cerebral vessels. J Neurosurg. 1974; 41(2):125–145

[22] Debrun G, Lacour P, Caron JP, et al. Experimental approach to the treatment of carotid cavernous fistulas with an inflatable and isolated balloon. Neuroradiology. 1975; 9(1):9–12

[23] Debrun G, Fox A, Drake C, Peerless S, Girvin J, Ferguson G. Giant unclippable aneurysms: treatment with detachable balloons. AJNR Am J Neuroradiol. 1981; 2(2):167–173

[24] Debrun G, Lacour P, Caron JP, Hurth M, Comoy J, Keravel Y. Inflatable and released balloon technique experimentation in dog – application in man. Neuroradiology. 1975; 9(5):267–271

[25] Berenstein A, Ransohoff J, Kupersmith M, Flamm E, Graeb D. Transvascular treatment of giant aneurysms of the cavernous carotid and vertebral arteries. Functional investigation and embolization. Surg Neurol. 1984; 21(1):3–12

[26] Higashida RT, Halbach VV, Hieshima GB, Weinstein PR, Hoyt WF. Treatment of a giant carotid ophthalmic artery aneurysm by intravascular balloon embolization therapy. Surg Neurol. 1988; 30(5):382–386

[27] Higashida RT, Halbach VV, Barnwell SL, et al. Treatment of intracranial aneurysms with preservation of the parent vessel: results of percutaneous balloon embolization in 84 patients. AJNR Am J Neuroradiol. 1990; 11(4):633–640

[28] Hieshima GB, Grinnell VS, Mehringer CM. A detachable balloon for therapeutic transcatheter occlusions. Radiology. 1981; 138(1):227–228

[29] Moret J, Boulin A, Mawad M, et al. Endovascular treatment of berry aneurysms by endosaccular balloon occlusion. Neuroradiology. 1991; 33-S:135–S136

[30] Moret J, Cognard C, Weill A, Castaings L, Rey A. The "remodelling technique" in the treatment of wide neck intracranial aneurysms: angiographic results and clinical follow-up in 56 cases. Interv Neuroradiol. 1997; 3(1):21–35

[31] Byrne JV. Endovascular Treatment of Intracranial Aneurysms. Berlin: Springer; 1998

[32] Matsumoto AH, Teitelbaum GP, Barth KH, Carvlin MJ, Savin MA, Strecker EP. Tantalum vascular stents: in vivo evaluation with MR imaging. Radiology. 1989; 170(3, Pt 1):753–755

[33] Strecker EP, Liermann D, Barth KH, et al. Expandable tubular stents for treatment of arterial occlusive diseases: experimental and clinical results. Work in progress. Radiology. 1990; 175(1):97–102

[34] Wakhloo AK, Schellhammer F, de Vries J, Haberstroh J, Schumacher M. Self-expanding and balloon-expandable stents in the treatment of carotid aneurysms: an experimental study in a canine model. AJNR Am J Neuroradiol. 1994; 15(3):493–502

[35] Geremia G, Haklin M, Brennecke L. Embolization of experimentally created aneurysms with intravascular stent devices. AJNR Am J Neuroradiol. 1994; 15(7):1223–1231

[36] Wakhloo AK, Shellhammer F,, De Vries J, et al. Coated and Non-Coated Stents for Vessel Reconstruction and Treatment of Aneurysms and AV-Fistulas: An Experimental Study. XVIIIth Congress of the European Society of Neuroradiology. Stockholm, Sweden; 1992

[37] Varsos V, Heros RC, DeBrun G, Zervas NT. Construction of experimental "giant" aneurysms. Surg Neurol. 1984; 22(1):17–20

[38] Turjman F, Acevedo G, Moll T, Duquesnel J, Eloy R, Sindou M. Treatment of experimental carotid aneurysms by endoprosthesis implantation: preliminary report. Neurol Res. 1993; 15(3):181–184

[39] Turjman F, Massoud TF, Ji C, Guglielmi G, Viñuela F, Robert J. Combined stent implantation and endosaccular coil placement for treatment of experimental wide-necked aneurysms: a feasibility study in swine. AJNR Am J Neuroradiol. 1994; 15(6):1087–1090

[40] Perktold K, Gruber K, Kenner T, Florian H. Calculation of pulsatile flow and particle paths in an aneurysm-model. Basic Res Cardiol. 1984; 79(3):253–261

[41] Steiger HJ, Poll A, Liepsch D, Reulen H-J. Basic flow structure in saccular aneurysms: a flow visualization study. Heart Vessels. 1987; 3(2):55–65

[42] Graves VB, Strother CM, Partington CR, Rappe A. Flow dynamics of lateral carotid artery aneurysms and their effects on coils and balloons: an experimental study in dogs. AJNR Am J Neuroradiol. 1992; 13(1):189–196

[43] Wakhloo AK, Tio FO, Lieber BB, Schellhammer F, Graf M, Hopkins LN. Self-expanding nitinol stents in canine vertebral arteries: hemodynamics and tissue response. AJNR Am J Neuroradiol. 1995; 16(5):1043–1051

[44] Kallmes DF, Ding YH, Dai D, Kadirvel R, Lewis DA, Cloft HJ. A new endoluminal, flow-disrupting device for treatment of saccular aneurysms. Stroke. 2007; 38(8):2346–2352

[45] Sadasivan C, Cesar L, Seong J, et al. An original flow diversion device for the treatment of intracranial aneurysms: evaluation in the rabbit elastase-induced model. Stroke. 2009; 40(3):952–958

[46] Lieber BB, Sadasivan C. Endoluminal scaffolds for vascular reconstruction and exclusion of aneurysms from the cerebral circulation. Stroke. 2010; 41(10) Suppl:S21–S25

[47] Lieber BB, Gounis MJ. The physics of endoluminal stenting in the treatment of cerebrovascular aneurysms. Neurol Res. 2002; 24 Suppl 1:S33–S42

[48] Tähtinen OI, Vanninen RL, Manninen HI, et al. Wide-necked intracranial aneurysms: treatment with stent-assisted coil embolization during acute (<72 hours) subarachnoid hemorrhage–experience in 61 consecutive patients. Radiology. 2009; 253(1):199–208

[49] Aenis M, Stancampiano AP, Wakhloo AK, Lieber BB. Modeling of flow in a straight stented and nonstented side wall aneurysm model. J Biomech Eng. 1997; 119(2):206–212

[50] Lieber BB, Stancampiano AP, Wakhloo AK. Alteration of hemodynamics in aneurysm models by stenting: influence of stent porosity. Ann Biomed Eng. 1997; 25(3):460–469

[51] Lieber BB, Livescu V, Hopkins LN, Wakhloo AK. Particle image velocimetry assessment of stent design influence on intra-aneurysmal flow. Amm Biomed Eng. 2002; 30(6):768–777

[52] Lieber BB, Livescu V, Hopkins LN, Wakhloo AK. Particle image velocimetry assessment of stent design influence on intra-aneurysmal flow. Ann Biomed Eng. 2002; 30(6):768–777

[53] Lieber BB, Sadasivan C, Gounis MJ, Seong J, Miskolczi L, Wakhloo AK. Functional angiography. Crit Rev Biomed Eng. 2005; 33(1):1–102

[54] Sadasivan C, Cesar L, Seong J, Wakhloo AK, Lieber BB. Treatment of rabbit elastase-induced aneurysm models by flow diverters: development of quantifiable indexes of device performance using digital subtraction angiography. IEEE Trans Med Imaging. 2009; 28(7):1117–1125

[55] Raymond J, Darsaut TE, Makoyeva A, Bing F, Salazkin I. Endovascular treatment with flow diverters may fail to occlude experimental bifurcation aneurysms. Neuroradiology. 2013; 55(11):1355–1363

[56] Kallmes DF, Ding YH, Dai D, Kadirvel R, Lewis DA, Cloft HJ. A second-generation, endoluminal, flow-disrupting device for treatment of saccular aneurysms. AJNR Am J Neuroradiol. 2009; 30(6):1153–1158

[57] Marosfoi M, Langan ET, Strittmatter L, et al. In situ tissue engineering: endothelial growth patterns as a function of flow diverter design. J Neurointerv Surg. 2016:neurintsurg-2016-012669

[58] Ionita CN, Natarajan SK, Wang W, et al. Evaluation of a second-generation self-expanding variable-porosity flow diverter in a rabbit elastase aneurysm model. AJNR Am J Neuroradiol. 2011; 32(8):1399–1407

[59] Ding Y, Dai D, Kallmes DF, et al. Preclinical testing of a novel thin film nitinol flow-diversion stent in a rabbit elastase aneurysm model. AJNR Am J Neuroradiol. 2016; 37(3):497–501

[60] Higashida RT, Smith W, Gress D, et al. Intravascular stent and endovascular coil placement for a ruptured fusiform aneurysm of the basilar artery. Case report and review of the literature. J Neurosurg. 1997; 87(6):944–949

[61] Lylyk P, Ceratto R, Hurvitz D, Basso A. Treatment of a vertebral dissecting aneurysm with stents and coils: technical case report. Neurosurgery. 1998; 43(2):385–388

[62] Sekhon LH, Morgan MK, Sorby W, Grinnell V. Combined endovascular stent implantation and endosaccular coil placement for the treatment of a wide-necked vertebral artery aneurysm: technical case report. Neurosurgery. 1998; 43(2):380–383, discussion 384

[63] Mericle RA, Lanzino G, Wakhloo AK, Guterman LR, Hopkins LN. Stenting and secondary coiling of intracranial internal carotid artery aneurysm: technical case report. Neurosurgery. 1998; 43(5):1229–1234

[64] Lanzino G, Wakhloo AK, Fessler RD, Hartney ML, Guterman LR, Hopkins LN. Efficacy and current limitations of intravascular stents for intracranial internal carotid, vertebral, and basilar artery aneurysms. J Neurosurg. 1999; 91(4):538–546

[65] Henkes H, Bose A, Felber S, Miloslavski E, Berg-Dammer E, Kühne D. Endovascular coil occlusion of intracranial aneurysms assisted by a novel self-expandable nitinol microstent (neuroform). Interv Neuroradiol. 2002; 8(2):107–119

[66] Wakhloo AK, Lanzino G, Lieber BB, Hopkins LN. Stents for intracranial aneurysms: the beginning of a new endovascular era? Neurosurgery. 1998; 43 (2):377–379

[67] Becske T, Kallmes DF, Saatci I, et al. Pipeline for uncoilable or failed aneurysms: results from a multicenter clinical trial. Radiology. 2013; 267 (3):858–868

[68] De Vries J, Boogaarts J, Van Norden A, Wakhloo AK. New generation of Flow Diverter (surpass) for unruptured intracranial aneurysms: a prospective single-center study in 37 patients. Stroke. 2013; 44(6):1567–1577

[69] Wakhloo AK, Lylyk P, de Vries J, et al. Surpass Study Group. Surpass flow diverter in the treatment of intracranial aneurysms: a prospective multicenter study. AJNR Am J Neuroradiol. 2015; 36(1):98–107

[70] Nelson PK, Lylyk P, Szikora I, Wetzel SG, Wanke I, Fiorella D. The pipeline embolization device for the intracranial treatment of aneurysms trial. AJNR Am J Neuroradiol. 2011; 32(1):34–40

[71] Kulcsár Z, Ernemann U, Wetzel SG, et al. High-profile flow diverter (silk) implantation in the basilar artery: efficacy in the treatment of aneurysms and the role of the perforators. Stroke. 2010; 41(8):1690–1696

[72] Lubicz B, Collignon L, Raphaeli G, et al. Flow-diverter stent for the endovascular treatment of intracranial aneurysms: a prospective study in 29 patients with 34 aneurysms. Stroke. 2010; 41(10):2247–2253

[73] Byrne JV, Beltechi R, Yarnold JA, Birks J, Kamran M. Early experience in the treatment of intra-cranial aneurysms by endovascular flow diversion: a multicentre prospective study. PLoS One. 2010; 5(9):5

[74] Möhlenbruch MA, Herweh C, Jestaedt L, et al. The FRED flow-diverter stent for intracranial aneurysms: clinical study to assess safety and efficacy. AJNR Am J Neuroradiol. 2015; 36(6):1155–1161

[75] Poncyljusz W, Sagan L, Safranow K, Rać M. Initial experience with implantation of novel dual layer flow-diverter device FRED. Wideochir Inne Tech Malo Inwazyjne. 2013; 8(3):258–264

[76] Fischer S, Aguilar-Pérez M, Henkes E, et al. Initial experience with p64: a novel mechanically detachable flow diverter for the treatment of intracranial saccular sidewall aneurysms. AJNR Am J Neuroradiol. 2015; 36 (11):2082–2089

[77] Akgul E, Onan HB, Akpinar S, Balli HT, Aksungur EH. The DERIVO embolization device in the treatment of intracranial aneurysms: short- and mid-term results. World Neurosurg. 2016; 95:229–240

[78] Zhou Y, Yang PF, Fang YB, et al. A novel flow-diverting device (Tubridge) for the treatment of 28 large or giant intracranial aneurysms: a single-center experience. AJNR Am J Neuroradiol. 2014; 35(12):2326–2333

[79] Marosfoi M, Langan E, King R, et al. E-005 aneurysm treatment with a new generation flow diverter. J Neurointerv Surg. 2016; 8(Suppl 1):A47

2 THEORETICAL BASIS OF FLOW DIVERSION

DAVID FIORELLA

Abstract

Flow-diverting devices induce a mechanical disruption of flow into and out of aneurysms which then induces physiological phenomena which lead to aneurysm thrombosis and endothelial overgrowth. Ultimately, these processes culminate in the anatomical reconstruction of the parent artery. These processes are directly affected by a complex interaction between the physical properties of the implanted flow diverter, the geometry of the parent artery–aneurysm complex, and the status of the coagulation system. We examine the existing data describing these interactions in reference to clinical practice.

Keywords: aneurysm, flow diverter, pore density, porosity, thrombosis

2.1 Introduction

Flow diverters are fine-mesh stents that are implanted in cerebral arteries at the site of aneurysms. They are so named because their primary function is to "divert" blood flow away from the aneurysm into the parent artery (strictly speaking, they reduce flow into and out of the aneurysm). The theoretical sequence of phenomena governing flow diversion treatment of aneurysms can be listed as follows: (1) the placement of a fine-mesh screen at the aneurysm neck reduces blood flow through the aneurysm, (2) the sluggish flow promotes clot formation within the aneurysm, (3) the fine-mesh screen is paved over by a new arterial wall lining, and (4) the thrombosed aneurysm is resorbed by the body's wound healing mechanisms—the end result of which is a remodeled vessel returned to its normal physiological state. These events are schematically described in ▶ Fig. 2.1. While it is a relatively straightforward list, needless to mention, the actual interplay of the various processes involved is quite complex. This chapter gives a brief overview of the therapeutic mechanism of flow diversion.

2.2 Device Mesh Structure

The mesh structure of flow diverters is crucial to their effective function; therefore, at the very least, a flow diverter's mesh needs to be far finer than that of a stent (▶ Fig. 2.2a). Because the device acts as a porous screen at the aneurysm neck, the characteristics of this porous media are defined by the mesh structure. Porous media are studied in a wide variety of fields, such as hydrogeology, petroleum engineering, ceramics, concrete, and textiles. In general, these fields evaluate two fundamental characteristics of the medium—porosity and pore connectivity—to assess the overall permeability.[1,2,3] While permeability is dependent on the porosity measure, it does not rely only on this variable.[3] For flow diverters, the two variables effecting device permeability and, by extension, device treatment efficacy can be termed as *porosity* and *pore density*. Porosity is the percentage ratio of the metal-free surface area (total surface area–metal surface area) to the total surface area. This is alternately referred to as metal coverage (ratio of metal surface area to total surface area). Pore density is number of pores per unit surface area of the device. Flow diverters are manufactured by braiding (helically wrapping multiple metal wires into a tubular structure) and the fundamental variables governing device design are the device diameter, the wire diameter, and the angle that the wires make to the device axis (called *braiding angle*). The nominal or design porosity and pore density of a device can be mathematically expressed in terms of these variables.

Using these mathematical expressions, theoretical variations in porosity and pore density of a characteristic flow diverter as it is deployed in arteries of varying diameter can be plotted (▶ Fig. 2.2b). Braiding allows for the device wires to slip on each other and thus elongate longitudinally when deployed in arteries with smaller diameter than the device's in-air diameter and, vice versa, expand in diameter when compressed longitudinally (such device "packing" at the aneurysm neck section is

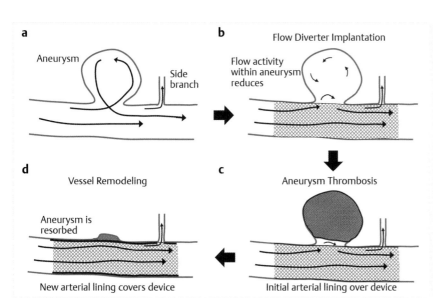

Fig. 2.1 Simplified schematic of the therapeutic mechanism of flow diversion treatment for aneurysms. **(a)** An aneurysm is **(b)** treated by implantation of a flow diverter, which reduces flow activity within the aneurysm, which **(c)** promotes clot formation within the aneurysm over hours to days; concurrently, a new arterial lining, called neointima, starts growing over the device. **(d)** Over weeks to months, the vessel remodels itself by resorbing the aneurysm along with completion of neointimal coverage of the device. While the aneurysm is essentially a "dead-end" clots off, the natural pressure gradient maintains blood flow through side branches covered by the mesh.

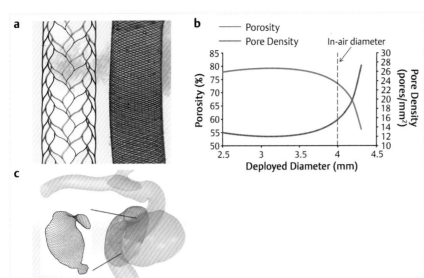

Fig. 2.2 **(a)** The different mesh structures of a flow diverter (Pipeline, right) and an intracranial stent (Enterprise, left) contribute to the difference in function of the devices. **(b)** Theoretical variation of porosity and pore density based on deployment diameter for a "typical" flow diverter with 48 wires, about 30-μm wire diameter, in-air device diameter (*dashed line*) of 4 mm, and approximately 70% porosity. These plots are characteristic of braided flow diverters. **(c)** Numerical simulation of a flow diverter deployed across a cavernous aneurysm shows the local variability that can exist in the pore structure at the aneurysm neck (inset; black border demarcates the aneurysm neck).

common practice when deploying some commercial flow diverters). While this feature allows for superior wall apposition in cerebral vessels of varying diameter, the deployed pore structure of a braided device, and hence its permeability at the aneurysm neck, will vary depending on parent vessel diameter, curvature, aneurysm neck size, etc. (▶ Fig. 2.2c). As the plots show, device oversizing can cause a maximal change (relative to designed values) in porosity and pore density of around 20 to 25% for most braided flow diverters. Whether this range effects aneurysm treatment efficacy is not yet clear, but a preliminary study[4] suggests that just a 3% absolute difference (~ 12% relative difference) in deployed device porosity can result in different aneurysm outcomes. The point of minimal efficacy (highest porosity and lower pore density) occurs when the angle between the wires is 90 degrees. On the other hand, radial expansion of the devices by longitudinal compression results in decreased device porosity and increased pore density.

2.3 Intra-aneurysmal Flow Alterations

Detailed evaluations of the changes in intra-aneurysmal hemodynamics due to flow diverters have mostly been conducted via in vitro and numerical studies.[5,6,7,8,9,10,11] The traditional or theoretical view of flow patterns in untreated idealized sidewall aneurysms holds that the parent artery flow divides or impinges at the distal neck of the aneurysm, follows the distal wall to the dome, and exits the aneurysm near the proximal neck (▶ Fig. 2.3a). This forms a vortex within the aneurysm that rotates opposite to the direction of flow in the parent vessel. Given the complexity and variability of patient aneurysm geometries, this flow pattern can vary substantially with the pulsatility and strength of the parent artery flow, aneurysm geometry and its orientation with respect to the parent vessel, and the presence of side branches at or near the aneurysm neck. Depending on these parameters, for example, there may be a single vortex with its center undulating (with the cardiac cycle) within the aneurysm and transiently entering the parent

vessel,[5,6] or the flow may divide after it enters the aneurysm and form regions with both clockwise and counterclockwise flow.[7,12] In general, and based mostly on numerical simulations, peak velocities ranging from 10 to 150% of the parent vessel velocity and average wall shear stress (shearing force per unit area exerted by fluid motion along the wall) values ranging from 10 to 220 dynes/sq.cm have been reported within aneurysms.[13]

The placement of a flow diverter across the aneurysm neck breaks up the in- and out-flow patterns. Intra-aneurysmal flow activity (optimally) becomes restricted to the neck region (▶ Fig. 2.3a, Pipeline device) and is generally in the direction of parent artery flow, entering near the proximal neck and exiting near the distal neck.[5,7,14,15] Most flow studies thus far have involved sparse, low sample sizes because of the computational expense required to numerically simulate flow fields in flow diverted aneurysms or the device expense involved with benchtop studies. Several intra-aneurysmal hemodynamic parameters have been evaluated, but the most common ones are related to flow velocity or its derivatives (inflow rate, average velocity, maximum velocity, kinetic energy [proportional to velocity squared], vorticity, and hydrodynamic circulation [velocity measures of rotational/vortical motion]); wall shear stress, a function of velocity gradient and viscosity, is another common parameter. Aggregating the results from about 20 flow studies on idealized, in vivo, and patient geometries (87 patient cases, half of which are from two studies[10,11]) suggests a spectrum of flow diversion response. Flow diversion reduces intra-aneurysmal flow activity in idealized/simplified sidewall-type geometries by about 75 to 95%,[7,16,17,18,19] in simplified bifurcation-type geometries by about 20 to 40%,[16,20] and in an in vivo aneurysm model by around 60%.[21,22] Reduction in intra-aneurysmal flow activity in clinical cases runs the entire gamut from around 20 to 30% in bifurcation geometries to around 80 to 90% in sidewall geometries with an average reduction of around 50 to 60%.[9,10,11,23,24,25,26,27,28,29,30]

While this class of studies measure detailed intra-aneurysmal velocity fields with the concomitant experimental or computational expense associated with trying to simulate reality,

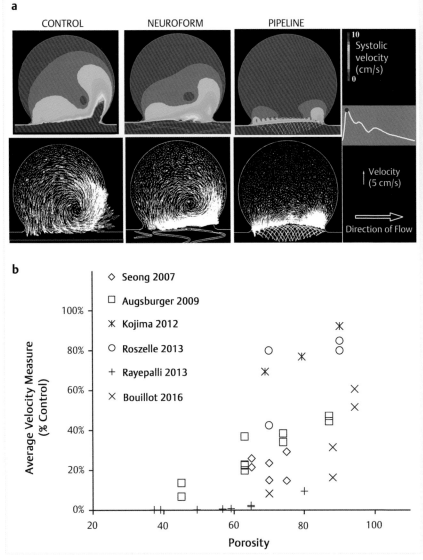

Fig. 2.3 (a) Computational fluid dynamic results (velocity magnitudes on top and vectors on bottom) of intra-aneurysmal flow during systole in a simplified sidewall aneurysm. The flow enters the distal neck in the un-stented (Control) case and forms a vortex within the aneurysm. Flow activity progressively reduces after implantation of a high-porosity stent (Neuroform) and a low-porosity stent (Pipeline). **(b)** Average velocity measures (as percentage of un-stented cases) from a few literature reports. Decreasing porosity is seen to reduce flow activity; data toward the bottom of the plot are from sidewall-type geometries, while those toward the top are from bifurcation-type geometries.

another category[31,32,33,34] evaluates the intra-aneurysmal transport of angiographic contrast from the images already being acquired during the endovascular procedure; these studies also note significant increases in contrast residence time measures after flow diversion. As a side consequence of this sluggish flow after flow diversion, intra-aneurysmal blood viscosity increases, especially near the aneurysm dome. Because blood is a non-Newtonian fluid, its viscosity increases with decreasing shear rate[35] (velocity gradient or change in velocity over a distance). A numerical simulation considering non-Newtonian effects in a simplified geometry suggests a threefold increase in blood viscosity in more than half of the aneurysm sac as compared to the nonstented case.[36] Another noteworthy phenomenon is that there is essentially no change in intra-aneurysmal pressure due to the deployment of a flow diverter.[37]

2.3.1 Effect of Pore Structure

The pore structure of a flow diverter primarily controls device-induced intra-aneurysmal flow alterations. As can be expected,

reducing device porosity can substantially reduce flow activity within the aneurysm as has been confirmed by numerous studies over the past two decades.[6,7,16,18,20,27,38,39] The numerical simulation results (▶ Fig. 2.3a) show an example of dampened flow activity within a simplified sidewall aneurysm from the deployment of devices with decreasing porosity. The vortical flow structure (and velocity magnitude) is slightly reduced after the deployment of a high-porosity stent (Neuroform), but is severely diminished after deployment of a flow diverter (Pipeline). ▶ Fig. 2.3b shows the collated results from a few studies evaluating the effect of porosity on aneurysmal velocities. While decreasing porosity clearly reduces flow activity, there is generally a wide spread in the degree of reduction depending on the geometry of the aneurysm–parent vessel complex. Flow diverter–equivalent porosities can induce near-stagnant flows in sidewall and/or low flow aneurysms, while the flow reductions in bifurcation and/or high-flow patient geometries are comparatively less. Increasing pore density of device while maintaining a constant porosity also results in reduced intra-aneurysmal flow activity.[7,14,39,40,41] Again, there is a wide variation in the results thus far and a very loose extrapolation from these studies on simplified geometries suggests that doubling the pore density (at constant porosity) can result in reduction of flow activity ranging anywhere between 20 and 150%.

It is unclear whether a "one-size-fits-all" porosity or pore density threshold exists that will result in successful occlusion of all aneurysms, but given that 1-year aneurysm occlusion rates after flow diversion are reasonably high (~ 90%), porosities and pore densities of current commercial devices can be considered to be more or less in the correct range. Needless to mention, any theoretical considerations of minimizing porosity and/or maximizing pore density need to be balanced against practical considerations such as additional metal-to-artery burden resulting in in-stent thrombosis, increased device stiffness resulting in difficulties with navigating tortuous vessels, as well as coverage of side-branch ostia resulting in perforator occlusions. As shown in ▶ Fig. 2.1, the physiological pressure gradient across perforators jailed by flow diverters maintains flow through these side branches and the rate of perforator infarction is thus only about 3%.[42] This is also supported by results from flow studies that have evaluated flow through side branches[7,17,43,44,45]; at maximum, flow diverters reduced the mean flow rate through the studied branches by 20%.

While the practice of "packing" flow diverter wires together at the aneurysm neck by longitudinal compression can theoretically improve flow diversion effects, there are precautions that must be considered during device deployment. In general, a uniform distribution of the pore structure covering the aneurysm neck will provide the most favorable flow diversion behavior. Marked differences in the pore structure can occur[46] and cause flow to preferentially enter the aneurysm through device segments with looser, more open pores and potentially lead to unfavorable results. The worst of these scenarios occurs when devices are mal-apposed to the arterial wall at the aneurysm neck resulting in a "jet"-type flow entry into the aneurysm from the gap between the device and the wall.[10,39] While more significant with stents,[20] flow diverters deployed across aneurysms at the outer curvature of vessels can have their pores spread open leading to increased flow activity within the aneurysm. A similar effect can occur when devices bulge into the aneurysm during device packing, causing pore structures to open up and increase intra-aneurysmal flow activity,[47] thus counteracting any beneficial effects of packing.

2.3.2 Predicting Aneurysm Occlusion

The primary goal of all these studies measuring intra-aneurysmal flow alterations is to derive flow-related parameters that can predict long-term aneurysm occlusion after flow diversion. If successful, such studies could facilitate optimal device selection prior to treatment and (the angiographic studies) could help modulate the treatment by assessing device efficacy in near-real time during the procedure. For example, ▶ Fig. 2.4 shows device-induced flow alterations in two right carotid aneurysms; the aneurysm with the 99% kinetic energy (KE) reduction was completely occluded at 6 months of follow-up, while the one

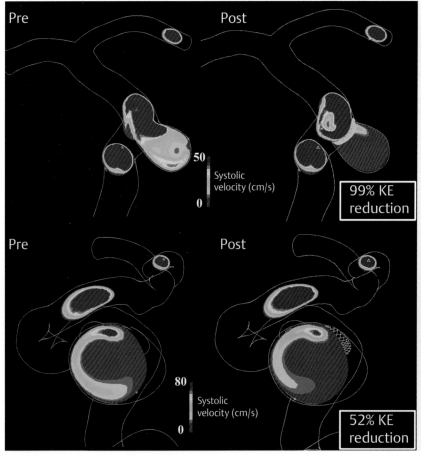

Fig. 2.4 Systolic velocity magnitudes in a right carotid superior hypophyseal (top) and a right carotid cavernous (bottom) aneurysm before (Pre) and after (Post) flow diversion treatment; the reductions in mean intra-aneurysmal kinetic energy (KE) are noted for each case.

with 52% KE reduction still had minimal residual filling at 6 months of follow-up. Sample sizes are, again, sparse but both in vivo[21,22,31,48] and clinical studies[9,10,23,49,50,51] have noted that the reduction in intra-aneurysmal flow activity (based on whichever variable the study chose to quantify) after flow diversion can be significantly different between aneurysms that remained patent at follow-up versus those that occluded at follow-up. Unfortunately, each research group chooses, even prefers, to define their own variable to define flow activity, and until some standard variables are evaluated by all laboratories on their patient datasets, it may be difficult to establish the index (indices) that is (are) able to predict long-term aneurysm occlusion after flow diversion. Such standardization will be required of both dominant paths of evaluation—angiographic analysis and numerical simulations—to establish a predictive index. Data are, however, being collected; for example, an aggregate of 95 patient cases (60 angiographic analysis[50,51] and 35 numerical simulations[10,23]) suggests a reasonably high predictive value of chosen indices, with specificity and sensitivity of around 75 to 90%.

While these results are promising, whether or not a purely flow-derived parameter will be able to predict aneurysm occlusion without the consideration of biological/biochemical parameters is unclear at this point. The incorporation of biochemical factors into flow studies is in the incipient stages.[52,53]

2.4 Vessel Remodeling

When arterial injury occurs, a series of molecular and cellular mechanisms is initiated to restore physiological function. This wound healing process is usually demarcated into four stages—thrombosis, inflammation, proliferation, and remodeling. Exposure of the sub-endothelial matrix causes a hemostatic thrombus plug to form at the site of injury via the extrinsic/tissue-factor pathway of coagulation. Thrombus constituents recruit leukocytes (e.g., by cell adhesion molecules on activated platelets), most notably neutrophils and monocytes, to the injury site to protect against infection. Monocytes differentiate into macrophages, which phagocytize thrombus constituents and apoptotic neutrophils, release anti-inflammatory cytokines toward the end of the inflammatory phase, and release cytokines along with platelets (such as transforming growth factor-β and fibroblast growth factor) that are involved in recruitment and proliferation of fibroblasts. Fibroblasts secrete collagen and other extracellular matrix components (such as glycosaminoglycans, proteoglycans, and fibronectin), thereby generating a scaffold for cell migration and organization. Differentiated fibroblasts, called *myofibroblasts*, can also exert traction (by expression of α-smooth muscle actin) and are thus crucial for wound contraction. Platelets, macrophages, and fibroblasts promote angiogenesis and neovascularization (such as by releasing platelet-derived growth factor and vascular endothelial growth factor). Macrophages and fibroblasts express metalloproteases that degrade the cellular/fibrous tissue in the remodeling or maturation phase. The tissue becomes increasingly acellular by apoptosis and migration and increasingly organized with replacement of immature collagen type III with collagen type I to eventually form a scar.

It should be noted that this is a brief and coarse description and the actual sequence of events involves a complex, coordinated interplay of overlapping feedback systems.[54,55,56,57] While the curative remodeling of the aneurysm–parent vessel complex following flow diverter implantation may not be identical to classical wound healing (especially the thrombosis and intra-aneurysmal organization stages[58,59]), it serves as a good guideline to explain the process.[60,61,62]

2.4.1 Changes within the Aneurysm

Within a period of hours to days after flow diverter deployment, the aneurysm is filled with acute thrombus (▶ Fig. 2.5a).

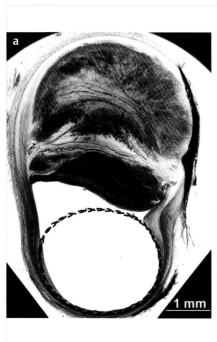

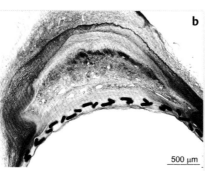

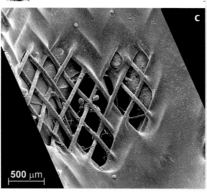

Fig. 2.5 Images from a rabbit aneurysm model showing **(a)** acute intra-aneurysmal thrombus at 21 days posttreatment; **(b)** by 180 days, the thrombus has organized to fibrous vascularized tissue with a complete neointimal lining covering the aneurysm ostium; **(c)** side-branch ostia are maintained patent with preferential coverage of the device struts.

While the mechanisms leading to aneurysm thrombosis are not entirely clear, the classical Virchow's triad requires the involvement of disrupted static flow, blood components, and dysfunctional wall, and a combination of these factors may very well be present in aneurysms after flow diversion. Separated flows (which occur when bulk flow cannot conform to the wall boundary) and/or stagnant/sluggish flow zones with concomitant low shear rates and long residence times are known to be prothrombotic. Thrombosis related to stagnant flow is observed in several vascular scenarios, such as atrial appendage thrombosis in patients with atrial fibrillation,[63] venous thromboembolism,[64] intraluminal thrombus in abdominal aortic aneurysms,[65] and spontaneous thrombosis of large/giant intracranial aneurysms.[66] Platelet aggregation at low shear rates is primarily due to cross-linkage of platelet surface integrins mediated by soluble fibrinogen,[67] and aggregation is preferentially seen in the separated flow region distal to arterial stenosis.[68] In vitro studies on flow past sudden expansions (causing separated flow) show increased adsorption of fibrinogen in the separated flow region[69] and increased thrombin production.[70] In vitro studies show significantly higher clot production at low shear rates than at high shear rates[71,72] and initiation of coagulation only below a threshold shear rate value[73]; shear rate amplitudes also seem to be statistically lower in cerebral aneurysms with spontaneous thrombosis than those without thrombosis.[66] To the extent that intracranial aneurysms are formed due to arterial wall degradation, the wall and endothelial lining can be dysfunctional,[74] predisposing the wall to thrombosis.[66] Putatively, activated platelets and/or prothrombotic factors generated at the flow diverter mesh covering the aneurysm neck can be washed into the aneurysm body, where the high residence time facilitates coagulation.

Over a period of weeks to months, the thrombus undergoes organization to fibrous scar tissue (▶ Fig. 2.5b) via mechanisms similar to those described earlier for wound healing and the aneurysmal structure is eventually resorbed. This organization proceeds from the periphery/wall of the aneurysm toward the center.[59] Myofibroblasts, for example, are seen to emanate from the periphery to infiltrate the thrombus[59,75]; myofibroblasts may be involved in the retraction of the aneurysm sac similar to their function in wound contraction.[76] Depending on the aneurysm–parent vessel complex, especially with large or giant aneurysms, thrombus organization may not occur as long as 1 year after flow diverter treatment.[77] Mechanically scraping the endothelial lining of venous pouch aneurysm models before parent vessel stenting has shown a four times greater aneurysm occlusion rate as compared to stenting only without denudation.[78]

2.4.2 Changes in the Parent Artery

A sequence of molecular and cellular interactions occurs on the luminal surface of the flow diverter, culminating in the formation of a new intimal lining (neointima) that covers the metallic surface (▶ Fig. 2.5b). The reactivity to the deployed foreign body depends on device surface characteristics at the molecular level that are a function of the crystallographic structure, surface defects, the metal finishing process, trace contaminants, and oxidation.[79,80] Initial interaction of the metal surface is via transient polar interactions with serum proteins, which alters protein conformation to expose and form more permanent nonpolar/hydrophobic interactions with other serum proteins that have intact structures and ligand sites to allow for cell interactions.[79,81] This protein layer develops over a period of seconds, as per the Vroman effect, through sequential adsorption and desorption of proteins with progressively higher affinity: albumin to globulin, fibrinogen, fibronectin, factor XII, and to high-molecular-weight kininogen, for example.[80,82,83] Depending on the magnitude and types of proteins adsorbed (of which fibrinogen may be the most important) as well as the conformational changes in the proteins, platelets as well as neutrophils adhere to the protein layer.[83,84] Activated factor XII initiates the coagulation cascade through the contact-activation or intrinsic pathway and along with common pathway interactions on activated platelet membranes,[82,85] and an amorphous platelet fibrin thrombus irregularly covers the metal surface over subsequent minutes.[79] Inflammatory, proliferative, and remodeling phases then occur similar to the description given earlier.[86] Growth factors released during the proliferative phase initiate the proliferation and migration of smooth muscle cells from the media into the developing neointima.[62,86] Endothelialization of the luminal surface of the neointima begins within days of device implantation with immature amorphous endothelial cells progressing to increasing coverage with fully mature, elongated cells oriented in the direction of flow over weeks to months.[87] Endothelial cell migration and proliferation is facilitated by growth factors (such as transforming growth factor, vascular endothelial growth factor) and occurs from sites with preserved endothelial lining toward sites of injury preferentially in the direction of flow[88,89]; thus, if the endothelial layer under the flow diverter is markedly degraded, reendothelialization must progress from the proximal and distal nontreated segments, delaying the healing process. Circulating (smooth muscle and endothelial) progenitor cells may be involved in neointimal endothelialization of the device as well as intra-aneurysmal thrombus organization,[90,91,92,93] but this is not yet clear.[94,95] The final neointimal thickness in rabbit arteries treated with flow diverters is around 100 to 200 μm.[96,97,98] Although the constituents of the neointima and its sequential organization are the same in animals as in humans, the time course to endothelialization and maturity may be significantly higher in humans (as much as five to six times longer, possibly in proportion to species longevity).[99]

The amount of thrombus deposited within the device is dependent on parent artery flow and more thrombus generated under lower flow is correlated with higher neointimal thickness; parent artery flow reduction by 25% has been shown to increase neointimal thickness by 50 to 100%.[100] Higher neointimal thickness has been observed on the slower flow inner curvature of stented arteries when compared to the higher flow outer curvatures,[101] and regions of higher neointimal thickness within stented regions correlate with regions of low wall shear.[102,103] Disturbed flow, low shear rate regions around stent struts can induce platelet aggregation[104] and thus poor apposition of stent struts to the vessel wall can result in acute to subacute stent thrombosis.[105] Stent thrombosis is of particular concern when devices are implanted in small arteries where the increased metal-to-artery burden may overwhelm the regular process of neointima formation and excessive thrombus occludes the vessel.[106]

Several in vivo and clinical studies have shown that, in general, side branches jailed by flow diverter implantation in the parent artery remain patent.[43,97,98,107] Although the incidence of reduced flow through side branches and ostial narrowing can be relatively high,[108] the rate of perforator infarction is reasonably low at about 3%.[42] Device struts covering side branch ostia are preferentially covered by endothelial cells in continuity with the neointimal lining (▶ Fig. 2.5c).[87,97,98] A similar process occurs at the aneurysm ostium where endothelialization (over a smooth muscle layer) of device struts proceeds from the adjacent parent artery.[94] Based on the deployed pore size at the ostium and low flow conditions created by the pressure gradient across the device struts, a complete neointimal lining occludes aneurysm ostia while the patency of side branch ostia is maintained.[109] Flow diversion treatment is then complete and the aneurysm parent–vessel complex is restored to a near-preaneurysmal state.

References

[1] Dullien FAL, Batra VK. Determination of the structure of porous media. Indust Engineer Chem. 1970; 62(10):25–53

[2] Koponen A, Kataja M, Timonen J. Permeability and effective porosity of porous media. Phys Rev E. 1997; 56(3):3319–3325

[3] Neithalath N, Sumanasooriya MS, Deo O. Characterizing pore volume, sizes, and connectivity in pervious concretes for permeability prediction. Materials Characterization. 2010; 61(8):802–813

[4] Jou LD, Chintalapani G, Mawad ME. Metal coverage ratio of pipeline embolization device for treatment of unruptured aneurysms: reality check. Interv Neuroradiol. 2016; 22(1):42–48

[5] Aenis M, Stancampiano AP, Wakhloo AK, Lieber BB. Modeling of flow in a straight stented and nonstented side wall aneurysm model. J Biomech Eng. 1997; 119(2):206–212

[6] Lieber BB, Stancampiano AP, Wakhloo AK. Alteration of hemodynamics in aneurysm models by stenting: influence of stent porosity. Ann Biomed Eng. 1997; 25(3):460–469

[7] Seong J, Wakhloo AK, Lieber BB. In vitro evaluation of flow diverters in an elastase-induced saccular aneurysm model in rabbit. J Biomech Eng. 2007; 129(6):863–872

[8] Stuhne GR, Steinman DA. Finite-element modeling of the hemodynamics of stented aneurysms. J Biomech Eng. 2004; 126(3):382–387

[9] Kulcsár Z, Augsburger L, Reymond P, et al. Flow diversion treatment: intra-aneurismal blood flow velocity and WSS reduction are parameters to predict aneurysm thrombosis. Acta Neurochir (Wien). 2012; 154(10):1827–1834

[10] Mut F, Raschi M, Scrivano E, et al. Association between hemodynamic conditions and occlusion times after flow diversion in cerebral aneurysms. J Neurointerv Surg. 2015; 7(4):286–290

[11] Larrabide I, Geers AJ, Morales HG, Aguilar ML, Rüfenacht DA. Effect of aneurysm and ICA morphology on hemodynamics before and after flow diverter treatment. J Neurointerv Surg. 2015; 7(4):272–280

[12] Liou TM, Liou SN, Chu KL. Intra-aneurysmal flow with helix and mesh stent placement across side-wall aneurysm pore of a straight parent vessel. J Biomech Eng. 2004; 126(1):36–43

[13] Sadasivan C, Fiorella DJ, Woo HH, Lieber BB. Physical factors effecting cerebral aneurysm pathophysiology. Ann Biomed Eng. 2013; 41(7):1347–1365

[14] Lieber BB, Livescu V, Hopkins LN, Wakhloo AK. Particle image velocimetry assessment of stent design influence on intra-aneurysmal flow. Ann Biomed Eng. 2002; 30(6):768–777

[15] Yu SC, Zhao JB. A steady flow analysis on the stented and non-stented side-wall aneurysm models. Med Eng Phys. 1999; 21(3):133–141

[16] Seshadhri S, Janiga G, Beuing O, Skalej M, Thévenin D. Impact of stents and flow diverters on hemodynamics in idealized aneurysm models. J Biomech Eng. 2011; 133(7):071005

[17] Trager AL, Sadasivan C, Lieber BB. Comparison of the in vitro hemodynamic performance of new flow diverters for bypass of brain aneurysms. J Biomech Eng. 2012; 134(8):084505

[18] Bouillot P, Brina O, Ouared R, et al. Computational fluid dynamics with stents: quantitative comparison with particle image velocimetry for three

commercial off the shelf intracranial stents. J Neurointerv Surg. 2016; 8 (3):309–315

[19] Dennis KD, Rossman TL, Kallmes DF, Dragomir-Daescu D. Intra-aneurysmal flow rates are reduced by two flow diverters: an experiment using tomographic particle image velocimetry in an aneurysm model. J Neurointerv Surg. 2015; 7(12):937–942

[20] Roszelle BN, Gonzalez LF, Babiker MH, Ryan J, Albuquerque FC, Frakes DH. Flow diverter effect on cerebral aneurysm hemodynamics: an in vitro comparison of telescoping stents and the Pipeline. Neuroradiology. 2013; 55 (6):751–758

[21] Cebral JR, Mut F, Raschi M, et al. Analysis of hemodynamics and aneurysm occlusion after flow-diverting treatment in rabbit models. AJNR Am J Neuroradiol. 2014; 35(8):1567–1573

[22] Huang Q, Xu J, Cheng J, Wang S, Wang K, Liu JM. Hemodynamic changes by flow diverters in rabbit aneurysm models: a computational fluid dynamic study based on micro-computed tomography reconstruction. Stroke. 2013; 44(7):1936–1941

[23] Ouared R, Larrabide I, Brina O, et al. Computational fluid dynamics analysis of flow reduction induced by flow-diverting stents in intracranial aneurysms: a patient-unspecific hemodynamics change perspective. J Neurointerv Surg. 2016:neurintsurg-2015-012154

[24] Jing L, Zhong J, Liu J, et al. Hemodynamic effect of flow diverter and coils in treatment of large and giant intracranial aneurysms. World Neurosurg. 2016; 89:199–207

[25] Karmonik C, Chintalapani G, Redel T, et al. Hemodynamics at the ostium of cerebral aneurysms with relation to post-treatment changes by a virtual flow diverter: a computational fluid dynamics study. Conf Proc IEEE Eng Med Biol Soc. 2013; 2013:1895–1898

[26] Tsang AC, Lai SS, Chung WC, et al. Blood flow in intracranial aneurysms treated with Pipeline embolization devices: computational simulation and verification with Doppler ultrasonography on phantom models. Ultrasonography. 2015; 34(2):98–108

[27] Kojima M, Irie K, Fukuda T, Arai F, Hirose Y, Negoro M. The study of flow diversion effects on aneurysm using multiple enterprise stents and two flow diverters. Asian J Neurosurg. 2012; 7(4):159–165

[28] Janiga G, Daróczy L, Berg P, Thévenin D, Skalej M, Beuing O. An automatic CFD-based flow diverter optimization principle for patient-specific intracranial aneurysms. J Biomech. 2015; 48(14):3846–3852

[29] Shobayashi Y, Tateshima S, Kakizaki R, Sudo R, Tanishita K, Viñuela F. Intra-aneurysmal hemodynamic alterations by a self-expandable intracranial stent and flow diversion stent: high intra-aneurysmal pressure remains regardless of flow velocity reduction. J Neurointerv Surg. 2013; 5 Suppl 3: iii38–iii42

[30] Augsburger L, Reymond P, Rufenacht DA, Stergiopulos N. Intracranial stents being modeled as a porous medium: flow simulation in stented cerebral aneurysms. Ann Biomed Eng. 2011; 39(2):850–863

[31] Sadasivan C, Cesar L, Seong J, Wakhloo AK, Lieber BB. Treatment of rabbit elastase-induced aneurysm models by flow diverters: development of quantifiable indexes of device performance using digital subtraction angiography. IEEE Trans Med Imaging. 2009; 28(7):1117–1125

[32] Grunwald IQ, Kamran M, Corkill RA, et al. Simple measurement of aneurysm residual after treatment: the SMART scale for evaluation of intracranial aneurysms treated with flow diverters. Acta Neurochir (Wien). 2012; 154 (1):21–26, discussion 26

[33] Joshi MD, O'Kelly CJ, Krings T, Fiorella D, Marotta TR. Observer variability of an angiographic grading scale used for the assessment of intracranial aneurysms treated with flow-diverting stents. AJNR Am J Neuroradiol. 2013; 34 (8):1589–1592

[34] Struffert T, Ott S, Kowarschik M, et al. Measurement of quantifiable parameters by time-density curves in the elastase-induced aneurysm model: first results in the comparison of a flow diverter and a conventional aneurysm stent. Eur Radiol. 2013; 23(2):521–527

[35] Cho YI, Kensey KR. Effects of the non-Newtonian viscosity of blood on flows in a diseased arterial vessel. Part 1: Steady flows. Biorheology. 1991; 28(3–4):241–262

[36] Ohta M, Wetzel SG, Dantan P, et al. Rheological changes after stenting of a cerebral aneurysm: a finite element modeling approach. Cardiovasc Intervent Radiol. 2005; 28(6):768–772

[37] Tateshima S, Jones JG, Mayor Basto F, Vinuela F, Duckwiler GR. Aneurysm pressure measurement before and after placement of a Pipeline stent: feasibility study using a 0.014 inch pressure wire for coronary intervention. J Neurointerv Surg. 2016; 8(6):603–607

[38] Augsburger L, Farhat M, Reymond P, et al. Effect of flow diverter porosity on intraaneurysmal blood flow. Klin Neuroradiol. 2009; 19(3):204–214

[39] Rayepalli S, Gupta R, Lum C, Majid A, Koochesfahani M. The impact of stent strut porosity on reducing flow in cerebral aneurysms. J Neuroimaging. 2013; 23(4):495–501

[40] Yu CH, Kwon TK. Study of parameters for evaluating flow reduction with stents in a sidewall aneurysm phantom model. Biomed Mater Eng. 2014; 24 (6):2417–2424

[41] Lee CJ, Srinivas K, Qian Y. Three-dimensional hemodynamic design optimization of stents for cerebral aneurysms. Proc Inst Mech Eng H. 2014; 228 (3):213–224

[42] Brinjikji W, Murad MH, Lanzino G, Cloft HJ, Kallmes DF. Endovascular treatment of intracranial aneurysms with flow diverters: a meta-analysis. Stroke. 2013; 44(2):442–447

[43] Cebral JR, Raschi M, Mut F, et al. Analysis of flow changes in side branches jailed by flow diverters in rabbit models. Int J Numer Methods Biomed Eng. 2014; 30(10):988–999

[44] Hu P, Qian Y, Zhang Y, et al. Blood flow reduction of covered small side branches after flow diverter treatment: a computational fluid hemodynamic quantitative analysis. J Biomech. 2015; 48(6):895–898

[45] Tang AY, Chung WC, Liu ET, et al. Computational fluid dynamics study of bifurcation aneurysms treated with pipeline embolization device: Side Branch Diameter Study. J Med Biol Eng. 2015; 35(3):293–304

[46] Makoyeva A, Bing F, Darsaut TE, Salazkin I, Raymond J. The varying porosity of braided self-expanding stents and flow diverters: an experimental study. AJNR Am J Neuroradiol. 2013; 34(3):596–602

[47] Karunanithi K, Lee CJ, Chong W, Qian Y. The influence of flow diverter's angle of curvature across the aneurysm neck on its haemodynamics. Proc Inst Mech Eng H. 2015; 229(8):560–569

[48] Chung B, Mut F, Kadirvel R, Lingineni R, Kallmes DF, Cebral JR. Hemodynamic analysis of fast and slow aneurysm occlusions by flow diversion in rabbits. J Neurointerv Surg. 2015; 7(12):931–935

[49] Chong W, Zhang Y, Qian Y, Lai L, Parker G, Mitchell K. Computational hemodynamics analysis of intracranial aneurysms treated with flow diverters: correlation with clinical outcomes. AJNR Am J Neuroradiol. 2014; 35 (1):136–142

[50] Pereira VM, Bonnefous O, Ouared R, et al. A DSA-based method using contrast-motion estimation for the assessment of the intra-aneurysmal flow changes induced by flow-diverter stents. AJNR Am J Neuroradiol. 2013; 34 (4):808–815

[51] Gölitz P, Struffert T, Rösch J, Ganslandt O, Knossalla F, Doerfler A. Cerebral aneurysm treatment using flow-diverting stents: in-vivo visualization of flow alterations by parametric colour coding to predict aneurysmal occlusion: preliminary results. Eur Radiol. 2015; 25(2):428–435

[52] Malaspinas O, Turjman A, Ribeiro de Sousa D, et al. A spatio-temporal model for spontaneous thrombus formation in cerebral aneurysms. J Theor Biol. 2016; 394:68–76

[53] Peach TW, Ngoepe M, Spranger K, Zajarias-Fainsod D, Ventikos Y. Personalizing flow-diverter intervention for cerebral aneurysms: from computational hemodynamics to biochemical modeling. Int J Numer Methods Biomed Eng. 2014; 30(11):1387–1407

[54] Sindrilaru A, Scharffetter-Kochanek K. Disclosure of the culprits: macrophages-versatile regulators of wound healing. Adv Wound Care (New Rochelle). 2013; 2(7):357–368

[55] Tracy LE, Minasian RA, Caterson EJ. Extracellular matrix and dermal fibroblast function in the healing wound. Adv Wound Care (New Rochelle). 2016; 5(3):119–136

[56] Yamaguchi Y, Yoshikawa K. Cutaneous wound healing: an update. J Dermatol. 2001; 28(10):521–534

[57] Zielins ER, Atashroo DA, Maan ZN, et al. Wound healing: an update. Regen Med. 2014; 9(6):817–830

[58] Rouchaud A, Johnson C, Thielen E, et al. Differential gene expression in coiled versus flow-diverter-treated aneurysms: RNA sequencing analysis in a rabbit aneurysm model. AJNR Am J Neuroradiol. 2016; 37(6):1114–1121

[59] Lee D, Yuki I, Murayama Y, et al. Thrombus organization and healing in the swine experimental aneurysm model. Part I. A histological and molecular analysis. J Neurosurg. 2007; 107(1):94–108

[60] Darsaut T, Salazkin I, Ogoudikpe C, Gevry G, Bouzeghrane F, Raymond J. Effects of stenting the parent artery on aneurysm filling and gene expression of various potential factors involved in healing of experimental aneurysms. Interv Neuroradiol. 2006; 12(4):289–302

[61] Edelman ER, Rogers C. Pathobiologic responses to stenting. Am J Cardiol. 1998; 81 7A:4E–6E

[62] Virmani R, Farb A. Pathology of in-stent restenosis. Curr Opin Lipidol. 1999; 10(6):499–506

[63] Watson T, Shantsila E, Lip GY. Mechanisms of thrombogenesis in atrial fibrillation: Virchow's triad revisited. Lancet. 2009; 373(9658):155–166

[64] Walton BL, Byrnes JR, Wolberg AS. Fibrinogen, red blood cells, and factor XIII in venous thrombosis. J Thromb Haemost. 2015; 13 Suppl 1:S208–S215

[65] Basciano C, Kleinstreuer C, Hyun S, Finol EA. A relation between near-wall particle-hemodynamics and onset of thrombus formation in abdominal aortic aneurysms. Ann Biomed Eng. 2011; 39(7):2010–2026

[66] Ribeiro de Sousa D, Vallecilla C, Chodzynski K, et al. Determination of a shear rate threshold for thrombus formation in intracranial aneurysms. J Neurointerv Surg. 2016; 8(8):853–858

[67] Maxwell MJ, Westein E, Nesbitt WS, Giuliano S, Dopheide SM, Jackson SP. Identification of a 2-stage platelet aggregation process mediating shear-dependent thrombus formation. Blood. 2007; 109(2):566–576

[68] Nesbitt WS, Westein E, Tovar-Lopez FJ, et al. A shear gradient-dependent platelet aggregation mechanism drives thrombus formation. Nat Med. 2009; 15(6):665–673

[69] Mandrusov E, Puszkin E, Vroman L, Leonard EF. Separated flows in artificial organs. A cause of early thrombogenesis? ASAIO J. 1996; 42(5):M506–M513

[70] Fallon AM, Dasi LP, Marzec UM, Hanson SR, Yoganathan AP. Procoagulant properties of flow fields in stenotic and expansive orifices. Ann Biomed Eng. 2008; 36(1):1–13

[71] Schultz JS, Lindenauer SM, Penner JA, Barenberg S. Determinants of thrombus formation on surfaces. Trans Am Soc Artif Intern Organs. 1980; 26:279–283

[72] Spaeth EE, Roberts GW, Yadwadkar SR, Ng PK, Jackson CM. The influence of fluid shear on the kinetics of blood coagulation reactions. Trans Am Soc Artif Intern Organs. 1973; 19:179–187

[73] Shen F, Kastrup CJ, Liu Y, Ismagilov RF. Threshold response of initiation of blood coagulation by tissue factor in patterned microfluidic capillaries is controlled by shear rate. Arterioscler Thromb Vasc Biol. 2008; 28 (11):2035–2041

[74] Frösen J, Tulamo R, Paetau A, et al. Saccular intracranial aneurysm: pathology and mechanisms. Acta Neuropathol. 2012; 123(6):773–786

[75] Dai D, Ding YH, Kadirvel R, et al. A longitudinal immunohistochemical study of the healing of experimental aneurysms after embolization with platinum coils. AJNR Am J Neuroradiol. 2006; 27(4):736–741

[76] Brinjikji W, Kallmes DF, Kadirvel R. Mechanisms of healing in coiled intracranial aneurysms: a review of the literature. AJNR Am J Neuroradiol. 2015; 36(7):1216–1222

[77] Szikora I, Turányi E, Marosfoi M. Evolution of flow-diverter endothelialization and thrombus organization in giant fusiform aneurysms after flow diversion: a histopathologic study. AJNR Am J Neuroradiol. 2015; 36 (9):1716–1720

[78] Darsaut T, Bouzeghrane F, Salazkin I, et al. The effects of stenting and endothelial denudation on aneurysm and branch occlusion in experimental aneurysm models. J Vasc Surg. 2007; 45(6):1228–1235

[79] Palmaz JC. Intravascular stents: tissue-stent interactions and design considerations. AJR Am J Roentgenol. 1993; 160(3):613–618

[80] Palmaz JC. The 2001 Charles T. Dotter lecture: understanding vascular devices at the molecular level is the key to progress. J Vasc Interv Radiol. 2001; 12(7):789–794

[81] Simon C, Palmaz JC, Sprague EA. Protein interactions with endovascular prosthetic surfaces. J Long Term Eff Med Implants. 2000; 10(1–2):127–141

[82] Basmadjian D, Sefton MV, Baldwin SA. Coagulation on biomaterials in flowing blood: some theoretical considerations. Biomaterials. 1997; 18 (23):1511–1522

[83] Rao GHR, Chandy T. Role of platelets in blood-biomaterial interactions. Bull Mater Sci. 1999; 22(3):633–639

[84] Milleret V, Buzzi S, Gehrig P, et al. Protein adsorption steers blood contact activation on engineered cobalt chromium alloy oxide layers. Acta Biomater. 2015; 24:343–351

[85] Vogler EA, Siedlecki CA. Contact activation of blood-plasma coagulation. Biomaterials. 2009; 30(10):1857–1869

[86] Chaabane C, Otsuka F, Virmani R, Bochaton-Piallat ML. Biological responses in stented arteries. Cardiovasc Res. 2013; 99(2):353–363

[87] Schatz RA, Palmaz JC, Tio FO, Garcia F, Garcia O, Reuter SR. Balloon-expandable intracoronary stents in the adult dog. Circulation. 1987; 76 (2):450–457

[88] Sprague EA, Luo J, Palmaz JC. Endothelial cell migration onto metal stent surfaces under static and flow conditions. J Long Term Eff Med Implants. 2000; 10(1–2):97–110

[89] Stemerman MB, Spaet TH, Pitlick F, Cintron J, Lejnieks I, Tiell ML. Intimal healing. The pattern of reendothelialization and intimal thickening. Am J Pathol. 1977; 87(1):125–142

[90] Tesfamariam B. Endothelial repair and regeneration following intimal injury. J Cardiovasc Transl Res. 2016; 9(2):91–101

[91] Li ZF, Fang XG, Yang PF, et al. Endothelial progenitor cells contribute to neo-intima formation in rabbit elastase-induced aneurysm after flow diverter treatment. CNS Neurosci Ther. 2013; 19(5):352–357

[92] O' Brien ER, Ma X, Simard T, Pourdjabbar A, Hibbert B, ER OB. Pathogenesis of neointima formation following vascular injury. Cardiovasc Hematol Disord Drug Targets. 2011; 11(1):30–39

[93] Moldovan NI, Asahara T. Role of blood mononuclear cells in recanalization and vascularization of thrombi: past, present, and future. Trends Cardiovasc Med. 2003; 13(7):265–269

[94] Kadirvel R, Ding YH, Dai D, Rezek I, Lewis DA, Kallmes DF. Cellular mechanisms of aneurysm occlusion after treatment with a flow diverter. Radiology. 2014; 270(2):394–399

[95] Raymond J, Guilbert F, Metcalfe A, Gévry G, Salazkin I, Robledo O. Role of the endothelial lining in recurrences after coil embolization: prevention of recanalization by endothelial denudation. Stroke. 2004; 35(6):1471–1475

[96] Kallmes DF, Ding YH, Dai D, Kadirvel R, Lewis DA, Cloft HJ. A new endoluminal, flow-disrupting device for treatment of saccular aneurysms. Stroke. 2007; 38(8):2346–2352

[97] Sadasivan C, Cesar L, Seong J, et al. An original flow diversion device for the treatment of intracranial aneurysms: evaluation in the rabbit elastase-induced model. Stroke. 2009; 40(3):952–958

[98] Dai D, Ding YH, Kadirvel R, Rad AE, Lewis DA, Kallmes DF. Patency of branches after coverage with multiple telescoping flow-diverter devices: an in vivo study in rabbits. AJNR Am J Neuroradiol. 2012; 33(1):171–174

[99] Virmani R, Kolodgie FD, Farb A, Lafont A. Drug eluting stents: are human and animal studies comparable? Heart. 2003; 89(2):133–138

[100] Richter GM, Palmaz JC, Noeldge G, Tio F. Blood flow and thrombus formation determine the development of stent neointima. J Long Term Eff Med Implants. 2000; 10(1–2):69–77

[101] Wakhloo AK, Tio FO, Lieber BB, Schellhammer F, Graf M, Hopkins LN. Self-expanding nitinol stents in canine vertebral arteries: hemodynamics and tissue response. AJNR Am J Neuroradiol. 1995; 16(5):1043–1051

[102] LaDisa JF, Jr, Olson LE, Molthen RC, et al. Alterations in wall shear stress predict sites of neointimal hyperplasia after stent implantation in rabbit iliac arteries. Am J Physiol Heart Circ Physiol. 2005; 288(5):H2465–H2475

[103] Wentzel JJ, Krams R, Schuurbiers JC, et al. Relationship between neointimal thickness and shear stress after Wallstent implantation in human coronary arteries. Circulation. 2001; 103(13):1740–1745

[104] Eto K, Goto S, Shimazaki T, et al. Two distinct mechanisms are involved in stent thrombosis under flow conditions. Platelets. 2001; 12(4):228–235

[105] Baim DS, Carrozza JP, Jr. Stent thrombosis. Closing in on the best preventive treatment. Circulation. 1997; 95(5):1098–1100

[106] Duprat G, Jr, Wright KC, Charnsangavej C, Wallace S, Gianturco C. Self-expanding metallic stents for small vessels: an experimental evaluation. Radiology. 1987; 162(2):469–472

[107] Neki H, Caroff J, Jittapiromsak P, et al. Patency of the anterior choroidal artery covered with a flow-diverter stent. J Neurosurg. 2015; 123 (6):1540–1545

[108] Gascou G, Lobotesis K, Brunel H, et al. Extra-aneurysmal flow modification following pipeline embolization device implantation: focus on regional branches, perforators, and the parent vessel. AJNR Am J Neuroradiol. 2015; 36(4):725–731

[109] Darsaut TE, Bing F, Makoyeva A, Gevry G, Salazkin I, Raymond J. Flow diversion to treat aneurysms: the free segment of stent. J Neurointerv Surg. 2013; 5(5):452–457

3 REVIEW OF CURRENT LITERATURE AND OCCLUSION RESULTS

PHILIP G. R. SCHMALZ, PAUL M. FOREMAN, AVRA LAARAKKER and MARK R. HARRIGAN

Abstract

Flow diversion is the most significant new development in the endovascular management of intracranial aneurysms. Multiple devices exist, but the Pipeline Embolization Device (PED) is the most-studied and is currently the only device with United States FDA approval. The PED is approved for treating large or giant wide-necked aneurysms of the internal carotid artery from the petrous through superior hypophyseal regions. In this chapter, occlusion rates of the most common flow diverters for both on-label and off-label applications are reviewed.

Flow diversion treatment of large, wide-necked aneurysms of the internal carotid artery below the circle of Willis is associated with favorable results, with occlusion rates greater than 90% in most reports. Though the literature is limited, successful treatment with flow diversion is also reported for small aneurysms of the internal carotid artery with complete occlusion ranging from 72-86%. Reports of flow diversion for ruptured or dissecting aneurysms, or those located in the posterior circulation are less favorable. Overall occlusion rates for posterior circulation aneurysms, such as giant fusiform vertebrobasilar aneurysms, appear lower than for more conventional lesions of the internal carotid artery. Ischemic complications, particularly perforator infarction, are higher than those reported for aneurysms of the internal carotid artery.

Flow diversion for large, wide-necked internal carotid artery aneurysms below the circle of Willis appears to be both effective and safe. Off-label results are not as favorable. Given the natural history of some posterior circulation aneurysms, flow diversion may be appropriate in select cases but should be approached with caution.

Keywords: aneurysm, endovascular, flow diversion, flow-diverting stent, occlusion

3.1 Introduction

Flow diversion is the technique of endoluminal reconstruction of the parent artery with a low-porosity stent leading to aneurysm thrombosis followed by neointimal growth across the aneurysm neck. It represents the latest technique in the cerebrovascular specialist's armamentarium for the treatment of complex and difficult-to-treat aneurysms, particularly wide-neck aneurysms, giant aneurysms, and aneurysms with fusiform morphology. The majority of flow diverters have received CE mark and Food and Drug Administration (FDA) approval for the treatment of aneurysms of the internal carotid artery (ICA) below the circle of Willis. In addition, there is a growing body of literature investigating flow diversion for the treatment of anterior and middle cerebral artery aneurysms and aneurysms involving the posterior circulation. In this chapter, we discuss the current regulatory approval status of flow diverters, as well as published occlusion rates for on-label and off-label applications.

3.2 Brief Overview of Flow Diverters—Approval Status and Indications

Flow diversion is one of the fastest growing areas in neurointervention, and new or updated devices are in constant development. This chapter focuses on four principal flow diverters: the Pipeline Embolization Device (PED; ev3/Covidien, Irving, CA), the SILK/SILK + (SFD; Balt Extrusion, Montmorency, France), the Flow Redirection Endoluminal Device (FRED; MicroVention, Tustin, CA), and the Surpass flow-diverting stent (SUR; Stryker Neurovascular, Fremont, CA).

Currently, the PED is the only flow diverter approved by the FDA for use in the United States. The PED and the other devices discussed have received CE-mark approval for use in the European Union. A detailed overview of the technical specifications of these devices may be found in Chapter 9. The approval status and indications for these devices are summarized in ▸ Table 3.1.

Table 3.1 Approval status of flow-diverting stents

Device	FDA	CE mark
Pipeline Embolization Device (PED; ev3/Covidien, Irving, CA)	FDA-approved in 2011 for treatment of large, giant, wide-neck aneurysms of the internal carotid artery from the petrous through the superior hypophyseal segments in patients aged 22 years or older. Pipeline Flex FDA approved in 2015	Approved for the treatment of intracranial aneurysms arising from a parent vessel with a diameter of 2–5.3 mm. Pipeline Flex CE mark approved in 2015
SILK/SILK + (SFD; Balt Extrusion, Montmorency, France)	Unavailable in the United States	Approved in 2008 for the treatment of intracranial aneurysms with adjunctive coil embolization (recommendation added in 2010)
Flow Redirection Endoluminal Device (FRED; MicroVention, Tustin, CA)	Unavailable in the United States	Approved for the treatment of intracranial aneurysms
Surpass (SUR: Stryker Neurovascular, Fremont, CA)	Unavailable in the United States	Approved for treatment of intracranial aneurysms arising from a parent vessel with a diameter of 2–5.3 mm

3.3 Literature Review and Analysis of Occlusion Rates

Various grading schemes have been published to evaluate the degree of occlusion for aneurysms treated with endovascular techniques.[1,2,3] Several new grading scales specific to flow diversion have been proposed and are discussed in Chapter 13. At present, no one system is in universal use. The reports reviewed in this chapter use variously the Roy and Raymond scale, the O'Kelley-Marotta scale, Kamran-Byrne scale, or simply the authors' own evaluation of complete versus incomplete occlusion. Owing to variability across studies as well as degrees of partial aneurysm occlusions across reports and devices, using a unified scale is not possible. Thus, only complete occlusion rates are presented in this review.

3.4 Anterior Circulation—Internal Carotid Artery Below the Circle of Willis

Three landmark trials have established the role of flow diverters, in particular the PED, for the treatment of giant, wide-neck, and fusiform aneurysms of the ICA: Pipeline for the Intracranial Treatment of Aneurysms (PITA), Lylyk and colleagues' "Buenos Aires Experience," and the Pipeline for Uncoilable and Failed Aneurysms trial (PUFs).[4,5,6] The study by Lylyk et al, termed the *Buenos Aires experience*, was a prospective, all-inclusive case series of 63 predominantly anterior circulation aneurysms of the ICA, though 8 aneurysms were located in the posterior circulation. Approximately half of aneurysms studied were large or giant, wide-neck (dome-to-neck ratio of < 2 or neck ≥ 4 mm) lesions of the cavernous and paraophthalmic region. Sixty-three percent of aneurysms treated were unruptured and untreated lesions, while the remainder had previously been treated with subsequent recanalization. Seven previously ruptured and previously treated aneurysms were included.

Seventy percent of aneurysms were treated with a single PED, while 30% were treated with multiple devices. Only four patients were treated with adjunctive coil embolization, all of whom had only a single PED placed. At 6-month follow-up angiography, 93% of patients demonstrated complete occlusion.

This successful trial was affirmed with two subsequent prospective single-arm trials: PITA and PUFs.[4,6] PITA included 31 patients harboring mostly sidewall aneurysms of the ICA with an average size of 11.5 mm. Fifty-two percent of aneurysms underwent adjunctive coil embolization. PUFs were more restrictive in aneurysm location and morphology, including 106 wide-neck (≥ 4 mm) aneurysms of the ICA at least 10 mm in diameter. Aneurysm location was limited to the ICA from the petrous segment to the superior hypophyseal segment. Only a single patient underwent combined flow diversion and coil embolization within the study, though six aneurysms had been previously coiled. A median of three PEDs were used per aneurysm. Both the PITA and PUFs trials demonstrated occlusion rates at 6-month follow-up of 93.3 and 73.6%, respectively. The occlusion rate in PUFs increased to 86% at 12 months, suggesting that angiographic cure may be prolonged in patients who undergo flow diversion alone without adjunctive coil embolization. These studies are summarized in ▶ Table 3.2.

Many additional studies have evaluated efficacy of the PED in the anterior circulation.[7,8,9,10,11] Most published studies to date have not excluded patients based on aneurysm location, and as a result, many publications include a small number of aneurysms either in the posterior circulation or aneurysms distal to the superior hypophyseal artery. Occlusion results from these trials are generally favorable with complete angiographic occlusion ranging from 55.7 to 92% (▶ Table 3.3).[7,9]

While the PED remains the most popular flow diverter in use in the United States, several trials have evaluated the Silk/Silk + (SFD), Surpass (SUR), and FRED for aneurysms of the ICA.

Eight major studies investigating the SFD have been published to date.[12,13,14,15,16,17,18,19] Most studies included aneurysms in an "all-comers" fashion, though most aneurysms were previously ruptured and coiled or unruptured, untreated, large,

Table 3.2 Details of the Buenos Aires Experience, PITA, and PUFs Trials (PED)

Author	Device	Indication	Adjunctive coiling	N (patients)	N (aneurysms)	Follow-up	Complete occlusion at follow-up
Lylyk et al 2009 Buenos Aires Experience	PED	Unruptured giant, wide-neck, anterior and posterior circulation	Yes, 52%	53	63	3–12 mo, mean 5.9 mo	93%
Nelson et al 2011 Pipeline for the Intracranial Treatment of Aneurysms (PITA)	PED	Wide-neck, most < 10 mm, 93% anterior circulation with 48% paraophthalmic	Yes, 52%	31	31	6 mo	93.3%
Becske et al 2013 Pipeline for Uncoilable or Failed Aneurysms (PUFs)	PED	Unruptured ICA aneurysms of petrous to superior hypophyseal segments, 10 mm or greater, with neck of 4 mm or greater	Single patient	104	106	6 mo	73.6% at 6 mo, 86% at 12 mo

Abbreviation: PED, Pipeline Embolization Device.

Table 3.3 Selected studies of the PED for predominantly anterior circulation large or giant, wide-neck aneurysms of the internal carotid artery

Author	Device	Indication	Adjunctive coiling	N (patients)	N (aneurysms)	Follow-up	Complete occlusion at follow-up
McAuliffe et al 2012[7]	PED	Unruptured large, wide-neck, and fusiform, previously coiled with recanalization	Yes (6 patients)	54	57	6 mo	85.7% at 6 mo, 92.5% for previously untreated aneurysms
Saatci et al 2012[8]	PED	Wide-neck, blister, recurrent sidewall	Yes (11 patients)	191	251	6 mo	91.2%
Yu et al 2012[9]	PED	Saccular and fusiform, both anterior and posterior circulation, previously treated	Yes (9 patients)	143	178	6, 12, 18 mo	55.7% at 6 mo, 81% at 12, and 92.2% at 18 mo. Combination of DSA, MRA, and CTA used to evaluate occlusion
Çinar et al 2013[10]	PED	Wide-neck, fusiform, prior treatment failures, anterior and posterior circulation	No	45	55	6 mo	85.3%
O'Kelly et al 2013[11]	PED	Unruptured, large or giant wide-neck	Yes	97	97	Mean 15 mo, range 3–30 mo	68.4% occluded, 84.2% "near occlusion"

Abbreviation: PED, Pipeline Embolization Device.

or giant aneurysms of the ICA. Most series also contain a minority of posterior circulation aneurysms. Many of the patients underwent adjuvant coil embolization due to a 2010 BALT safety advisory and update to the instructions for use (IFU) that warned of an increased risk of rupture with SFD deployment without adjunctive coil embolization. One study included patients treated with both the SFD and other conventional stents including coronary stents and the LEO stent (Balt Extrusion, Montmorency, France).[16] Occlusion rates for the SFD in the aforementioned applications ranged from 49% at 1 month to 87.8% complete occlusion at a mean follow-up of 17.8 months, reflecting the trend of higher occlusion rates with longer follow-up times.[12,13,14,15,16,17,18,19] Notably, one study reported a 23% recanalization rate of previously occluded aneurysms treated with flow diversion without adjuvant coil placement.[19] No aneurysms in this study treated with the SFD with adjuvant coiling recanalized. This observation confirmed the need for long-term angiographic follow-up and supported BALT's revised IFU, which instructs users to perform coil embolization in conjunction with stent placement. Details of the aforementioned studies are highlighted in ▶ Table 3.4.

While several reports of the FRED flow diverter have been published to date, only one study sufficiently limits inclusion criteria to include predominantly anterior circulation aneurysms isolated to the ICA.[20,21,22] Kocer et al reported a single-center experience with 33 patients with wide-neck, saccular, and fusiform aneurysms predominantly of the ICA proximal to the origin of the anterior choroidal artery; however, 2 patients with dissecting fusiform aneurysms of the vertebral arteries were included. They reported a complete occlusion rate of 67 and 80% at 3- and 6-month follow-up, respectively. This study is limited by incomplete follow-up, with only 8 of 33 patients

with 12-month follow-up. Of these eight, 100% of aneurysms were completely occluded at 12 months.[22]

Relative to the PED and SFD, published experience with the Surpass flow diverter for aneurysms of the ICA is limited. de Vries and coauthors published a prospective single-center study of 37 patients with aneurysms in the anterior and posterior circulation and the middle cerebral artery (MCA). The majority of cases consisted of saccular aneurysms located within the ICA from the cavernous through ophthalmic segments. Adjuvant coils were used in two patients. They reported a complete occlusion rate of 94% at 6 months.[23] The largest published series included 165 patients with wide-neck, saccular aneurysms of the cerebral circulation. In this series, 22% of aneurysms were distal to the circle of Willis and 14.5% in the posterior circulation. The authors reported a complete occlusion rate of 75%, which improved to 78% when only anterior circulation aneurysms were included.[24]

3.5 Posterior Circulation

In the United States, flow diversion for posterior circulation aneurysms remains an off-label application. Relative to anterior circulation aneurysms, there is relatively little data on posterior circulation aneurysm treatment with flow diversion. A recent literature review and meta-analysis of flow diversion for cerebral aneurysms found that only 12.5% of all published aneurysms treated by flow diversion were located in the posterior circulation.[25] Several series reporting flow diversion for aneurysms specifically in the posterior circulation are presented in ▶ Table 3.5.[26,27,28,29,30,31]

A 2011 study examined 32 patients with diverse posterior circulation lesions, including blister, wide-neck, dissecting, and

Table 3.4 Selected studies of the SFD stent for the treatment of predominantly anterior circulation aneurysms

Author	Device	Indication	Adjunctive coiling	N (patients)	N (aneurysms)	Follow-up	Complete occlusion at follow-up
Byrne et al 2010[12]	SFD	Saccular and wide-neck, fusiform, anterior and posterior circulation	Yes	70	70	1 mo for all, median 119 d	49% at 1 mo
Lubicz et al 2010[13]	SFD	Unruptured fusiform, giant, or wide neck	No	29	34	3–6 mo (12 patients at 3 mo, 12 patients at 6 mo)	69% for mixed time point
Berge et al 2012[14]	SFD	Unruptured and previously treated, saccular including large and giant, fusiform, anterior and posterior circulation	Yes (6 patients)	65	77	6 and 12	6.6% at deployment, 68% at 6 mo, 84% at 12 mo
Wagner et al 2012[15]	SFD	Symptomatic (no acute ruptures), predominantly ICA saccular aneurysms, 7 posterior circulations, one giant ICA with thrombus, one-third prior treatment	Yes (2 patients)	22	26	3, 6 (DSA), 12 mo (MRA)	68% complete occlusion at 6 mo, 86% complete occlusion at 12 mo
Maimon et al 2012[16]	SFD/adjuvant stents (LEO)	Previously ruptured, treated, saccular and fusiform, anterior and posterior circulation	Yes (aneurysms > 15 mm)	28	32	Cross-sectional 3–6 mo	83.3% "secured"
Tähtinen et al 2012[17]	SFD	Mixed, ruptured previously treated, anterior and posterior circulation	Yes (4 patients)	24	24	Mean 9 mo (range 2–17, median 8 mo)	80%
Velioglu et al 2012[18]	SFD	Wide neck or fusiform, no acute hemorrhages	No	76	87	Mean 17.5 (range: 2–48)	87.8%
Mpotsaris et al 2015[19]	SFD	Unruptured, wide-neck saccular, giant, and fusiform anterior and posterior circulation	Yes	25	28	Mean 14.9 mo	59% Recanalization seen in 23% of aneurysms without adjunctive coiling

Abbreviation: SFD, SILK/SILK + flow diverting.

basilar tip aneurysms. The authors reported complete occlusion with PED treatment in 86% of patients at 6 months, increasing to 96% at 12 months.[26] Notably, eight aneurysms were ruptured at the time of treatment. This series reported significant complications; 14% of PEDs placed within the basilar artery resulted in perforating artery territory infarctions.[26]

The risk of flow diversion within the basilar artery is corroborated by a 2010 report from Kulcsár and colleagues. In a series of 12 patients with basilar tip or trunk aneurysms treated with the SFD with and without adjunctive coiling, the authors reported complete aneurysm occlusion in 7 patients (58%) at a mean follow-up of 16 weeks. In this series, one patient suffered an acute stent thrombosis and three patients developed late infarctions for an overall ischemic complication rate of 33%.[31]

Toth et al published a series of six patients with fusiform and saccular aneurysms of the posterior circulation treated with either the PED or SFD. The authors reported a similar complete aneurysm occlusion rate to prior studies. In this series, 57% of aneurysms were occluded at a mean follow-up interval of 14.5 months. But again, significant complications were reported in

Table 3.5 Selected studies of flow diversion for posterior circulation aneurysms (PED and SFD)

Author	Device	Indication	Adjunctive coiling	N (patients)	N (aneurysms)	Follow-up	Complete occlusion at follow-up
Phillips et al 2012[26]	PED	Wide-neck (>4 mm), fusiform, dissecting, basilar tip and PCA, blister aneurysms, 8 ruptured	Yes	32	32	6, 12 mo	86% at 6 mo, 96% at 12 mo 14% of basilar stents caused perforator infarcts
Toth et al 2015[27]	PED/SFD	Fusiform and saccular aneurysms in posterior circulation	Yes (50%)	6	7	Mean 14.5 mo	57% 14% mortality
Siddiqui et al 2012[28]	PED (6)/SFD (1)	Large or giant fusiform vertebrobasilar	Yes	7	7		4/7 patients died, 1 mRS = 5
Chalouhi et al 2013[29]	PED	Posterior circulation, saccular or fusiform	No	7	7	6 mo	43%
Munich et al 2014[30]	PED	Posterior circulation fusiform	Yes	12	12	6 mo	90%
Kulcsár et al 2010[31]	SFD	Basilar tip and trunk, two ruptured	Yes (50%)	12	12	16 wk	58%

Abbreviations: PED, Pipeline Embolization Device; SFD, SILK/SILK + flow diverting.

this series, including one death and one patient with a modified Rankin scale (mRS) score of 5.[27]

Giant, fusiform aneurysms of the vertebrobasilar system remain one of the most difficult-to-treat aneurysms. Traditional treatment options for these aneurysms are associated with high complication and mortality rates. There has been great hope that flow diversion will offer a solution to this relatively rare and complex problem.

A handful of case series of fusiform vertebrobasilar aneurysms have been published.[28,29,30] In a 2014 study, Munich and colleagues reported a small series of 12 patients with giant fusiform vertebrobasilar aneurysms treated with the PED. Of the 10 patients evaluated, nine (90%) were found to have complete occlusion at 6-month follow-up.[30]

Despite this glowing report, less favorable results are more commonly reported for fusiform vertebrobasilar aneurysms. Two other small series reported occlusion rates less than 50%, and in one series four of seven patients died, while a fifth had an mRS of 5 at follow-up.[28,29]

Overall, occlusion rates for flow diversion of aneurysms within the posterior circulation are lower than for aneurysms at other sites. Additionally, treatment of these lesions is associated with a high complication rate. Flow diversion for these lesions remains off-label. Nevertheless, the natural history of posterior circulation aneurysms, including giant aneurysms with symptomatic compression of the brainstem, may warrant treatment with flow diverters in select cases.

3.6 Ruptured and Dissecting Aneurysms

Flow diversion for acutely ruptured aneurysms remains an off-label application. Many published studies of flow diversion include a small fraction of patients presenting with acute subarachnoid hemorrhage, and only a minority are specific to treatment of acutely ruptured or dissecting aneurysms. The majority of reports of flow diverter treatment of aneurysms described cases of unruptured aneurysms or previously ruptured and treated aneurysms. The use of flow diversion for acutely ruptured aneurysms has been less widely applied due to the need for antiplatelet therapy and consequent risk of re-rupture. Unlike surgical clipping or coil embolization, treatment with flow diversion alone does not provide immediate protection from aneurysmal re-rupture. Additionally, the possibility that these patients will require surgical procedures such as cerebrospinal fluid diversion or even craniotomy while taking antiplatelet agents has given pause to clinicians contemplating flow diversion for acutely ruptured aneurysms. Here, we review two reports of flow diversion treatment specific to patients presenting with acute subarachnoid hemorrhage.[32,33]

Cruz et al reported a single-center experience of 20 patients who underwent PED treatment for blister, saccular, and dissecting aneurysms presenting with acute subarachnoid hemorrhage. The majority of patients were treated in the acute phase, while one was treated in a delayed fashion. Adjunctive coil embolization was used in 5 patients, and 15 patients were treated with PED placement alone. The authors reported a 94% complete occlusion rate at 12-month follow-up; of note, aneurysm occlusion was assessed with computed tomography angiography and magnetic resonance angiography in some cases. Two patients were severely disabled due to procedure-related complications and one patient died from an intraparenchymal hematoma caused by aneurysm rerupture.[32]

A multicenter study by Lin et al included 26 patients presenting with acute subarachnoid hemorrhage from blister, saccular, and dissecting aneurysms predominantly of the ICA. This series included mostly Hunt-Hess grade I–III subarachnoid hemorrhage patients who underwent PED placement. Adjunctive coil embolization was performed in 12 of 26 patients. More than half of the patients were treated during the acute period after aneurysm rupture. The authors reported an occlusion rate of 78.3% at a mean follow-up of 5.9 months. Notably, of the eight patients with blister aneurysms, 100% had complete occlusion at angiographic follow-up.[33]

Only one study to date has focused exclusively on dissecting aneurysms.[34] These relatively rare lesions comprise less than 5% of intracranial aneurysms and have historically been challenging to treat by open or endovascular methods.[35] In a 2011 report, de Barros Faria and colleagues presented 23 patients with dissecting aneurysms, predominantly of the vertebrobasilar circulation, treated with the PED. Approximately half of all patients presented with subarachnoid hemorrhage, though only four were treated during the acute phase. At mean 6-month follow-up, the authors reported a 69.5% complete occlusion rate. This increased to 87.5% when only patients with follow-up duration longer than 3 months were included for analysis.[34]

3.7 Aneurysms of the Circle of Willis and Beyond

Most reports of flow diversion for the treatment of aneurysms focus on lesions of the ICA involving the cavernous and paraclinoid regions, as well as applications in the posterior circulation. Few studies have addressed the use of flow diversion for aneurysms of the circle of Willis and more distal vessels. Three studies to date have examined flow diversion for these common aneurysms, with a single study specific to aneurysms of the circle of Willis and beyond.[23,24,36] Pistocchi and colleagues reported a single-center experience of 26 patients with 30 aneurysms located predominantly at the anterior communicating artery, MCA, and pericallosal artery. The majority of aneurysms were unruptured and of either saccular or fusiform morphology. Patients were treated with flow diversion with either the PED or SFD and adjunctive coil embolization was used in 23% of aneurysms. The authors reported a complete occlusion rate of 78.9% with flow diverter placement alone at a mean follow-up of 13 months. Of aneurysms treated with flow diversion and coil embolization, 100% were occluded at follow-up.[36]

3.8 Small Aneurysms

Most aneurysms encountered in the general population are less than 10 mm.[37] These lesions may present difficulty for conventional endosaccular techniques, with an increased risk of procedural rupture or coil dislodgement.[38,39,40] Two studies specifically addressing flow diversion for the treatment of small aneurysms are included in this review.[41,42]

Lin et al reported a single-center experience with 41 patients harboring 44 unruptured aneurysms of the ICA measuring less than 10 mm. Most aneurysms were paraophthalmic and clinoidal and averaged 5 mm in size. All patients were treated with the PED, and adjunctive coiling was performed only in two cases. In 88% of cases, a single device was used. The authors reported a complete occlusion rate of 85.7% at 6-month follow-up.[41]

A second study focusing on small aneurysms has been reported by Chalouhi et al. The authors reported a single-center experience of 100 aneurysms of less than 7 mm treated with the PED. Eighty percent of aneurysms were treated with a single device and only two patients underwent placement of coils. The authors reported a 72% complete aneurysm occlusion at a mean follow-up of 6.3 months.[42]

3.9 Conclusion

Flow diverters allow for the endoluminal reconstruction of a parent artery for the treatment of complex and difficult-to-treat aneurysms. There are multiple devices on the market, but the PED is the most-studied and the only device with FDA approval. Published aneurysm occlusion rates are favorable with an acceptable adverse event rate when used for approved indications. The off-label use of flow diverters has been met with mixed results and should be approached with caution in only select cases.

References

[1] O'Kelly CJ, Krings T, Fiorella D, Marotta TR. A novel grading scale for the angiographic assessment of intracranial aneurysms treated using flow diverting stents. Interv Neuroradiol. 2010; 16(2):133–137

[2] Kamran M, Yarnold J, Grunwald IQ, Byrne JV. Assessment of angiographic outcomes after flow diversion treatment of intracranial aneurysms: a new grading schema. Neuroradiology. 2011; 53(7):501–508

[3] Grunwald IQ, Kamran M, Corkill RA, et al. Simple measurement of aneurysm residual after treatment: the SMART scale for evaluation of intracranial aneurysms treated with flow diverters. Acta Neurochir (Wien). 2012; 154 (1):21–26, discussion 26

[4] Nelson PK, Lylyk P, Szikora I, Wetzel SG, Wanke I, Fiorella D. The pipeline embolization device for the intracranial treatment of aneurysms trial. AJNR Am J Neuroradiol. 2011; 32(1):34–40

[5] Lylyk P, Miranda C, Ceratto R, et al. Curative endovascular reconstruction of cerebral aneurysms with the pipeline embolization device: the Buenos Aires experience. Neurosurgery. 2009; 64(4):632–642, discussion 642–643, quiz N6

[6] Becske T, Kallmes DF, Saatci I, et al. Pipeline for uncoilable or failed aneurysms: results from a multicenter clinical trial. Radiology. 2013; 267 (3):858–868

[7] McAuliffe W, Wycoco V, Rice H, Phatouros C, Singh TJ, Wenderoth J. Immediate and midterm results following treatment of unruptured intracranial aneurysms with the pipeline embolization device. AJNR Am J Neuroradiol. 2012; 33(1):164–170

[8] Saatci I, Yavuz K, Ozer C, Geyik S, Cekirge HS. Treatment of intracranial aneurysms using the pipeline flow-diverter embolization device: a single-center experience with long-term follow-up results. AJNR Am J Neuroradiol. 2012; 33(8):1436–1446

[9] Yu SC, Kwok CK, Cheng PW, et al. Intracranial aneurysms: midterm outcome of pipeline embolization device–a prospective study in 143 patients with 178 aneurysms. Radiology. 2012; 265(3):893–901

[10] Çinar C, Bozkaya H, Oran I. Endovascular treatment of cranial aneurysms with the pipeline flow-diverting stent: preliminary mid-term results. Diagn Interv Radiol. 2013; 19(2):154–164

[11] O'Kelly CJ, Spears J, Chow M, et al. Canadian experience with the pipeline embolization device for repair of unruptured intracranial aneurysms. AJNR Am J Neuroradiol. 2013; 34(2):381–387

[12] Byrne JV, Beltechi R, Yarnold JA, Birks J, Kamran M. Early experience in the treatment of intra-cranial aneurysms by endovascular flow diversion: a multicentre prospective study. PLoS One. 2010; 5(9):e12492

[13] Lubicz B, Collignon L, Raphaeli G, et al. Flow-diverter stent for the endovascular treatment of intracranial aneurysms: a prospective study in 29 patients with 34 aneurysms. Stroke. 2010; 41(10):2247–2253

[14] Berge J, Biondi A, Machi P, et al. Flow-diverter silk stent for the treatment of intracranial aneurysms: 1-year follow-up in a multicenter study. AJNR Am J Neuroradiol. 2012; 33(6):1150–1155

[15] Wagner A, Cortsen M, Hauerberg J, Romner B, Wagner MP. Treatment of intracranial aneurysms. Reconstruction of the parent artery with flow-diverting (Silk) stent. Neuroradiology. 2012; 54(7):709–718

[16] Maimon S, Gonen L, Nossek E, Strauss I, Levite R, Ram Z. Treatment of intracranial aneurysms with the SILK flow diverter: 2 years' experience with 28 patients at a single center. Acta Neurochir (Wien). 2012; 154(6):979–987

[17] Tähtinen OI, Manninen HI, Vanninen RL, et al. The silk flow-diverting stent in the endovascular treatment of complex intracranial aneurysms: technical aspects and midterm results in 24 consecutive patients. Neurosurgery. 2012; 70(3):617–623, discussion 623–624

[18] Velioglu M, Kizilkilic O, Selcuk H, et al. Early and midterm results of complex cerebral aneurysms treated with Silk stent. Neuroradiology. 2012; 54 (12):1355–1365

[19] Mpotsaris A, Skalej M, Beuing O, Eckert B, Behme D, Weber W. Long-term occlusion results with SILK flow diversion in 28 aneurysms: do recanalizations occur during follow-up? Interv Neuroradiol. 2015; 21(3):300–310

[20] Möhlenbruch MA, Herweh C, Jestaedt L, et al. The FRED flow-diverter stent for intracranial aneurysms: clinical study to assess safety and efficacy. AJNR Am J Neuroradiol. 2015; 36(6):1155–1161

[21] Diaz O, Gist TL, Manjarez G, Orozco F, Almeida R. Treatment of 14 intracranial aneurysms with the FRED system. J Neurointerv Surg. 2014; 6(8):614–617

[22] Kocer N, Islak C, Kizilkilic O, Kocak B, Saglam M, Tureci E. Flow re-direction endoluminal device in treatment of cerebral aneurysms: initial experience with short-term follow-up results. J Neurosurg. 2014; 120(5):1158–1171

[23] De Vries J, Boogaarts J, Van Norden A, Wakhloo AK. New generation of Flow Diverter (Surpass) for unruptured intracranial aneurysms: a prospective single-center study in 37 patients. Stroke. 2013; 44(6):1567–1577

[24] Wakhloo AK, Lylyk P, de Vries J, et al. Surpass Study Group. Surpass flow diverter in the treatment of intracranial aneurysms: a prospective multicenter study. AJNR Am J Neuroradiol. 2015; 36(1):98–107

[25] Briganti F, Leone G, Marseglia M, et al. Endovascular treatment of cerebral aneurysms using flow-diverter devices: a systematic review. Neuroradiol J. 2015; 28(4):365–375

[26] Phillips TJ, Wenderoth JD, Phatouros CC, et al. Safety of the pipeline embolization device in treatment of posterior circulation aneurysms. AJNR Am J Neuroradiol. 2012; 33(7):1225–1231

[27] Toth G, Bain M, Hussain MS, et al. Posterior circulation flow diversion: a single-center experience and literature review. J Neurointerv Surg. 2015; 7 (8):574–583

[28] Siddiqui AH, Abla AA, Kan P, et al. Panacea or problem: flow diverters in the treatment of symptomatic large or giant fusiform vertebrobasilar aneurysms. J Neurosurg. 2012; 116(6):1258–1266

[29] Chalouhi N, Tjoumakaris S, Dumont AS, et al. Treatment of posterior circulation aneurysms with the pipeline embolization device. Neurosurgery. 2013; 72(6):883–889

[30] Munich SA, Tan LA, Keigher KM, Chen M, Moftakhar R, Lopes DK. The Pipeline Embolization Device for the treatment of posterior circulation fusiform aneurysms: lessons learned at a single institution. J Neurosurg. 2014; 121 (5):1077–1084

[31] Kulcsár Z, Ernemann U, Wetzel SG, et al. High-profile flow diverter (silk) implantation in the basilar artery: efficacy in the treatment of aneurysms and the role of the perforators. Stroke. 2010; 41(8):1690–1696

[32] Cruz JP, O'Kelly C, Kelly M, et al. Pipeline embolization device in aneurysmal subarachnoid hemorrhage. AJNR Am J Neuroradiol. 2013; 34(2):271–276

[33] Lin N, Brouillard AM, Keigher KM, et al. Utilization of Pipeline embolization device for treatment of ruptured intracranial aneurysms: US multicenter experience. J Neurointerv Surg. 2015; 7(11):808–815

[34] de Barros Faria M, Castro RN, Lundquist J, et al. The role of the pipeline embolization device for the treatment of dissecting intracranial aneurysms. AJNR Am J Neuroradiol. 2011; 32(11):2192–2195

[35] Santos-Franco JA, Zenteno M, Lee A. Dissecting aneurysms of the vertebrobasilar system. A comprehensive review on natural history and treatment options. Neurosurg Rev. 2008; 31(2):131–140, discussion 140

[36] Pistocchi S, Blanc R, Bartolini B, Piotin M. Flow diverters at and beyond the level of the circle of Willis for the treatment of intracranial aneurysms. Stroke. 2012; 43(4):1032–1038

[37] Wiebers DO, Whisnant JP, Huston J, III, et al. International Study of Unruptured Intracranial Aneurysms Investigators. Unruptured intracranial aneurysms: natural history, clinical outcome, and risks of surgical and endovascular treatment. Lancet. 2003; 362(9378):103–110

[38] Brinjikji W, Lanzino G, Cloft HJ, Rabinstein A, Kallmes DF. Endovascular treatment of very small (3 mm or smaller) intracranial aneurysms: report of a consecutive series and a meta-analysis. Stroke. 2010; 41(1):116–121

[39] Mitchell PJ, Muthusamy S, Dowling R, Yan B. Does small aneurysm size predict intraoperative rupture during coiling in ruptured and unruptured aneurysms? J Stroke Cerebrovasc Dis. 2013; 22(8):1298–1303

[40] Nguyen TN, Raymond J, Guilbert F, et al. Association of endovascular therapy of very small ruptured aneurysms with higher rates of procedure-related rupture. J Neurosurg. 2008; 108(6):1088–1092

[41] Lin LM, Colby GP, Kim JE, Huang J, Tamargo RJ, Coon AL. Immediate and follow-up results for 44 consecutive cases of small (< 10 mm) internal carotid artery aneurysms treated with the pipeline embolization device. Surg Neurol Int. 2013; 4:114

[42] Chalouhi N, Zanaty M, Whiting A, et al. Safety and efficacy of the Pipeline Embolization Device in 100 small intracranial aneurysms. J Neurosurg. 2015; 122(6):1498–1502

4 COIL EMBOLIZATION VERSUS FLOW DIVERSION

JEFFREY A. STEINBERG, PETER ABRAHAM, J. SCOTT PANNELL, and ALEXANDER KHALESSI

Abstract

First attempts at flow diversion for the healing of intracranial aneurysms began with open surgical Hunterian ligation. Flow diverting embolization devices represent a recent endovascular treatment modality for cerebral aneurysms that allow in situ flow diversion with device reconstruction of the parent vessel. Current utilization focuses on large, giant, fusiform, and wide-neck aneurysms. Endovascular coil embolization with or without adjunctive devices and open surgical reconstruction represent the current standard of care. Although the goal of both flow diversion and coil embolization is exclusion of aneurysmal lesions from circulation, the method of exclusion differs between the two. Appropriate application of this technology requires understanding the basic deployment technique, physiology of aneurysm occlusion, rates of occlusion, and complication profile. This chapter provides the reader with a concise review of the current literature evaluating flow diversion versus coil embolization for treatment of intracerebral aneurysms. Additional considerations of cost and resource implications are addressed.

Keywords: benefits, coil embolization, comparison, complications, cost analysis, flow diverting stent

4.1 Introduction

The development of the Guglielmi detachable coil in the early 1990s[1] represented a major paradigm shift in the treatment of intracranial aneurysms, the first alternative to open surgical reconstruction. Further development of adjunct endovascular devices such as stents and balloons allowed for successful treatment of a wider range of aneurysms by stent-assisted coiling and balloon remodeling. These early stents were primarily utilized as a scaffold to contain coils, allowing for increased packing density within the aneurysm and preventing encroachment on the lumen of the parent vessel. However, even with these significant advancements in endovascular management of aneurysms, there remains a subset of lesions particularly difficult to treat. Specifically, large (> 10 mm), giant (> 25 mm), fusiform, and wide-neck (dome-to-neck ratio < 2) aneurysms still pose challenges to practitioners, as aneurysm remnant or recurrence rates remain high after treatment for these lesions.[1] Additionally, these types of aneurysms portend a much poorer natural history than small, saccular aneurysms. Giant aneurysms have a 5-year cumulative rupture risk of 40% in the anterior circulation and 50% in the posterior circulation. Additionally, morbidity and mortality with surgical treatment may be as high as 30%. Endovascular treatment of these lesions remains a challenge as well with occlusion rates of 57% and mortality rates of 7 to 11%.[1]

Flow diverting stents with lower porosity (higher metallic coverage) were recently developed with the intention of diverting blood flow away from the aneurysm, resulting in aneurysmal stasis and thrombosis, endothelialization across the aneurysm neck, and aneurysm regression.[1,2] This mechanistic strategy allows for remodeling of the diseased segment of the parent artery itself.[1] Theoretically, parent vessel reconstruction versus aneurysm occlusion and passive vessel healing may provide a more durable treatment.

There are multiple flow diverting stents in practice, including Surpass (Stryker), Silk (Balt), and FRED (Microvention). While all these devices have CE mark and are in various stages of U.S. Food and Drug Administration (FDA) approval, the Pipeline Embolization Device (Medtronic) was FDA approved (2011) for use in the United States. Currently, its FDA approval is for adults with large or giant, wide-neck intracranial aneurysms between the petrous and supraclinoid segment of the internal carotid artery (ICA) proximal to the anterior choroidal artery.[1] A brief comparison between coil embolization and flow diversion for aneurysm treatment is outline in ▶ Table 4.1.

4.2 Flow Diversion and Coil Embolization Technique: Benefits and Risks

To understand the benefits and risks of flow diverting stents, a brief understanding of the deployment procedure is necessary. Deployment of flow diverting stents entails passing a microcatheter distal to an aneurysm, deployment of the stent, and subsequent removal of the deployment device. As compared to coil embolization alone, deployment of flow diverting stents presents some technical challenges, including navigating a larger device through the intracranial circulation, achieving adequate device apposition against the parent vessel, and appropriate stent placement.[2] This entails choosing a suitable stent diameter and ensuring the stent covers both proximal and distal segments of the parent vessel, given that the stent foreshortens once deployed.[1] Additionally, care must be exercised to ensure that the distal catheter tip and deployment wire remain in the parent vessel and do not deviate into smaller perforators that may lead to complications. Balloon angioplasty may be required to fully appose the stent against the vessel wall, given that an endoleak will prevent complete aneurysm occlusion and obstruct endothelialization.[1] Multiple flow diverting stents may be placed. However, after a flow diverting stent is placed, the interventionalist permanently surrenders endovascular access to the aneurysm. Catheter-based treatment will now be restricted to further flow-diverter placement and commitment of an even greater hardware burden to the parent artery. This represents a significant limitation of flow diversion technology. Although most practitioners are well versed in stent deployment, this novel device does present new challenges and technical nuances that must be mastered for optimal patient outcome.

As discussed further, immediate aneurysm occlusion after treatment is rarely observed after flow diversion, with rates reported around 8 to 21%.[2] These flow diverting stents are utilized with the knowledge that aneurysm occlusion may take

Table 4.1 Brief comparison of coil embolization and flow diversion

	Coil embolization (GDC)	Flow diversion
Mechanism of action	Catheterization of aneurysm for placement of one or more coils that induce thrombus formation with immediate onset of action	Stent placement across aneurysm within parent artery, inducing gradual intra-aneurysmal flow stagnation, thrombosis, and subsequent remodeling (endothelialization) of the parent vessel, with regression of the aneurysm
Current use	Diverse usage ranging from small saccular aneurysms to giant fusiform aneurysms, often in conjunction with stent assistance and balloon remodeling. Utilized in both ruptured and unruptured setting	Large, wide-neck, or fusiform aneurysms, typically unruptured
Adjuvant technologies	Use of balloons and stents	Additional flow diversion stent placement
Complete occlusion percentage at 6 mo	Approximately 50%[6]	Approximately 75%[4]
Antiplatelet regimen	Not required. Single agent use may be utilized to decrease thromboembolic events	Dual agent required for 3–6 mo with aspirin continued indefinitely
Complications	Thromboembolic events, intraoperative rupture, aneurysm recurrence, failure to occlude	Non-aneurysmal IPH, perforator occlusion, in-stent stenosis/thrombosis, seclusion of aneurysm from future access
Unruptured aneurysm morbidity and mortality	Approximately 5 and 1%[13]	Approximately 5 and 1%[10,14]
Cost	Potential cost savings with smaller aneurysm volumes	Potential cost savings with larger aneurysm volumes

Abbreviations: GDC, Guglielmi detachable coil; IPH, intraparenchymal hemorrhage.

6 to 12 months. For this reason, flow diversion is primarily utilized for unruptured aneurysms,[2] given that the delayed occlusion may still allow for re-rupture after initial subarachnoid hemorrhage (SAH).

In contrast to flow diversion techniques, coil embolization involves catheterization of the aneurysm directly for placement of coils within the aneurysm. The coils induce thrombus formation and aneurysm occlusion in a more immediate manner as compared to flow diversion. As discussed, stent-assisted coiling (higher porosity stent) and balloon remodeling are techniques to enhance coil embolization methods. Because coil embolization is thrombogenic, coiling remains the first-line method for endovascular treatment of ruptured aneurysm.

The major procedural advantage in the placement of flow diverting stents is elimination of need for direct catheterization of the aneurysm. The advantage of not needing to catheterize the aneurysm becomes particularly apparent in non–flow-related aneurysms projecting inferiorly or laterally from the petrous or cavernous carotid.

4.3 Use of Antiplatelet

The process of endothelialization of flow diverting stents is incompletely understood resulting in variability in antiplatelet regimens employed by individual practitioners. Many practitioners pretreat with aspirin and clopidogrel prior to stent placement followed by 3 to 6 months of continued dual-antiplatelet use and single agent use indefinitely.[1,2,3] A clopidogrel assay is utilized by some practitioners to ensure adequate responsiveness prior to intervention.[1] Nonresponders to conventional antiplatelet agents require special consideration.

Coil embolization does not require use of antiplatelet agent. However, some practitioners do prescribe antiplatelet agents with coil embolization treatment, typically a single agent to prevent thromboembolic complications. Stent-assisted coiling requires use of dual antiplatelet similar to flow diversion stent placement.

Patients with bleeding risk factors, those who may require further surgical interventions, or those with poor compliance may be more amenable to coil embolization instead of flow diversion. Stopping antiplatelet agents, especially in the acute period after stent placement, has a high likelihood of complication related to thromboembolic events or stent thrombosis. Starting the antiplatelet regimen at least 1 week prior to placement of the flow diverter is recommended to elucidate which patients may encounter bleeding complications.

Additionally, patients with ruptured aneurysms must be started on dual-antiplatelet therapy if flow diversion stenting is to be utilized, a risk in the setting of known SAH. These factors must be considered during treatment planning.

4.4 Occlusion Rates with Flow Diversion Compared to Coil Embolization

Comparing outcomes subsequent to coil embolization versus flow diverting stent placement is challenging with much of the data on flow diverting stents primarily related to the treatment of complex aneurysms. However, there are meta-analyses and some comparison studies that do provide insight into outcomes and complications of flow diversion stents demonstrating the pros and cons of each modality. In a meta-analysis published in *Stroke* by Brinjikji et al,[4] the authors examined 29 studies assessing flow diverting stents for treatment of intracerebral aneurysms. Overall results represent a total of 1,451 patients. Complete aneurysmal occlusion was 76% at 6 months. This was further broken down according to aneurysm size, with small aneurysms achieving an occlusion rate of 80%, large aneurysms achieving an occlusion rate of 74%, and giant aneurysms achieving an occlusion rate of 76%. Similar results have been shown in other studies with occlusion rates of 80 to 85% between the 6- and 12-month periods.[5]

Coil embolization of aneurysms is associated with lower occlusion rates as compared to flow diverting stent placement. As discussed in the article by Siddiqui and coworkers, recent studies have demonstrated complete occlusion in 48% of aneurysms treated by coil embolization with a neck remnant of 22% and aneurysmal remnant of 30%.[6] In another study examining 501 aneurysms treated with detachable coils, the authors found an early follow-up (3–12 months) complete occlusion rate of 44.6% and late follow-up (> 12 months) complete occlusion rate of 38.3%. These studies indicate that complete occlusion rates are higher with flow diversion; however, they were discrete studies making direct comparison difficult.

In the study by Chalouhi et al, the authors compared flow diversion to coil embolization in a matched pair analysis for large saccular aneurysms treated with the Pipeline Embolization Device or coil embolization. Although the study was not randomized, and did include adjunctive coiling techniques such as stent-coiling and balloon-assisted coiling, trends can still be gleaned from the analysis. Complete aneurysm occlusion was higher in the flow diversion group at all time points with 86% in the flow diversion group and 41% in the coiled group at last follow-up.[7]

In another comparison study, Lanzino et al compared treatment of paraclinoid ICA aneurysms with flow diversion to a matched historic control treated with coil embolization. Again complete occlusion of aneurysms was higher in the flow diversion group.[8]

Because of the success found with flow diverting stents, some interventionalists have broadened the use to include smaller aneurysms traditionally treated with coil embolization. In the study by Chalouhi et al, the authors compared flow diverting stents to coil embolization for unruptured, saccular aneurysms of the anterior circulation. The authors found similar results between the two groups with regard to occlusion rates, complications, and clinical outcome. The study highlights the continued broadening of use of flow diversion.

4.5 Complication Profile: Flow Diversion versus Coil Embolization

Complications, morbidity, and mortality must be carefully evaluated when comparing flow diverting stents to coil embolization. One of the most unexpected and unique complications found with flow diversion is non-aneurysmal intraparenchymal hemorrhage (IPH), oftentimes distant to the treated lesion. Brinjikji et al demonstrated overall IPH occurrence of 3% with no correlation to aneurysm size.[4] Other flow diversion studies report similar intracerebral hemorrhage (ICH) occurrences

between 0 and 2%[1,5] Etiology for these non-aneurysmal parenchymal hemorrhages is unclear, with hypotheses including hemorrhagic transformation of thromboemboli, embolization of stent coating material, and hyperperfusion syndrome secondary to hemodynamic flow changes.[1] Although these events appear to occur only in a small percent of patients treated with flow diversion, IPH does carry significant morbidity and further studies are required to elucidate these causes and prevalence. Non-aneurysmal IPH has not been associated with coil embolization.

Another complication that is unique to flow diversion is perforator occlusion secondary to stent overlay of nearby vessels. In the meta-analysis by Brinjikji et al with 1,654 treated aneurysms by flow diversion, occurrence of perforator infarction was 3% overall, with posterior circulation aneurysms having an overall higher perforator occlusion occurrence.[4] In an expert review article, Eller et al suggested that perforators may occlude if greater than 50% of the perforator outlet is compromised. They further discussed a small case series of flow diversion stents utilized in posterior circulation giant vertebrobasilar fusiform aneurysms noting four of seven patients died, with two of these deaths secondary to brainstem strokes.[1] Posterior circulation aneurysm treatment with flow diversion is off-label and should be used judiciously in this vascular distribution especially with regard to multi-stent placement, given this risk of perforator occlusion.

In the same flow diversion meta-analysis study by Brinjikji et al, overall SAH rate was 4%, with patients harboring smaller aneurysms having a significantly lower occurrence of postprocedural SAH. No association between SAH and aneurysm location was found. Stroke occurrence was reported at 6% overall, with treatment of smaller aneurysms having a lower stroke rate. Additionally, treated anterior circulation aneurysms demonstrated a lower stroke occurrence as compared to posterior circulation aneurysms.[4] Other complication risks with flow diversion include in-stent stenosis and potential mass effect of giant aneurysms after treatment. Eller et al reported that the rates of stent thrombosis and stenosis were 1.9 and 5%, respectively.[1] Lylyk et al reported worsening mass effect after flow diversion treatment in three patients after treatment of giant aneurysms.[3] In the matched study by Chalouhi et al comparing coil embolization to flow diversion, the authors reported overall similar complication rates of less than 10% in both groups.[7]

Another reported complication with flow diverting stents is delayed rupture of large or giant aneurysms. In the study by Kulcsár et al, the authors reviewed 13 cases from 12 different medical centers of large or giant, wide-neck saccular or fusiform aneurysms treated with flow diversion. Each of these cases represents a report of delayed aneurysm rupture.[9] All aneurysms were symptomatic prior to treatment with mean diameter of 22 mm. The authors divided patients into two groups: early rupture (< 3 months) and late rupture (3–5 months). Ten of the patients were categorized as early rupture from treatment (mean time: 16 days) and three patients were categorized as late rupture from treatment (mean time: 132 days). The authors discussed this delayed rupture phenomenon in the study including postmortem dissection and histological analysis. Interestingly, all aneurysms demonstrated thrombus formation within the aneurysm, in some cases complete thrombosis. However, in cases of histological examination, the aneurysm wall was found to be extremely thin, containing areas of mural necrosis, loss of fibrous tissue and smooth muscle cells, and infiltration by inflammatory cells. This cascade of thrombotic events appears to have resulted in an autolysis phenomenon, which eventually lead to aneurysm rupture. It is unclear why intra-aneurysmal thrombosis led to delayed rupture in these aneurysms. The authors concluded with four features of these aneurysms that may predispose to rupture after flow diversion. Specifically, aneurysm characteristics included large or giant size, symptomatic, complex dome to neck morphology, and dynamic inflow characteristics.[9] Although only 13 occurrences are reported in this study, delayed aneurysm rupture appears to be a real complication of flow diversion, especially with complex aneurysmal features as discussed by these authors.

Again, looking at the large meta-analysis study by Brinjikji et al, the authors reported a permanent morbidity rate of 5% and mortality rate of 4%.[4] In a different study by Fargen et al, the authors presented seven studies evaluating use of the Pipeline Embolization Device and note an overall major complication rate of 5.3% and mortality rate of 1.3%.[10]

Although overall complication rate, morbidity, and mortality appear fairly similar to coil embolization, risks of non-aneurysmal IPH and perforator occlusion appear consistent between studies. These complications carry significant morbidity and may represent a persistent risk associated with the use of flow diversion stent.

4.6 Cost Analysis

Cost analysis is limited, given the recent development of flow diverters and few studies on the topic. Some data suggest cost savings with flow diversion as compared to other endovascular methods.[11] Other studies have suggested many coils would have to be utilized before equating the cost of flow diversion, with one study estimating 32 coils or more.[1] In a study by Chalouhi et al, the authors found a correlation with aneurysm size and break point cost. Specifically, aneurysms over 0.90 cm^3 treated with flow diversion stenting were associated with lower cost as compared to coil embolization. Below this volume, flow diversion was more costly. Additionally, use of multiple flow diversion stents negated the cost advantage with aneurysms over 0.90 cm^3.[12] Once the cost of these new flow diverting stent devices decreases, a direct cost advantage may become more apparent. However, cost savings must also include patient outcomes, need for further treatment, complications, and overall hospital cost. No study can evaluate all these factors, but if flow diversion allows for better occlusion rates resulting in more durable treatment, this may result in substantial cost benefits.

4.7 Conclusion

The data for flow diverting stents remain promising, especially when considered for large fusiform aneurysms that are otherwise challenging to treat. Flow diversion has shown significantly improved occlusion rates for these complex lesions in multiple studies. Complication rates appear similar to coil embolization; however, there are risks unique to flow diverting stents that must be considered, such as perforator occlusion

and non-aneurysmal ICH. Additionally, once a flow diverting stent is deployed, direct access to the aneurysm is lost because of the decreased porosity of the stent and subsequent inability to catheterize through the stent. Further treatment is limited to overlaying additional stents. However, given the unique challenge posed by large and giant intracranial aneurysms, flow diverting stents may become standard of care for unruptured giant and fusiform aneurysms. Unfortunately, ruptured giant or fusiform aneurysms present more difficult management considerations, given that flow diverting stents require dual-antiplatelet agents, increasing the risk of re-rupture and IPH associated with cerebrospinal fluid diversion procedures. Concomitantly, flow diversion with coil embolization has been employed in the setting of SAH; however, minimal data exist to date. Additionally, flow diversion for unruptured small, saccular aneurysms will be of increasing interest, as the data suggest that a more complete occlusion may be obtainable. Long-term studies will need to be completed, but it appears that flow diverting stents are a new endovascular technique, providing interventionalists with another tool in their armamentarium for the treatment of intracerebral aneurysms.

References

[1] Eller JL, Dumont TM, Sorkin GC, et al. The Pipeline embolization device for treatment of intracranial aneurysms. Expert Rev Med Devices. 2014; 11 (2):137–150

[2] D'Urso PI, Lanzino G, Cloft HJ, Kallmes DF. Flow diversion for intracranial aneurysms: a review. Stroke. 2011; 42(8):2363–2368

[3] Lylyk P, Miranda C, Ceratto R, et al. Curative endovascular reconstruction of cerebral aneurysms with the pipeline embolization device: the Buenos Aires experience. Neurosurgery. 2009; 64(4):632–642, discussion 642–643, quiz N6

[4] Brinjikji W, Murad MH, Lanzino G, Cloft HJ, Kallmes DF. Endovascular treatment of intracranial aneurysms with flow diverters: a meta-analysis. Stroke. 2013; 44(2):442–447

[5] Fargen KM, Hoh BL. Flow diversion technologies in evolution: a review of the first 4 generations of flow diversion devices. World Neurosurg. 2014; 81(3–4):452–453

[6] Krishna C, Sonig A, Natarajan SK, Siddiqui AH. The expanding realm of endovascular neurosurgery: flow diversion for cerebral aneurysm management. Methodist DeBakey Cardiovasc J. 2014; 10(4):214–219

[7] Chalouhi N, Tjoumakaris S, Starke RM, et al. Comparison of flow diversion and coiling in large unruptured intracranial saccular aneurysms. Stroke. 2013; 44(8):2150–2154

[8] Lanzino G, Crobeddu E, Cloft HJ, Hanel R, Kallmes DF. Efficacy and safety of flow diversion for paraclinoid aneurysms: a matched-pair analysis compared with standard endovascular approaches. AJNR Am J Neuroradiol. 2012; 33 (11):2158–2161

[9] Kulcsár Z, Houdart E, Bonafé A, et al. Intra-aneurysmal thrombosis as a possible cause of delayed aneurysm rupture after flow-diversion treatment. AJNR Am J Neuroradiol. 2011; 32(1):20–25

[10] Fargen KM, Velat GJ, Lawson MF, Mocco J, Hoh BL. Review of reported complications associated with the Pipeline Embolization Device. World Neurosurg. 2012; 77(3–4):403–404

[11] Colby GP, Lin L-M, Paul AR, Huang J, Tamargo RJ, Coon AL. Cost comparison of endovascular treatment of anterior circulation aneurysms with the pipeline embolization device and stent-assisted coiling. Neurosurgery. 2012; 71 (5):944–948, discussion 948–950

[12] el-Chalouhi N, Jabbour PM, Tjoumakaris SI, et al. Treatment of large and giant intracranial aneurysms: cost comparison of flow diversion and traditional embolization strategies. World Neurosurg. 2014; 82(5):696–701

[13] Montanera W. Editorial: Does physician specialty matter? J Neurosurg. 2016; 124(1):7

[14] Tse MMY, Yan B, Dowling RJ, Mitchell PJ. Current status of pipeline embolization device in the treatment of intracranial aneurysms: a review. World Neurosurg. 2013; 80(6):829–835

5 ON-LABEL USE (ILLUSTRATIVE CASES)

LYNN B. McGRATH JR., JOHN D. NERVA, and LOUIS J. KIM

Abstract

The Pipeline for Uncoilable or Failed Aneurysms (PUFS) trial helped define the on-label indications for use of the Pipeline Embolization Device (Covidien, Medtronic, Irvine, CA).[1] Indications include large or giant aneurysms of the petrous, cavernous, clinoidal, and/or ophthalmic internal carotid artery (ICA) segments (i.e., proximal to the posterior communicating artery [PCoA]) with a diameter of ≥ 10 mm and a neck diameter of ≥ 4 mm. Pipeline was approved by the Food and Drug Administration (FDA) in April 2011 and the next-generation Pipeline Flex was approved in February 2015. Other flow-diverting stents with the CE mark of approval include the Silk (Balt Extrusion; Montgomery, France), Surpass (Stryker Neurovascular, Fremont, CA), and FRED (Microvention, Terumo; Somerset, NJ). Surpass and FRED are undergoing trials for FDA approval in the United States.

Keywords: endovascular aneurysm treatment, flow-diverting stent, large or giant intracranial aneurysms, on-label use of Pipeline, Pipeline Embolization Device, unruptured intracranial aneurysms

5.1 Case 1: H3165540

5.1.1 Clinical Presentation

The patient, a 50-year-old woman, came to our attention while undergoing a workup for transient left-sided hearing loss. She underwent magnetic resonance imaging (MRI) of her brain, which incidentally demonstrated a 7-mm flow void within the R middle cerebral artery (MCA). She was then referred for computed tomography angiography, which revealed a 12-mm irregularly shaped aneurysm involving the cavernous and ophthalmic segments of the right internal carotid artery (ICA). She had no history of headache or neurological deficit apart from the transient hearing loss.

5.1.2 Radiologic studies

Cerebral angiography demonstrated a multilobulated, broad-based aneurysm extending from the distal cavernous segment of right ICA into the ophthalmic segment ICA. The dome measuregd 12 mm in maximum diameter with a neck diameter of 7 mm. The aneurysmal segment of artery involved greater than 180 degrees of the vessel circumference. The ophthalmic artery was demonstrated to be of cavernous origin and remote to the aneurysm. There was a normal variant early bifurcation of the MCA with a normal M1 branch and an accessory anterior temporal artery branch. In venous phase, there was no contrast stagnation within the aneurysm (▶ Fig. 5.1a–d).

5.1.3 Diagnosis

Large, unruptured, wide-necked multilobulated aneurysm of the right distal cavernous and ophthalmic ICA without involvement of the ophthalmic artery.

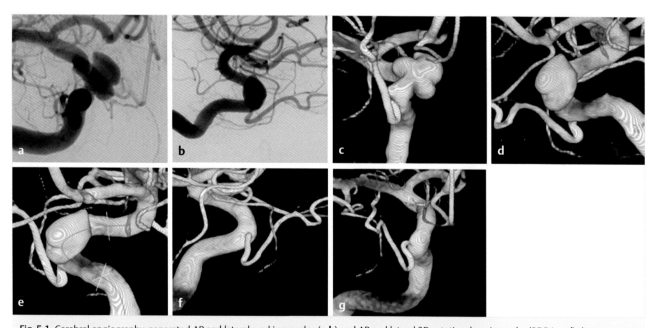

Fig. 5.1 Cerebral angiography-generated AP and lateral working angles (**a,b**) and AP and lateral 3D rotational angiography (3DRA; **c,d**) demonstrate a multilobulated, broad-based aneurysm extending from the distal cavernous segment of right internal carotid artery (ICA) into the ophthalmic segment ICA. Intraoperative 3DRA demonstrating measurements of the proximal and distal landing zones for the planned Pipeline stent (**e**). 6-month 3DRA demonstrates complete obliteration of the aneurysm (**f,g**).

5.1.4 Treatment

Equipment

- Standard 4F access and 4F catheter (VERT; Cook Medical; Bloomington, IN).
- 0.035" hydrophilic guidewire (GLIDEWIRE; Terumo; Somerset, NJ).
- 6F shuttle sheath catheter (KSAW; Cook Medical).
- 0.058" Navien catheter (Covidien, Irvine, CA).
- 0.027" Marksman microcatheter (Covidien).
- 0.014" Synchro II microwire (Stryker Neurovascular, Fremont, CA).
- Pipeline Embolization Device (Covidien); 4.75 mm × 18 mm.
- Exchange length Synchro II guidewire (Stryker Neurovascular).
- 6F closure device (Angio-Seal; St. Jude's Medical, St. Paul, MN).
- Intravenous heparin.

Description

The patient was loaded with aspirin and clopidogrel and taken electively to the angiography suite. The patient was intubated, and using Seldinger technique a 6F KSAW Shuttle catheter sheath was introduced. As per our protocol, the patient was then heparinized to an activated clotting time (ACT) of greater than 250 and less than 350, which was maintained throughout the entire procedure.

The KSAW Shuttle was then taken up into the proximal cervical segment of the right ICA. Introduced through this was a Navien 0.058 catheter with an internalized Marksman microcatheter and 0.14 Synchro II microwire. This coaxial construct was then used to pass the Navien catheter tip into the cavernous segment of the ICA. Angiography including three-dimensional (3D) workstation reconstructions was used to align our working angle views. Measurements were taken at the landing zones intended for the Pipeline device, demonstrating arterial calibers of 3.7 mm distally and 4.3 mm proximally with an intervening maximum diameter of 4.8 mm (▶ Fig. 5.1e).

At this point, the Marksman catheter was advanced into the M1 segment on the right. A premeasured 4.75 mm × 18 mm Pipeline Embolization Device was placed into the Marksman catheter and then deployed across the neck of the aneurysm with good overlap achieved proximal and distal to the neck. A high-resolution XperCT 3D angiogram was performed which demonstrated excellent apposition of the deployed Pipeline device to the normal surrounding parent vessel walls and no evidence of endoleak.

Final branch vessel and working angle views demonstrated good flow through the normal and parent vessels, no evidence of any thromboembolic event, and early stasis of flow in the large aneurysm. Flow through the ophthalmic artery and the choroidal blush of the retina remained intact both pre– and post–device placement. The microcatheters and guide catheters were then removed and the common femoral arteriotomy was sealed with a closure device.

5.1.5 Outcome

The patient was discharged home on postoperative day 1 without complication and maintained on dual-antiplatelet therapy.

Angiography at 6 months demonstrated almost total thrombosis and resolution of the aneurysm, which at this point appeared as a 0.7-mm irregularity on the sidewall of the otherwise normal-in-appearance parent vessel (▶ Fig. 5.1f, g). Angiography at 12 months demonstrated no residual aneurysm opacification (▶ Fig. 5.1g). Clopidogrel was discontinued, and aspirin was changed to 81 mg daily. Magnetic resonance angiography (MRA) obtained 2 years after treatment demonstrated stable result, and the patient was at her preoperative baseline.

5.1.6 Discussion

This patient was offered treatment for this unruptured aneurysm for several reasons. First, the aneurysm carried a 1 to 2% per year risk of rupture at minimum.[2,3] Second, the aneurysm was multilobulated and highly irregular in appearance which also has been shown to increase the risk of rupture.[3]

Placement of a flow-diverting stent was presented to this patient as the safest and most effective treatment for several reasons. The wide neck of the aneurysm would make coil embolization or balloon-assisted coil embolization difficult to perform safely due to the risk of coil herniation into the ICA. Performing stent-assisted coil embolization may have been effective in producing thrombosis in the dome of the aneurysm; however, the affected segment of the ICA appeared to demonstrate aneurysmal irregularity spanning more than half of the circumference of the parent artery. Thus, scaffold stent-assisted coil embolization would accept a high rate of recurrence in the long term.[4] This pathologic feature called for either open microsurgical clip reconstruction or flow diversion. The wide neck of the aneurysm and the pathologic dilatation of an extensive portion of the ICA made microsurgical clip reconstruction a less attractive option due to the high risk of parent vessel stenosis, need for prolonged brain retraction, and potential progression of dilatation into previously unaffected segments.

Fortunately, the origin of the ophthalmic artery was not involved in the aneurysmal segment. Persistent anterograde flow through large vessels, in proximity to or involved in the aneurysm, counteracts the flow diversion effect of the stent and portends a high risk of residual filling of the aneurysm on follow-up imaging.[5]

The ability of a flow diverting device to achieve endoluminal reconstruction of the vessel wall makes it ideal for the treatment of aneurysms involving large portions of the affected segment of the parent vessel.

5.2 Case 2: H3205881

5.2.1 Clinical Presentation

The patient was a 75-year-old woman, who presented with 2 years of progressive worsening of headaches and right-sided retro-orbital pain. She reported a 30-year smoking history, but was in otherwise excellent health. She underwent an MRI/MRA of the brain that demonstrated a 10-mm right ophthalmic ICA aneurysm. She was counseled that due to the large size of her aneurysm and her smoking history she faced a significant risk of rupture within her lifetime. Owing to her advanced age and the broad neck of the aneurysm, we recommended endovascular treatment with the Pipeline Embolization Device with coil embolization. She was started on aspirin 325 mg PO daily and clopidogrel 75 mg PO daily 1 week prior to treatment, and taken to the angiography suite for evaluation.

5.2.2 Radiologic Studies

Cerebral angiography demonstrated a 10-mm wide-necked saccular aneurysm of the ophthalmic segment of the right ICA. The neck measured 4.5 mm, while the dome measured 12 x 8 mm in maximum dimension. There was no significant stasis of contrast in the dome and filling downstream of the aneurysm appeared to be within normal limits (▶ Fig. 5.2a–c).

5.2.3 Diagnosis

Large, unruptured, wide-necked saccular aneurysm of the right ophthalmic ICA.

5.2.4 Treatment

Equipment

- Standard 4F access sheath (VERT, Cook Medical).
- 4F H1 catheter (GLIDECATH, Terumo).
- 0.035" hydrophilic guidewire (GLIDEWIRE, Terumo).
- Amplatz Super Stiff Guidewire (Boston Scientific, Marlborough, MA).
- Standard 8F access sheath (Envoy; Depuy Synthes, Raynham, MA).
- 6F shuttle sheath catheter (KSAW, Cook Medical).
- 0.027" Marksman microcatheter (Covidien).
- 0.058" ReVerse microcatheter (Reverse Med, Irvine, CA).
- SL-10 microcatheter (Excelsior, Stryker Neurovascular).
- 0.014" Synchro II microwire (Stryker Neurovascular).
- Presidio microcoil (Micrusphere, Depuy Synthes); 9 mm × 46 cm.

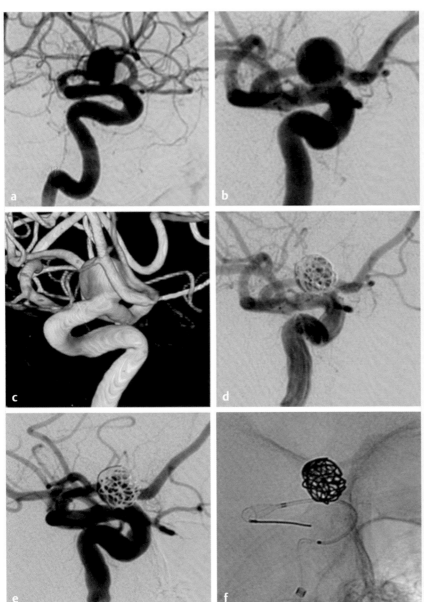

Fig. 5.2 Cerebral angiography-generated AP and lateral working angles (**a,b**) and 3D rotational angiography (3DRA; **c**) demonstrate a large, unruptured, wide-necked large aneurysm of the right ophthalmic internal carotid artery. Intraoperative runs demonstrating coil embolization pre–stent deployment (**d,e**). Successful coil embolization of the aneurysm, with active deployment of the flow diverter (**f**).

- 2 × Pipeline Embolization Device (Covidien); 5 mm × 20 mm, 5 mm × 18 mm.
- Exchange length Synchro II guidewire (Stryker Neurovascular).
- 6F closure device (Angio-Seal, St. Jude's Medical).

Description

The patient was loaded with aspirin and clopidogrel and taken electively to the angiography suite. The patient was intubated and under general anesthesia for the duration of the procedure. Using Seldinger technique, a 4F sheath was placed and a 4F H1 catheter was introduced into the patient over a 0.035-inch wire and manipulated gently into the right ICA. Diagnostic runs were performed including working angles and 3D reconstructions. At this point, the patient was heparinized to an ACT of greater than 250 and less than 350.

Once therapeutic heparin levels were achieved, the HI catheter was maneuvered into the external carotid artery and due to the patient's type 2 arch, an Amplatz Super Stiff wire was introduced. We exchanged the H1 catheter over this wire for an 8F sheath and a 6F shuttle. Once the shuttle was in place, a 0.058" ReVerse catheter was introduced and maneuvered into the right ICA. At this point, a Marksman microcatheter was passed through the ReVerse catheter into the cavernous carotid, allowing us to advance the ReVerse catheter over it and into the petrous segment. We removed the Marksman and introduced an SL-10 catheter over a 0.014" Synchro soft tip pre-shaped wire, which was used to catheterize the aneurysm. We then placed a 9 mm × 46 cm Presidio Micrus coil into the saccular aneurysm with no evidence of parent vessel herniation (▶ Fig. 5.2d, e). We performed pre- and postdetachment diagnostic runs, confirming that our coil mass was the appropriate density and well situated. The SL-10 catheter was then removed from the aneurysm. At this point, we reintroduced the Marksman catheter over a Synchro wire and passed it into the right MCA M3 segment. After measuring intended landing zones for our stent, a 4.5 × 14 mm diameter Pipeline Embolization Device was introduced into the Marksman and advanced until it sat tip to tip within the catheter in the MCA branch. Under fluoroscopic guidance, the Pipeline Embolization Device was deployed across the neck of the aneurysm, with the distal stent just at the distal ICA segment and the proximal segment in the cavernous segment of the ICA (▶ Fig. 5.2f). We confirmed appropriate apposition of the stent to the normal parent vessel walls both angiographically with catheter injection and with an angiographic spin and 3D reconstruction.

The Marksman catheter was removed along with the wire, and final working angle and branch vessel views demonstrated excellent placement of the coil and the Pipeline Embolization Device, with no evidence of any thromboembolic event or flow limitation. The catheters were then removed entirely without any evidence of dissection or arterial injury. The arteriotomy was then sealed with a femoral closure device.

5.2.5 Outcome

The patient was discharged home on postoperative day 1 without complication and maintained on dual-antiplatelet therapy. Angiography at 6 months demonstrated satisfactory appearance of the right ophthalmic segment carotid artery aneurysm with no recurrent filling of the aneurysm. Clopidogrel was discontinued, and the patient was transitioned to single antiplatelet therapy with 81 mg aspirin, on which the patient has remained.

5.2.6 Discussion

The patient was offered treatment for this unruptured aneurysm for several reasons. First, the aneurysm carried a 1 to 2% per year risk of rupture at minimum.[2,3] Second, the risk of aneurysmal rupture was increased due to her long history of smoking. Third, despite her advanced age and smoking status, she was otherwise a very healthy woman with a projected life expectancy robust enough to make the cumulative risk of aneurysmal rupture unacceptable.

Placement of a flow-diverting stent was presented to this patient as a safe and effective method of treatment given her age, the wide-necked morphology of the aneurysm, and her desire for the least invasive treatment method available. This patient had a wide-necked aneurysm that would make stand-alone coil embolization or balloon-assisted coil embolization difficult to perform effectively due to the risk of coil herniation into the ICA, as well as the relatively high rate of aneurysm recanalization. As before, stent-assisted coil embolization may have been effective in producing thrombosis in the dome of the aneurysm; however, the affected segment of the ICA appeared to demonstrate aneurysmal changes spanning more than half of the circumference of the vessel wall (▶ Fig. 5.2c). This pathologic feature called for either open microsurgical clip reconstruction or coil embolization with flow diverter–facilitated endoluminal reconstruction. The conditions for flow diversion were favorable given the origin of the ophthalmic artery was remote to the aneurysm and the patient had no contraindication to antithrombotic medications. We chose in this case to additionally coil the aneurysm due to the patient's progressively worsening headaches and the presence of an inflow jet into the aneurysm that pushed us toward more rapid occlusion of the aneurysm. In the absences of these concerns, we would not have placed coils simultaneously.

There are a few nuances involved in the decision to introduce supportive coils in addition to the stand-alone placement of a flow-diverting stent. Single flow-diverting stent placement has been associated with occlusion rates as low as 52% at 6 months, and even with placement of multiple devices the need for retreatment can be as high as 5.6 to 13.2%.[6] One method that has been explored for mitigating this risk is the introduction of concurrent aneurysm coiling. In this case, due to the patient's age and our reluctance to pursue further treatment for this wide-necked aneurysm, we chose to employ coil embolization to augment disruption of the inflow jet and support thrombosis of the aneurysm. Several factors led to our decision to coil rather than deploy multiple, overlapping devices. First, the complications inherent in laying down multiple devices may be significant and include misalignment of stents, early stent thrombosis, delayed in-stent stenosis, and decreased safety when operating in the vicinity of important perforators.[6] Supportive coil embolization appears to have a high rate of early aneurysm occlusion when compared with the use of multiple flow-diverting stents and eschews the cumulative risk inherent in layering devices.[7]

While there is no definitively superior method for performing coil embolization in conjunction with flow diversion, there are several principles that have been described in the literature that we have adhered to in our approach to this case. First, we decided preprocedurally to coil the aneurysm, thereby circumventing the risk inherent in jailing a microcatheter when the intention is to proceed with coiling after deployment of the flow diverter. Second, our objective in coiling the aneurysm is simply to disrupt the inflow jet into the dome which does not require a particularly dense coil mass. Third, a modest coil embolization mass can serve as a framework for thrombus formation and more rapid occlusion of the aneurysm. This is key, as flow diverters on rare occasion have been demonstrated to suffer catastrophic thrombosis and occlusion in association with a high-density coil mass, as well as postprocedural rupture of the aneurysm due to degradation of the endothelial layer.[8]

The ability of the flow diverters to achieve endoluminal reconstruction of the vessel wall and the versatility afforded by this class of device again made it uniquely suited for the treatment of this aneurysm which historically may have been treated utilizing an open approach.

5.3 Case 3: H3423163

5.3.1 Clinical Presentation

The patient was a 63-year-old female who presented with an unruptured intracranial aneurysm diagnosed 13 years prior after an episode of vertigo. She elected to have it treated conservatively at that time. Her mother recently died from aneurysmal subarachnoid hemorrhage, and her family urged her to seek consultation. She underwent an MRA at an outside hospital and was referred to our institution. She had a history of hypertension and hypercholesterolemia for which she was on medications and was neurologically intact. She was offered Pipeline placement and started 325 mg orally daily and clopidogrel 75 mg orally daily 1 week prior to treatment. Preoperative VerifyNow testing demonstrated therapeutic effect (ASA assay 393, P2Y12 reaction 154).

5.3.2 Radiologic Studies

Cerebral angiography demonstrated a multilobulated, broad-based aneurysm extending from the distal cavernous segment of left ICA into the ophthalmic segment and supraclinoid ICA. The dome measured 20 mm in maximum diameter with a neck diameter of 6 mm (▶ Fig. 5.3a–d). Intraluminal irregularities were present along the cavernous and ophthalmic segments. The A1 segments of the anterior cerebral artery were codominant, and there was a left fetal-type posterior cerebral artery. In venous phase, there was no contrast stagnation within the aneurysm.

5.3.3 Diagnosis

Large, unruptured, multilobulated aneurysm of the left distal and cavernous and paraclinoid ICA with evidence of collateral flow from the right ICA circulation.

5.3.4 Treatment

Equipment

- Standard 4F access and 4F catheter (VERT, Cook Medical).
- 0.035" hydrophilic guidewire (GLIDEWIRE, Terumo).
- Standard 6F access and 6F guiding catheter (Envoy, Depuy Synthes).

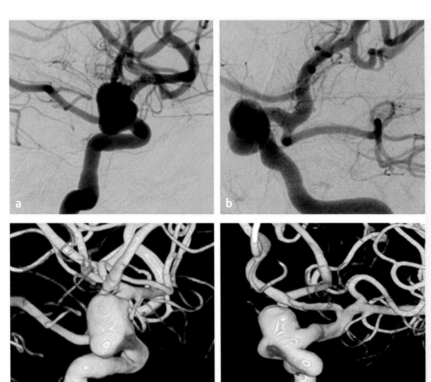

Fig. 5.3 Preoperative cerebral angiography demonstrates the large, multilobulated aneurysm of the left distal cavernous and paraclinoid internal carotid artery (ICA) in lateral and AP working angle projections (**a,b**) as well as lateral and AP 3D rotational angiography (3DRA; **c,d**).

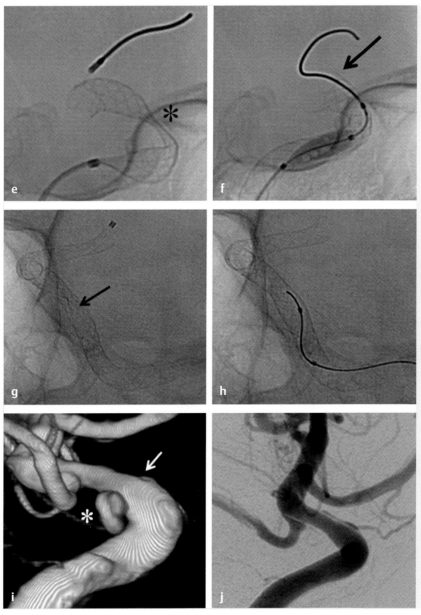

Fig. 5.3 (*contuned*) During deployment, the midportion (*) of the Pipeline was kinked, torqued, and did not fully open (lateral working angle, spot film; **e**). Balloon angioplasty was successful at opening the Pipeline, but the distal end migrated proximally (→, **f**). The midportion of the second Pipeline did not fully open (→, **g**) and was successfully opened with the HyperGlide balloon (**h**). 6-month angiography demonstrated small residual filling of the dome (*, **i**) with non–flow-limiting stenosis of the supraclinoid ICA (**j**).

- 0.027" Marksman microcatheter (Covidien).
- 0.014" Synchro II guidewire (Stryker Neurovascular).
- Pipeline Embolization Device (Covidien) 5 mm × 20 mm and 5 mm × 18 mm.
- Exchange length Synchro II guidewire (Stryker Neurovascular).
- Scepter XC balloon catheter (MicroVention, Tustin, CA) 4 mm × 11 mm.
- HyperGlide balloon occlusion system (Covidien) 4 mm × 10 mm.
- 6F closure device (Angio-Seal, St. Jude's Medical).
- Intravenous heparin.

Description

After diagnostic cerebral angiography confirmed the aneurysm seen on preoperative MRA, heparin IV was administered, and the 6F guiding catheter was placed into the distal cervical left ICA. Working angle projections were performed using the 3D rotational angiography images. The Marksman microcatheter over Synchro II microwire was navigated into the M2 segment to safely cross the aneurysm. The 5 × 20 mm Pipeline was introduced and a third of the device was unsheathed with the distal end initially proximal to the posterior communicating artery (PCoA). As deployment continued, there was kinking and torquing in the midportion, which prevented proper opening despite numerous attempts at wagging the stent (► Fig. 5.3e). The device was deployed with a plan for balloon angioplasty of the Pipeline, which was successfully performed after the Marksman was exchanged for a Scepter XC balloon catheter (► Fig. 5.3f). After angioplasty, the distal device had migrated to the distal neck of the aneurysm (► Fig. 5.3f).

Access was reobtained with the microcatheter/microwire, and a second Pipeline (5 mm × 18 mm) was deployed without difficulty with the distal end at the PCoA telescoping into the first Pipeline. However, the midportion of the stent failed to fully open, and this segment was angioplastied using the HyperGlide balloon without complication (▶ Fig. 5.3g, h). Intraprocedural stent-view flat-detector CT (XperCT; Philips Medical, Best, the Netherlands) was performed to detect stent positioning and endoleak demonstrating excellent wall apposition. Postembolization angiography demonstrated excellent flow through the ICA and distal branches without evidence of thromboembolic complications. Early stasis within the aneurysm was apparent. Heparin IV was not reversed and the groin site was closed with a 6F closure device.

5.3.5 Outcome

The patient was discharged home on postoperative day 1 without complication and maintained on dual-antiplatelet therapy. Angiography at 6 months demonstrated small arterial inflow at the inferior aspect of the aneurysm, leaving residual aneurysm approximately 4 mm in size with non–flow-limiting in-stent narrowing of the supraclinoid ICA and patency of the ophthalmic artery (▶ Fig. 5.3i). Angiography at 12 months demonstrated no residual aneurysm opacification and improvement of the in-stent narrowing (▶ Fig. 5.3j). Clopidogrel was discontinued, and aspirin was changed to 81 mg daily. MRA obtained 2 years after treatment demonstrated stable result, and the patient was at her preoperative baseline.

5.3.6 Discussion

This patient was offered treatment for this unruptured aneurysm for several reasons. First, the aneurysm carried a 3 to 4% per year risk of rupture based on size alone.[2,3] Second, the aneurysm was multilobulated containing one daughter sac, which also has been shown to increase the risk of rupture.[3] Third, the patient had a family history of aneurysmal subarachnoid hemorrhage, and a past medical history of hypertension further increasing the risk.[9]

Placement of a flow diverter was favored over stent-assisted coil embolization to allow for endoluminal reconstruction of the parent vessel. Coil embolization and balloon-assisted coil embolization may not have prevented coil herniation into the ICA. Owing to the wide neck of the aneurysm, microsurgical clip reconstruction was not advised due to the high likelihood of parent vessel narrowing and potential need for cerebral revascularization with severe clip-induced stenosis.

Early recognition of intraoperative technical complications enabled the technical success of the procedure. Failure of the device to fully deploy was managed by balloon angioplasty of the device. In each case, distal access was maintained, and an exchange length microwire was used to minimize the risk of navigating the balloon microcatheter through an inadequately deployed device. Balloon deployment caused foreshortening of the first device to the distal neck of the aneurysm, which required placement of a second device to ensure adequate neck coverage and prevent migration into the aneurysm dome. Balloon angioplasty was successful in both instances and improved the stent apposition to the ICA, which was confirmed via a stent-view CT.[10] Progressive obliteration of the aneurysm

occurred during follow-up without evidence of long-term complication.

5.4 Conclusion

The advent of flow-diverting stents has been a revolutionary force in the treatment of intracranial aneurysms. Aneurysms that previously represented some of the most challenging clinical entities confronting neurosurgeons have become eminently treatable, as the use of flow-diverting stents has become routine.[1,11,12,13] The device is not without flaws, and can be difficult to deploy, even with the introduction of the second generation of devices. Nonetheless, flow diversion technology is efficacious for the treatment of complex aneurysms when applied appropriately and is a superior alternative to earlier endovascular technology that produced less durable results.

References

[1] Becske T, Kallmes DF, Saatci I, et al. Pipeline for uncoilable or failed aneurysms: results from a multicenter clinical trial. Radiology. 2013; 267(3):858–868

[2] Wiebers DO, Whisnant JP, Huston J, III, et al. International Study of Unruptured Intracranial Aneurysms Investigators. Unruptured intracranial aneurysms: natural history, clinical outcome, and risks of surgical and endovascular treatment. Lancet. 2003; 362(9378):103–110

[3] Morita A, Kirino T, Hashi K, et al. UCAS Japan Investigators. The natural course of unruptured cerebral aneurysms in a Japanese cohort. N Engl J Med. 2012; 366(26):2474–2482

[4] Hauck EF, Welch BG, White JA, et al. Stent/coil treatment of very large and giant unruptured ophthalmic and cavernous aneurysms. Surg Neurol. 2009; 71(1):19–24, discussion 24

[5] Tsang ACOFA, Fung AM, Tsang FC, Leung GK, Lee R, Lui WM. Failure of flow diverter treatment of intracranial aneurysms related to the fetal-type posterior communicating artery. Neurointervention. 2015; 10(2):60–66

[6] Nossek E, Chalif DJ, Chakraborty S, Lombardo K, Black KS, Setton A. Concurrent use of the Pipeline Embolization Device and coils for intracranial aneurysms: technique, safety, and efficacy. J Neurosurg. 2015; 122(4):904–911

[7] Park MS, Nanaszko M, Sanborn MR, Moon K, Albuquerque FC, McDougall CG. Re-treatment rates after treatment with the Pipeline Embolization Device alone versus Pipeline and coil embolization of cerebral aneurysms: a single-center experience. J Neurosurg. 2016; 125(1):137–144

[8] Siddiqui AH, Kan P, Abla AA, Hopkins LN, Levy EI. Complications after treatment with pipeline embolization for giant distal intracranial aneurysms with or without coil embolization. Neurosurgery. 2012; 71(2):E509–E513, discussion E513

[9] Thompson BG, Brown RD, Jr, Amin-Hanjani S, et al. American Heart Association Stroke Council, Council on Cardiovascular and Stroke Nursing, and Council on Epidemiology and Prevention, American Heart Association, American Stroke Association. Guidelines for the management of patients with unruptured intracranial aneurysms: a guideline for healthcare professionals from the American Heart Association/American Stroke Association. Stroke. 2015; 46(8):2368–2400

[10] Levitt MR, Cooke DL, Ghodke BV, Kim LJ, Hallam DK, Sekhar LN. "Stent view" flat-detector CT and stent-assisted treatment strategies for complex intracranial aneurysms. World Neurosurg. 2011; 75(2):275–278

[11] Dumont TM, Mokin M, Snyder KV, Siddiqui AH, Levy EI, Hopkins LN, III. A paradigm-shifting technology for the treatment of cerebral aneurysms: the pipeline embolization device. World Neurosurg. 2013; 80(6):800–803

[12] Fischer S, Vajda Z, Aguilar Perez M, et al. Pipeline embolization device (PED) for neurovascular reconstruction: initial experience in the treatment of 101 intracranial aneurysms and dissections. Neuroradiology. 2012; 54 (4):369–382

[13] Sahlein DH, Fouladvand M, Becske T, et al. Neuroophthalmological outcomes associated with use of the Pipeline Embolization Device: analysis of the PUFS trial results. J Neurosurg. 2015; 123(4):897–905

6 OFF-LABEL USE

DENNIS J. RIVET II, JOHN REAVEY-CANTWELL, and CHRISTOPHER J. MORAN

Abstract

Flow diversion has been demonstrated to be an effective treatment for cerebral aneurysms as well as a variety of other cerebrovascular lesions. Aneurysms and other lesions, which were previously considered untreatable or treated only with significant rates of morbidity and mortality, are now treated on a routine basis and with greatly reduced neurological sequela. The Pipeline Embolization Device (PED) received Food and Drug Administration (FDA) approval in 2011 for relatively narrow range of indications. FDA approved uses or "on-label" indications are restricted to large cerebral aneurysms from the petrous segment through the superior hypophyseal segment in adults. However, the application of flow diversion techniques has great value in lesions which do not fit strictly within this classification and in fact, the majority of cases that are treated with flow diversion currently are classified as "off-label" for one or multiple reasons. Some of the most common clinical situations where flow diversion is used in this manner include recurrent aneurysms previously treated with alternative endovascular means; aneurysms located in the posterior circulation or segments distal to the original proximal-indicated segment; and pathologies such as dissecting, fusiform, and blister-type aneurysms. Given that some of these conditions and specific lesions are subjected to treatment with this technology, the complexity and breadth of treatment possibilities has expanded greatly. In this chapter, we highlight some of the most common off-label indications and provide illustrative cases as examples.

Keywords: blister-type aneurysm, dissecting aneurysm, flow diversion, off-label, Pipeline device, recurrent aneurysms

6.1 Introduction

The Pipeline Embolization Device (PED) was approved by the U.S. Food and Drug Administration (FDA) for use in the United States on April 6, 2011, with labeling indications that specified its use for the treatment of wide-necked, large (≥ 10 mm), or giant intracranial aneurysms in the internal carotid artery (ICA), from the petrous segment through the superior hypophyseal segment, in adults 22 years of age or greater. This chapter focuses on the clinical use of these stents for indications outside the original FDA approval or "off-label" use as initially designated for the PED. At the time of this writing, no other flow diversion technologies are approved for use in the United States. It is noteworthy that the majority of cases performed with the PED are off-label. For instance, 53% of the 893 aneurysm treatments included in the IntrePED registry were performed for an off-label indication.[1]

6.2 Recurrent Aneurysms

The recurrence rate after initial aneurysm coiling is not insignificant with rates reported in the range of 15 to 20%.[2,3,4] Furthermore, the recurrence rate for recoiling of previously coiled aneurysms may be as high as 50%.[5] This makes these lesions a potentially attractive target for the off-label use of flow diversion devices. Daou et al utilized the PED in a series of recurrent aneurysms and of 30 previously coiled aneurysms with angiographic follow-up, and they found a rate of complete occlusion of 76.7% and near-complete ($\geq 90\%$) occlusion of 86.7%.[6] Of the aneurysms treated with a PED, only 6.7% required retreatment.

Another frequent off-label application of flow diversion is, as a rescue strategy after treatment failure, using a stent-assisted coiling with a nitinol self-expanding stent (▶ Fig. 6.1). Recurrent aneurysms that have been previously treated with stent-assisted coiling can be difficult to access with a microcatheter due to endothelialization of the coils and stents. Flow diversion offers the advantage of avoiding the need to access the aneurysm through the hardware. However, this application is often challenging technically due to the difficulty in navigation of the microcatheter and flow diverter through the existing stent, obtaining adequate vessel wall apposition, or successful expansion of the flow diversion device if it becomes entangled in the preexisting stent(s) and coil construct. It is also worth noting that in the labeling indications (▶ Table 6.1), one of the four listed contraindications for use is the presence of a preexisting stent in the parent artery at the target aneurysm location.

The use of a PED, however, has been reported in conjunction with the Neuroform stent, Enterprise stent, and the Leo + stent. Heiferman et al reported a series[7] of 25 aneurysms for which prior stent-assisted coiling had failed. Twenty-four of the 25 aneurysms were able to be treated and at 12-month follow-up, angiography showed Raymond class I obliteration in 38% (9 aneurysms) with all treated cases demonstrating decreased filling on follow-up imaging. Daou et al also reported a series of 21 patients with recurrent aneurysms initially treated with stent-assisted coiling.[8] The complete occlusion rate was 55.6%, which was a significantly lower obliteration rate than their own series of recurrent aneurysms that were originally treated with coiling alone. The retreatment (11.1%) and complication rates (14.3%) were also higher.

The majority of the cases treated in the aforementioned series involved aneurysms in the anterior circulation only. In addition, the reported complication rates (6–9%) are slightly higher in these series than the complication rates reported for recoiling procedures (1–3%). These results point to a potential cost for the higher occlusion rates when using flow diverters following stent-assisted coiling.

6.3 Ruptured Aneurysms

The treatment of ruptured aneurysms was traditionally believed to be contraindicated, given the gradual rate of aneurysm thrombosis resulting from flow diversion. It was believed that the risk of short-term morbidity and mortality, principally from re-rupture, would be too great to justify flow diversion as a protective strategy. In addition, the requirement for dual

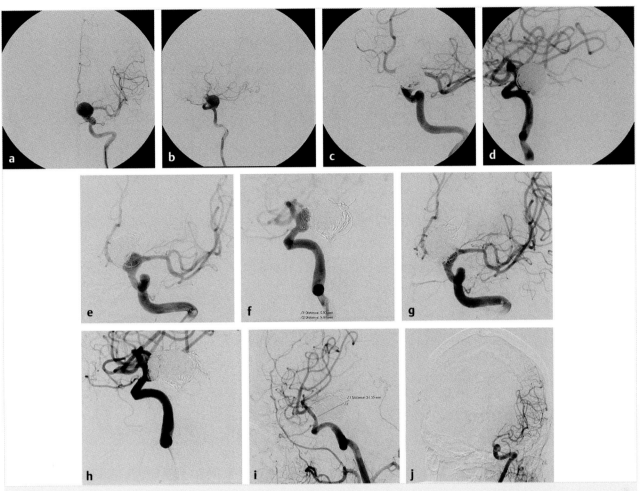

Fig. 6.1 A 59-year-old woman with an incidentally discovered left internal carotid artery (ICA) aneurysm (**a,b**) measuring 18 × 19 × 16.5 mm with a wide neck. Patient underwent stent coiling with Guglielmi detachable coils and a 4.5 × 28 mm Enterprise VRD in 2009 (**c,d**). Patient was lost to follow-up until August 2015 when she returned with headaches. Angiography demonstrated a recurrent very wide-necked aneurysm in the left ICA posterior wall and posterior communicating artery segment with a 9 × 5 mm neck (**e,f**). The Enterprise stent extended from the cavernous ICA to the left M1 segment of the middle cerebral artery. Retreatment was performed with a Pipeline Flex 4.25 mm × 35 mm device supplemented by Axium coils. Initial posttreatment angiography is shown (**g,h**) with marked reduction in the opacification of the aneurysm and the neck. Six-month follow-up angiography showed complete obliteration of the aneurysm with the left A1 patent but with slow flow (**i,j**).

Table 6.1 Pipeline Embolization Device—FDA-approved indications and contraindications

Indications
Large or giant intracranial, wide-necked aneurysms
Anterior circulation, from petrous segment of ICA to superior hypophyseal artery
Adults aged 22 or older

Contraindications
Patients with active bacterial infection
Patients in whom dual antiplatelet therapy (aspirin and clopidogrel) is contraindicated
Patients who have not received dual antiplatelet agents prior to the procedure
Patients in whom a preexisting stent is in place in the parent artery at the target aneurysm location

Abbreviation: ICA, internal carotid artery.

antiplatelet therapy complicated any additional surgical interventions for the patient, that is, the management of hydrocephalus with external ventricular drainage and/or shunt placement. However, as experience has accumulated, it has been increasingly recognized that flow diversion may be a reasonable option and can be accomplished with an acceptable outcome rate for a subset of ruptured aneurysms, with a particularly challenging morphology (▶ Fig. 6.2).[9,10] Lin et al[9] published a series of 26 patients treated with PED in the setting of subarachnoid hemorrhage (SAH). Eight of the 26 patients were treated in a delayed fashion and all but 4 patients had dissecting, fusiform, or blister aneurysms. In addition, 12 of the 26 patients were treated with adjunctive coiling along with flow diversion to accomplish a more immediate and complete aneurysm occlusion. Perioperative complications were seen in 19.2% of patients with three mortalities. Follow-up angiography was available for 23 of the patients with a 78.2% rate of aneurysm occlusion. A more complete review of flow diversion for ruptured aneurysms is covered elsewhere in this book.

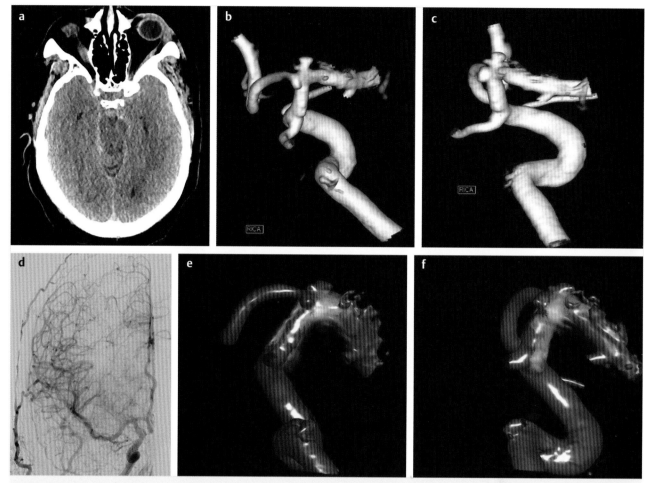

Fig. 6.2 A 41-year-old woman with a mild headache 1 day prior to presentation that acutely became worst headache of life while using the bathroom. Head CT (**a**) showed a subarachnoid hemorrhage. Catheter angiography including 3D rotational angiography (**b–d**) shows two small, irregular aneurysms at the right internal carotid artery (ICA) terminus and proximal middle cerebral artery. Endovascular treatment was elected and the aneurysm was treated with a single Pipeline 3 mm × 18 mm device deployed from the distal ICA into the M1 segment. Post–placement angiography showed coverage over both aneurysms and (**e,f**) increased cross-filling of the anterior cerebral artery (ACA) from the left (**g,h**) (continued).

6.4 Distal Anterior Circulation and Posterior Circulation Aneurysms

There are currently ongoing clinical trials which may expand the approved indications, if confirmed to have similar outcomes as the original studies that were the basis for FDA approval. The Pipeline Premier Trial expanded the indications to include aneurysms located throughout the intracranial course of the ICA up to the terminus, the vertebral artery up to and including the posterior inferior cerebellar artery (PICA), and aneurysms ≤ 12 mm in dimension. The follow-up collection period for the Premier Trial concluded in late 2016 with the hopes that these data may lead to broadening of indications to include the current clinical practice within the FDA-approved indications. It is also possible that if and when additional flow diversion devices are approved for use, the approved indications will be broader than the PED.

Currently, flow diversion with a PED can be an excellent, albeit, off-label solution for posterior circulation aneurysms (▶ Fig. 6.3, ▶ Fig. 6.4, ▶ Fig. 6.5). A proximal location of posterior circulation aneurysms reduces, but does not eliminate, the risk of occlusion of a perforating vessel. Additionally, an endovascular treatment may eliminate the risks for what can be a challenging surgical approach. However, perforators are oftentimes not visualized during the procedure and the rate of complications may rise with the use of multiple overlapping devices.[11] Patency of large branch vessels such as the PICA has been reported in multiple series and is presumed to occur due to downstream demand maintaining anterograde flow. In a small series of vertebral artery aneurysms located on the V4 segment, 8 of 11 patients maintained PICA patency despite coverage with the PED at follow-up without evidence of clinical sequela.[12]

Flow diversion has also been used effectively in more distal posterior circulation segments, where other treatment options

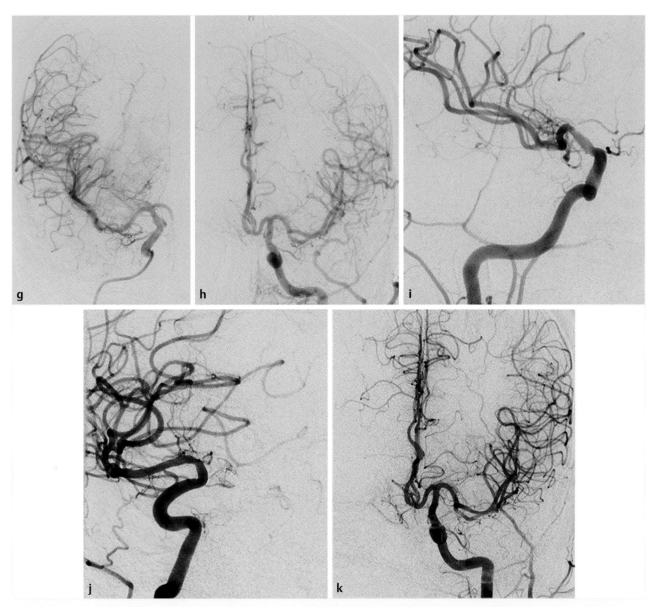

Fig. 6.2 (*continued*) Post–placement angiography showed coverage over both aneurysms and (**e,f**) increased cross-filling of the anterior cerebral artery (ACA) from the left (**g,h**). Follow-up angiography at 1 year showed complete aneurysm occlusion, absent right A1 filling (**i, j**), and bilateral ACA filling from the left carotid injection (**k**).

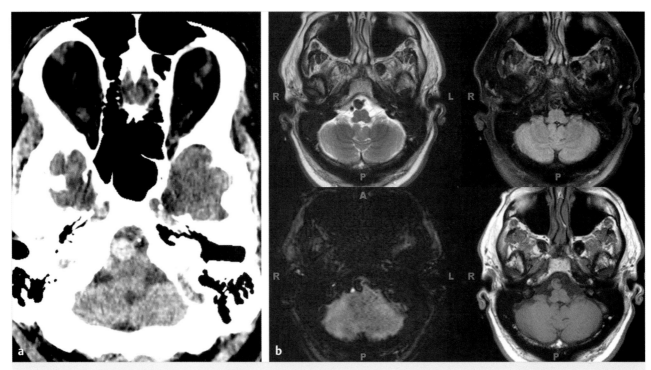

Fig. 6.3 A 69-year-old man with a 1-week history of severe headaches. CT head (**a**) showed no SAH but a hyperdense lesion anterior to the brainstem. MRI (**b,c**) and MRA (**d,e**) were performed and showed a left vertebral artery aneurysm at the pontomedullary junction, projecting posteriorly and superiorly (*continued*).

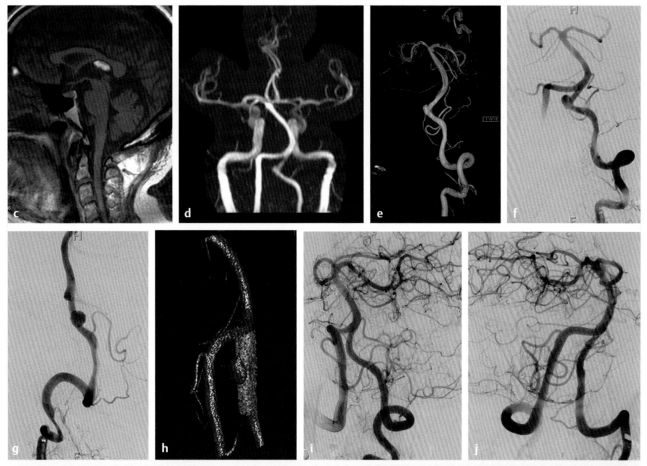

Fig. 6.3 (*continued*) MRI (**b,c**) and MRA (**d,e**) were performed and showed a left vertebral artery aneurysm at the pontomedullary junction, projecting posteriorly and superiorly. Cerebral angiography (**f,g**) showed the lesion was located at the terminal left vertebral artery and measured 7.5 mm. This was treated with a single Pipeline device placed proximal to the vertebrobasilar junction (**h**). One-year follow-up angiography (**i,j**) showed complete aneurysm occlusion.

would have distinct disadvantages (▶ Fig. 6.6). However, the initial experience with posterior circulation flow diversion, particularly with fusiform aneurysms, was filled with significant morbidity and mortality from both perforator infarcts and delayed ruptures.[13]

Albuquerque et al,[14] however, published a series of 17 cases with more than 90% complete or near-complete occlusion. Only one patient experienced a significant complication related to a ventriculostomy hemorrhage. Munich et al[11] reported a series of 12 fusiform vertebrobasilar aneurysms treated with PED and reported one death and two significant new neurological complications, both of which improved significantly at follow-up. At follow-up, 90% of the cases were angiographically occluded. In a subsequent reanalysis of the treatment indication after their initial cautionary report, the University of Buffalo group published[15] a series of 12 patients with fusiform vertebrobasilar aneurysms treated with flow diversion with 50% of the cases treated with adjunctive coiling. At last radiological follow-up (14-month average), all 12 patients had patent devices and complete aneurysm occlusion. Two patients did require a second treatment with a PED to achieve complete occlusion. Only one patient suffered a perforator infarct. In these and other reports,[16] multiple factors are cited which may have improved the outcomes and make posterior circulation aneurysm viable treatment targets. These strategies included adjunctive coiling to limit delayed rupture, limiting the number of devices utilized as longer Pipeline device lengths became available, and meticulous attention to dual antiplatelet efficacy and adherence. Although this represents small retrospective case series, the results lend support to the use of flow diversion in cases where alternatives, such as stent-assisted coiling, clip reconstruction, or deconstructive procedures with or without bypass, are not feasible or carry similar substantial risks.

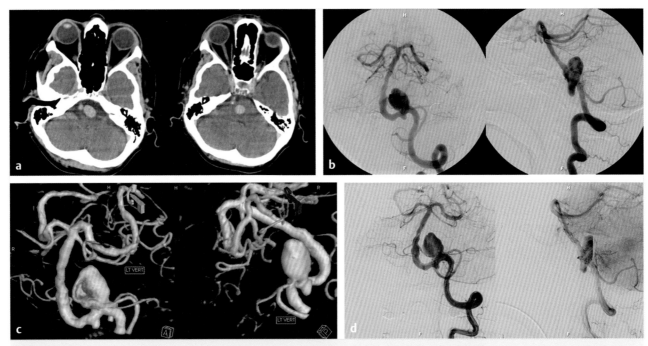

Fig. 6.4 A 62-year-old woman with multiple medical problems referred for treatment of an incidentally detected left vertebral artery fusiform aneurysm discovered on a contrast-enhanced CT scan of the head (**a**). Angiography demonstrated a fusiform aneurysmal dilation of the left vertebral artery at the site of the left posterior inferior cerebellar artery (PICA) origin as well as a 14-mm saccular portion to the aneurysm adjacent to this (**b,c**). This was treated with a 4.5 mm × 20 mm Pipeline device (**d**). These intraoperative images show stasis of contrast within the saccular component of the aneurysm and no change in filling of the PICA (*continued*).

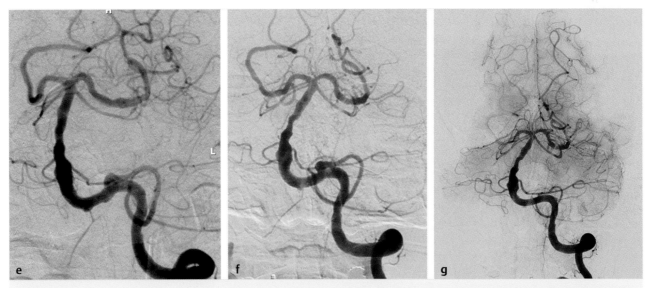

Fig. 6.4 (*continued*) Follow-up angiography at 6 months showed a small residual component to the saccular aneurysm and improvement in the fusiform portion (**e**). At 2-year follow-up, only a small portion of the saccular portion remained (**f**). This was completely occluded at 3-year follow-up and the PICA remained patent (**g**).

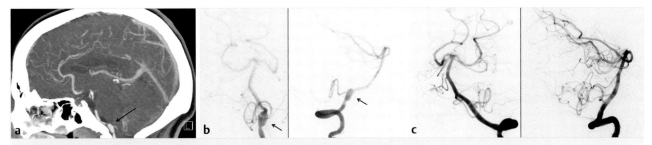

Fig. 6.5 A 51-year-old woman who presented to an outside hospital in a delayed manner after the worst headache of her life, which initially began as severe posterior neck pain. The patient used medications for the symptoms for 8 days and then presented to medical attention. CT scan and lumbar puncture were negative for evidence of hemorrhage. CT angiography (**a**, *arrow*) demonstrated a left vertebral artery aneurysm and the patient was transferred for treatment. Angiography confirmed a 11 × 9 × 7 mm dissecting left vertebral artery aneurysm spanning the origin of the posterior inferior cerebellar artery (PICA; **b**, *arrows*). After treatment with dual antiplatelet therapy, the patient was treated with flow diversion using a single 4 mm × 20 mm Pipeline device. Follow-up angiography 2.9 years after treatment demonstrated no in-stent stenosis, occlusion of the aneurysm, normal caliber to the vertebral artery, and antegrade filling of the PICA (**c**).

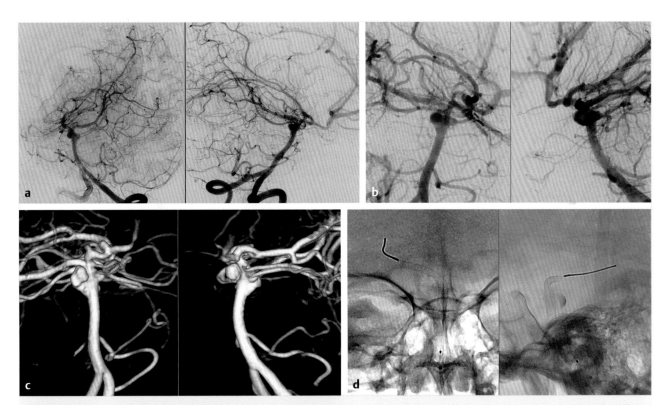

Fig. 6.6 A 15-year-old female with a history of chronic headaches presented with a 2-week history of severe headaches. Head CT showed a diffuse SAH, intraventricular hemorrhage, and mild hydrocephalus. The date that the hemorrhage occurred was unknown based on history. A ventriculostomy was placed and a cerebral angiography was performed. This showed an atypical basilar artery aneurysm, consistent with a dissecting-type aneurysm, just below the superior cerebellar artery (SCA) origins with a duplicated left SCA (**a–c**). She was treated with CSF drainage for 11 days and the ventriculostomy was weaned and then removed. She was then loaded with dual antiplatelet therapy and treated with a 3.0 × 18 mm Pipeline which was advanced into the right posterior cerebral artery (PCA) and deployed from the proximal R PCA to the distal basilar artery. (**d**) Intraoperative single series fluoroscopic views after placement of the device with stasis of contrast within the aneurysm (*continued*).

The distal anterior circulation is another area of off-label use that has expanded as experience has been gained (▶ Fig. 6.7, ▶ Fig. 6.8, ▶ Fig. 6.9). Initial published reports[17,18] did not seem to validate concerns regarding coverage of A1 and M1 segments and perforators. Additionally, the technical feasibility of navigating devices into smaller distal vessels has been well documented. Lin et al[18] reported successful treatment of 27 distal anterior circulation aneurysms with PEDs in a series that included fusiform (15), dissecting (5), and saccular (8) aneurysms. They reported a perioperative complication rate of 10.7% and complete aneurysm occlusion in almost 80% at an average follow-up of 10.7 months. It is noteworthy that 10 of the 27 cases had failed previous treatment with either clipping or coiling.

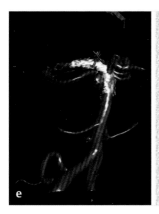
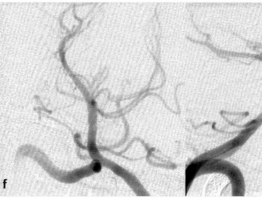

Fig. 6.6 (*continued*) (**e**) Dual volume 3D angiography, depicting the relationship of the stent to the aneurysm and terminal basilar artery. Angiography at 1 year (**f**) showed no evidence of residual aneurysm and anterograde filling of the bilateral PCA and superior cerebellar artery arteries.

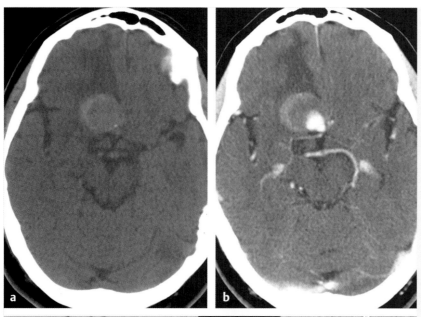

Fig. 6.7 A 66-year-old left-handed man presents with altered mental status. Head CT showed a spherical hyperdensity in the region of the anterior communicating artery with adjacent vasogenic edema (**a**). Contrast-enhanced CT showed a partially thrombosed anterior communicating artery aneurysm (**b**). Cerebral angiography confirmed a large partially thrombosed anterior communicating artery aneurysm supplied by the left A1 only (**c**) (*continued*).

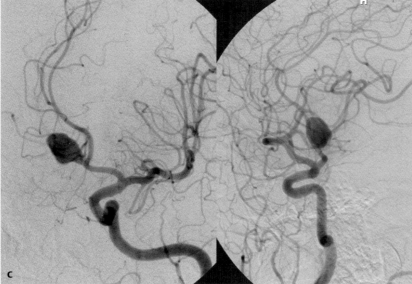

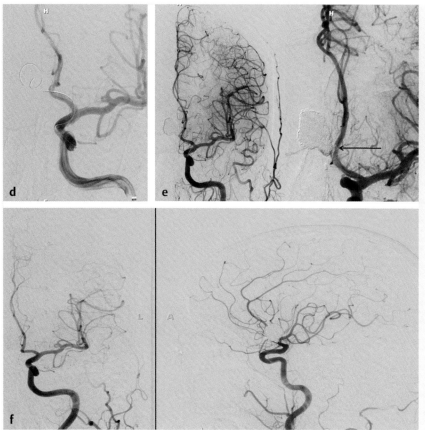

Fig. 6.7 (*continued*) This was treated with placement of a 2.5 × 14 mm PED in the left anterior cerebral artery (ACA) from the A2 segment back into the distal A1, with an Echelon microcatheter jailed in the aneurysm (**d**) and then coiling of the aneurysm with 23 Axium coils. There was complete occlusion of the aneurysm. The procedure was complicated by the development of intra-arterial thrombus formation, within the Pipeline device (**e**, *arrow*), noted at the completion of the coiling. This responded to intra-arterial abciximab infusion, followed by 12 hours of postoperative intravenous abciximab infusion without neurological complication. At 23-month follow-up, there was patency of the left ACA, no recurrence of the aneurysm (**f**), and no filling of the aneurysm from the right internal carotid artery (not shown).

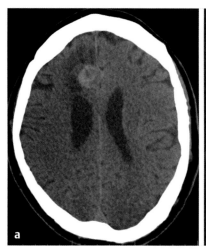
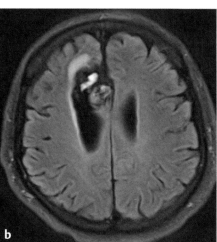

Fig. 6.8 A 49-year-old man who suffered a right frontal traumatic intraparenchymal hematoma after a motorcycle collision 3 months prior to presentation. He then had a fall and underwent CT of the head which revealed a right frontal lesion concerning for an anterior cerebral artery (ACA) aneurysm (**a**). MRI was performed (**b**) which showed right frontal lobe posttraumatic encephalopathy with an adjacent rounded focus of signal abnormality, most likely a pseudoaneurysm, and an additional area of chronic intraparenchymal hemorrhage surrounding the pseudoaneurysm (*continued*).

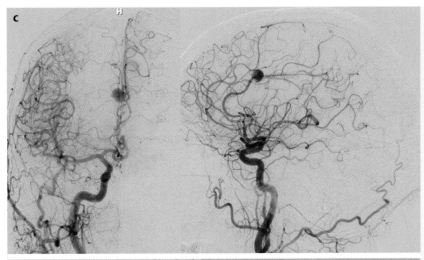

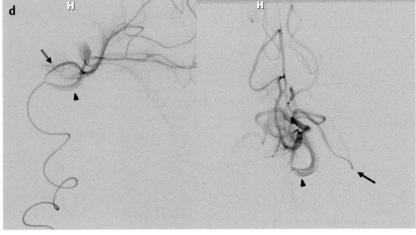

Fig. 6.8 (*continued*) Angiography showed a 9-mm pseudoaneurysm of the left A2 segment which better opacifies from the right carotid injection (**c**), and a relatively avascular area in the right ACA territory from the hematoma and encephalomalacia. A microcatheter run (**d**) in the left A2 demonstrated a right callosomarginal artery (*double line arrow*) originating from the left A2 as well as the left pericallosal (*arrow*) artery originating from the left A2 (*arrowhead*), which gives rise to the aneurysm. At treatment, an initial 2.5 × 10 mm PED device was deployed distal to the aneurysm neck; therefore, a second 2.75 × 10 mm device was placed at the proximal end and overlapping the first (*continued*).

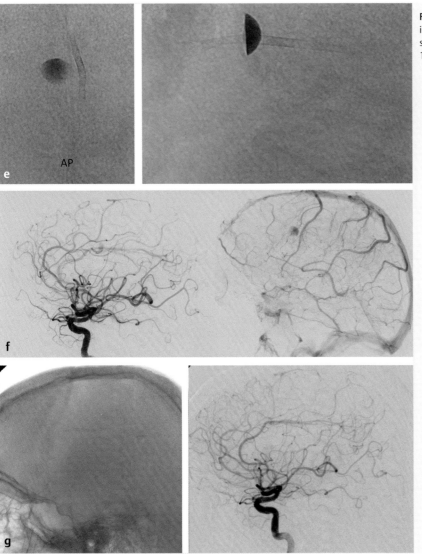

Fig. 6.8 (*continued*) There was stasis of contrast in the aneurysm after PED placement (**e,f**) and stable occlusion of the pseudoaneurysm at the 1-year follow-up (**g**).

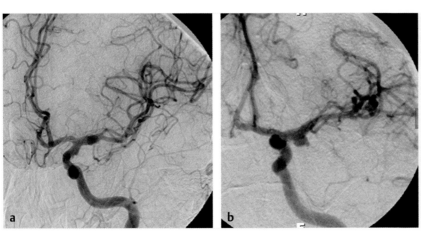

Fig. 6.9 A 53-year-old woman originally presented with a Hunt-Hess Grade 2 SAH. She was found to have a left middle cerebral artery aneurysm with adjacent fusiform dilatation in the M1 segment (**a,b**). She underwent craniotomy and clipping (*continued*).

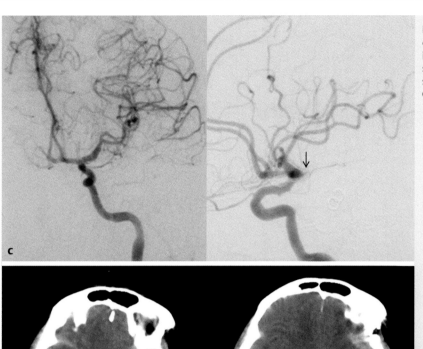

Fig. 6.9 (*continued*) Intraoperative angiography demonstrated a small dog-ear remnant (*arrow* on lateral projection, **c**). The patient lived out of state and was lost to follow-up. Two years later, she re-presented with a recurrent Hunt-Hess Grade 2 SAH (**d**) (*continued*).

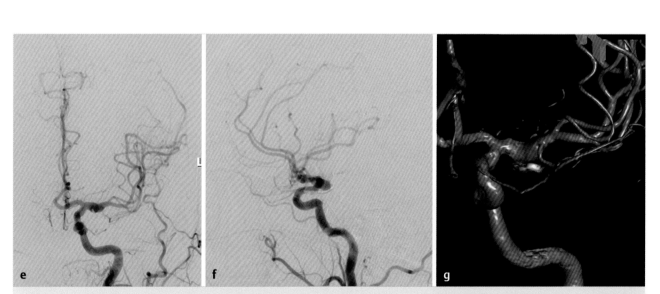

Fig. 6.9 (*continued*) Angiography showed a recurrence of the aneurysm and progression of the fusiform changes in the left M1 segment (**e–g**). She was loaded with aspirin and clopidogrel and treated with flow diversion the day following presentation. An Echelon microcatheter was jailed in the aneurysm by deploying a Pipeline 4 × 20 mm device from the M1 segment back into the internal carotid artery (*continued*).

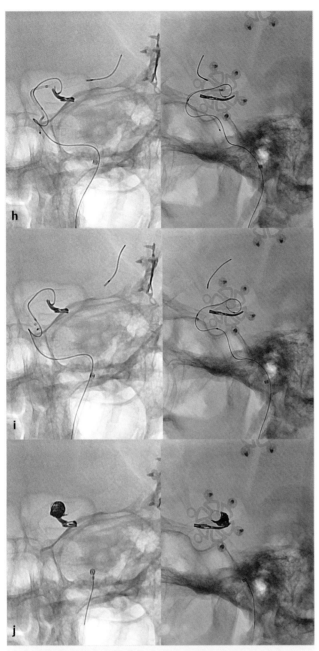

Fig. 6.9 (*continued*) **(h)** The device during deployment with the microcatheter in the aneurysm. A microwire was left within the microcatheter for stability. **(i)** The device immediately after deployment. There was no residual filling of the aneurysm after completion of coiling and placement of the Pipeline **(j,k)** (*continued*).

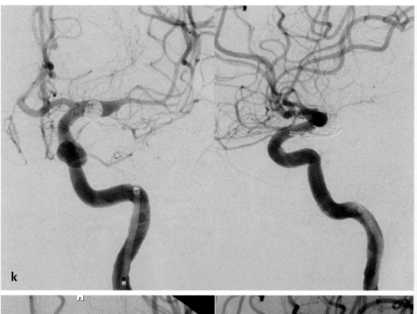

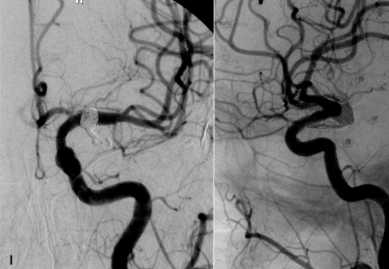

Fig. 6.9 (*continued*) There was no residual filling of the aneurysm after completion of coiling and placement of the Pipeline (**j,k**). Angiography performed 6 months later showed interval decrease in the fusiform dilatation of the M1 segment and no recurrence of the aneurysm (**l**).

6.5 Blister Aneurysms

Blister aneurysms are another type of aneurysm which have been effectively treated with flow diversion with PED (▶ Fig. 6.10, ▶ Fig. 6.11). The increasing utilization of flow diversion for these lesions, as in our previous examples, stems from the particular difficulty with which they are managed with other techniques, such as stent-assisted coiling and open wrapping with or without clip assistance. Additionally, there is a general lack of consensus on the preferred treatment of these very difficult lesions. Rouchaud et al's[19] review of the endovascular treatment of blister aneurysms in the literature compared deconstructive to reconstructive strategies. Deconstructive procedures, which represented less than 10% of published cases, had a higher rate of initial occlusion, but with a higher rate of perioperative stroke (29.1 vs. 5%). Of the reconstructive cases reported, flow diversion represented 25.8% and had higher rates of long-term, complete occlusion than other techniques (90.8 vs. 67.9%). Multiple other small series[20,21,22] reported

successful outcomes, though short-term re-rupture has also been reported.[23]

6.6 Carotid Cavernous Fistulas

Carotid cavernous fistulas (CCF) have been reported both as a complication of flow diversion and as a successful treatment strategy for flow diversion (▶ Fig. 6.12).[24] Most of these reports involve flow diversion (transarterial) of the ICA supplemented with transvenous coil embolization to further obliterate the fistula.[25,26] This strategy has been more commonly applied to posttraumatic fistulas rather than spontaneous fistulas as a sequela of a cavernous segment ICA aneurysm rupture.

Another related and rare application of flow diversion relates to iatrogenic carotid injuries, typically in the setting of endonasal surgery. A recently published series of endovascular treatments of carotid injuries found 5 cases treated with flow diversion out of 105 cases.[27] There was only one case of a minor technical complication without permanent neurological

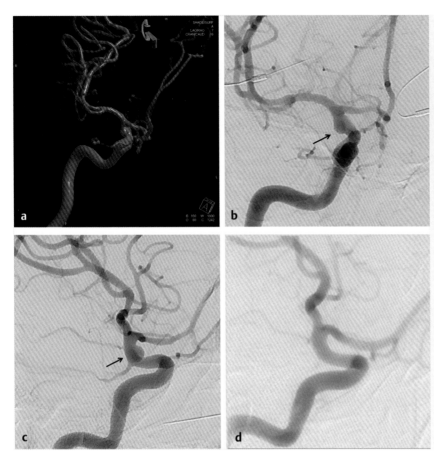

Fig. 6.10 A 40-year-old man presented with sudden-onset severe headache superimposed on an episode of urolithiasis. Initial CT scan without contrast was performed which was negative for evidence of hemorrhage. He was discharged from the emergency department with pain medications. After returning with persistence of headaches, repeat CT scan remained negative for evidence of hemorrhage. Lumbar puncture was performed which demonstrated 51,000 red blood cells. CT angiography and diagnostic angiography showed a 4.3 mm × 4.1 mm blister-type aneurysm of the dorsal right internal carotid artery. The lesion had a classic blister-type aneurysm appearance with a broad base and mild focal stenosis just proximal to the aneurysm (**a-c**, *arrow*). Endovascular treatment with coiling was attempted at outside hospital but abandoned. The patient was transferred to our medical center and loaded with aspirin and clopidogrel. He was treated with placement of a single 3.75 × 14 mm Pipeline embolization device without supplemental coils, 7 days following his hemorrhage. The remainder of his hospital course was unremarkable. Follow-up angiography demonstrated no evidence of recurrence after 22 months (**d**).

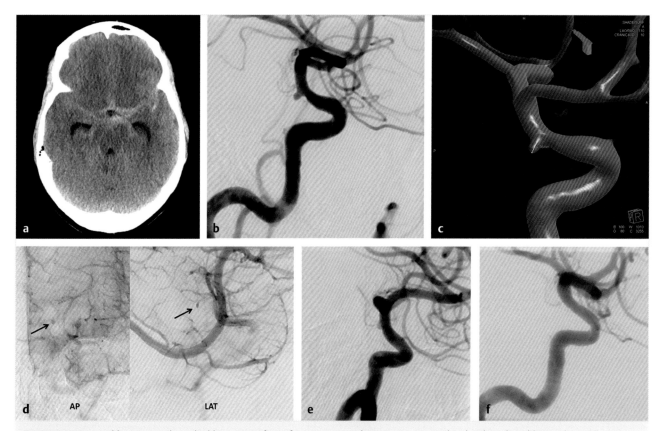

Fig. 6.11 A 47-year-old woman with medical history significant for metastatic colon cancer presented with subarachnoid hemorrhage (**a**). CT angiography did not demonstrate any aneurysm or other lesion to account for the patient's hemorrhage. Cerebral arteriography demonstrated a blister-type aneurysm of the left internal carotid artery (**b, c**). After loading with dual antiplatelet agents intraoperatively, the lesion was treated with a single 3.75 × 14 mm Pipeline Flex embolization device which resulted in stasis within the aneurysm (**d**, *arrows*). Angiography performed 1 week later (**e**) demonstrated decrease in size of the aneurysm and increased degree of contrast stasis compared to initial posttreatment angiography. Repeat angiography 6 weeks later (**f**) demonstrated no filling of the aneurysm. No further follow-up studies were performed because the patient succumbed to colorectal cancer 7 months after her hemorrhage.

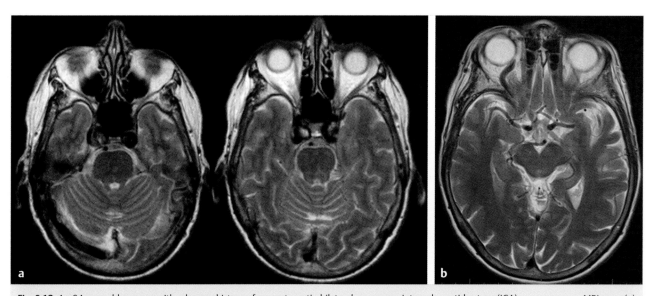

Fig. 6.12 An 84-year-old woman with a known history of asymptomatic bilateral cavernous internal carotid artery (ICA) aneurysms on MRI scan (**a**) presented with months of ptosis, swelling, and injection involving the right eye, as well as noticing a pulsatile "whooshing" sound. Physical exam was significant for left-sided ptosis. Repeat MRI showed proptosis and interval enlargement of the right superior ophthalmic vein (**b**). Diagnostic angiography demonstrated bilateral cavernous carotid ICA aneurysms and a right carotid to cavernous fistula (CCF) fed directly from the ruptured right cavernous ICA aneurysm. Venous outflow of the fistula was via dilated right ophthalmic veins, the inferior petrosal sinus, and retrograde cortical venous drainage (RCVD) via the right Sylvian vein (*continued*).

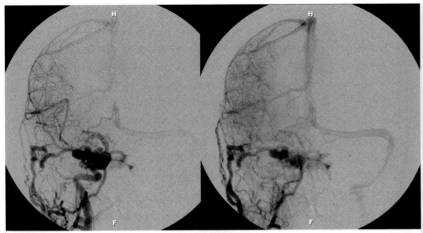

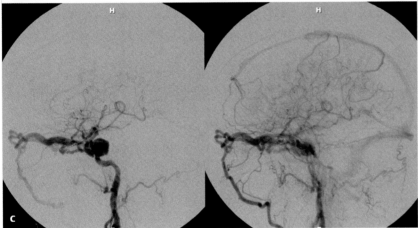

Fig. 6.12 (*continued*) There was also flow across circular sinus to the left cavernous sinus (**c,d**). Attempts at accessing the cavernous sinus via retrograde transvenous approach through the inferior petrosal sinus, as well as by transiting the direct connection from the cavernous aneurysm to the cavernous sinus were all unsuccessful. Eventually, it was possible to navigate retrograde through the facial vein, the angular branch, and then superior ophthalmic vein, into the confluence of the ophthalmic veins and the cavernous sinus. Transvenous coil embolization was performed in this region (*continued*).

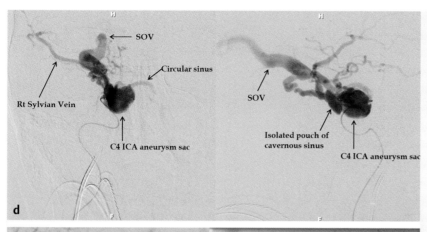

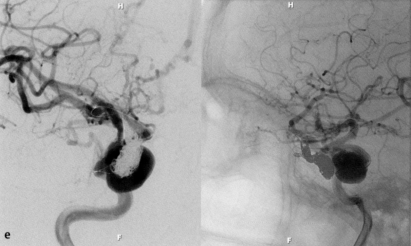

Fig. 6.12 (*continued*) However, after coiling, there was still retrograde cortical venous drainage in the Sylvian vein and persistent filling of the isolated lateral sac of the fistula (**e**). Transvenous embolization was therefore attempted with 6% ethylene vinyl alcohol (EVO) copolymer (Onyx 18) (*continued*).

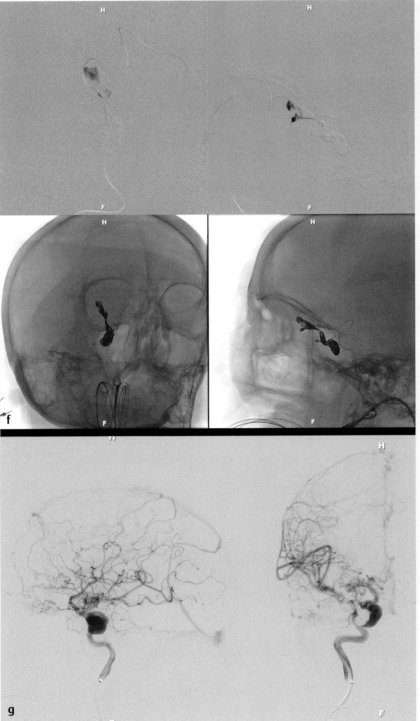

Fig. 6.12 (*continued*) This progressed partially into the residual lateral sac but then also began to reflux into the ophthalmic veins; therefore, the injection was discontinued (**f**). The coiling and EVO embolization eliminated the orbital drainage (**g**), but there was persistence of RCVD and the lateral cavernous sinus sac. Flow diversion across the site of the fistula was then performed (*continued*).

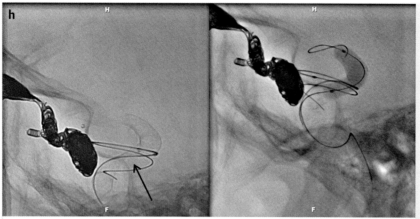

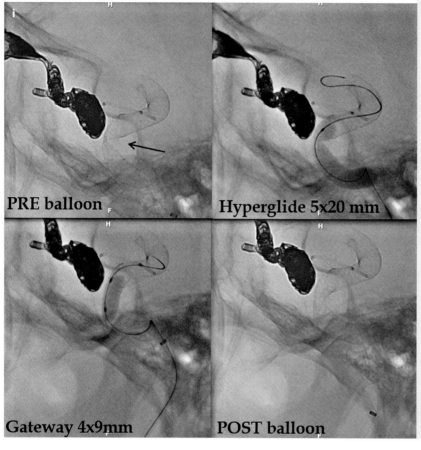

PRE balloon

Hyperglide 5x20 mm

Gateway 4x9mm

POST balloon

Fig. 6.12 (*continued*) First, the aneurysm was catheterized with an Echelon 10 microcatheter. Then, a 4.75 mm × 20 mm device was deployed in the right ICA, "jailing" the microcatheter. Post-deployment angiography (**h**) showed that the stent was not fully apposed to the parent artery (*arrow*) due to a kink in the midportion. Angioplasty was performed using a Hyperglide 5 mm × 20 mm balloon at the distal landing zone and within a narrowed middle segment of the device to achieve optimal wall apposition. After correction of the kinking, there was excellent wall apposition and stasis of flow in the aneurysm sac, though persistent filling of the CCF. A second Pipeline device (5 mm × 25 mm) was placed proximal and slightly overlapping the first device. Again, the device did not fully appose the vessel wall (**i**, *arrow*) and required angioplasty. A Hyperglide 5 mm × 20 mm balloon was unsuccessful; therefore, a second angioplasty with a Gateway 4 mm × 9 mm balloon successfully opened the device (**i**, POST balloon) (*continued*).

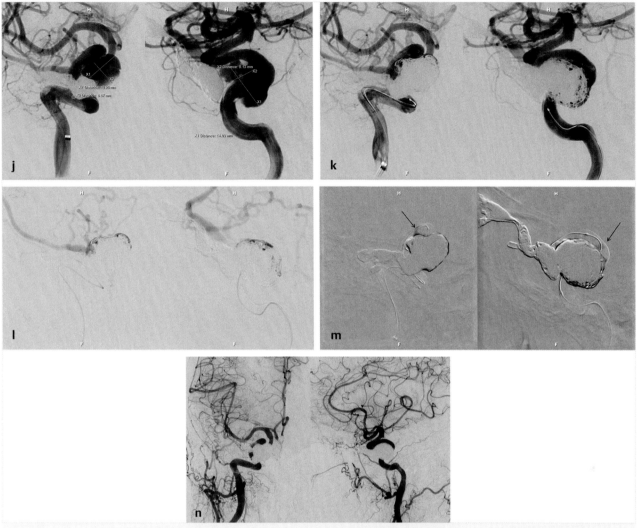

Fig. 6.12 (*continued*) The residual aneurysm was then coiled with a total of 16 Axium helix microcoils (**j**, pre-coiling). Post-coiling angiography (**k**) demonstrated no residual filling of the cavernous aneurysm, cavernous sinus, or ophthalmic venous confluence. However, there was persistent arteriovenous shunting into the right Sylvian vein with retrograde cortical flow to the right cerebral hemisphere. A contrast injection was performed through the microcatheter trapped in the cavernous aneurysm that confirmed that this arteriovenous shunting was via the direct CC fistula. (**l**). In a further attempt to eliminate the cortical venous reflux, embolization with 20% EVO copolymer (Onyx 500) of the fistula from a transarterial approach was attempted. This decreased but did not eliminate the amount of fistulous flow into the Sylvian vein, but the injection was discontinued after 2.8 mL was injected when the EVO was seen to migrate around the outside of the PED (**m**, *arrows*). Final posttreatment arteriography showed persistent arteriovenous shunting into the right Sylvian vein through the fistula with retrograde cortical venous drainage, however markedly reduced flow through the fistula compared to baseline. This had resolved by 3-month follow-up imaging. At follow-up angiography 2.5 years after treatment, there was no residual fistula or RCVD and normal filling of the right middle cerebral artery and anterior cerebral artery, without in-stent stenosis (**n**).

sequelae. In many instances, these injuries can be characterized by life-threatening intraoperative hemorrhage and were historically treated with parent vessel sacrifice, with a significant risk of ischemic infarction. Treatment with coil embolization, with or without stent assistance, or endoluminal reconstruction with a covered stent also carried significant risk of complications. Flow diversion, with or without coil embolization of the pseudoaneurysm, offered the advantage of parent vessel preservation (▶ Fig. 6.13). As with ruptured aneurysms, potential disadvantages of this treatment strategy included the need for dual antiplatelet therapy in the setting of a recent hemorrhage and the often delayed nature of the pseudoaneurysm occlusion.

6.7 Flow Diversion in the Young

Another off-label use of Pipeline flow diversion relates to the use in patients 21 years of age or younger. Aneurysms are particularly rare in the pediatric population and may be associated with genetic syndromes which predispose to both aneurysms and other systemic vasculopathies contributing to the complexity of treatment. However, there are instances where flow diversion has been used successfully in this patient population (▶ Fig. 6.6). A recent report detailed the treatment of three unruptured aneurysms with one case involving a patient as young as 4 years of age.[28] Other series have also reported acceptable outcomes in this population.[29,30]

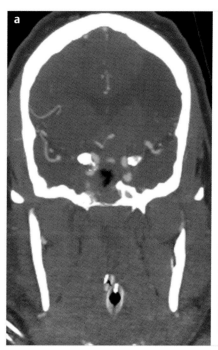
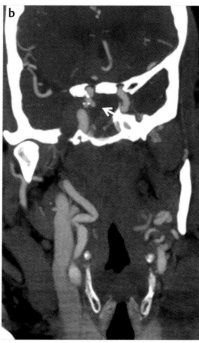

Fig. 6.13 A 51-year-old woman underwent elective repeat transsphenoidal resection of a recurrent nonsecretory pituitary macroadenoma. Besides the previous transsphenoidal resection 9 years prior, the patient's history was significant for a left hemispheric cerebral infarct of unknown etiology with residual right-sided weakness. Intraoperatively, brisk bleeding was encountered and controlled easily with gel foam and tamponade. Gross total resection of the tumor was then completed and postoperatively CT scan and CT angiography were performed. This demonstrated no evidence of hemorrhage in the tumor bed and no evidence of pseudoaneurysm or other vascular abnormality (**a**). The patient was discharged home on postoperative day 9 but 4 days later was awakened from sleep with severe epistaxis. She presented to an outside hospital emergency department where her nose was packed and she was intubated. She was transferred to our medical center for treatment. CT angiography demonstrated a 5-mm pseudoaneurysm of the right internal carotid artery (**b**, *arrow*), confirmed on digital subtraction angiography (*continued*).

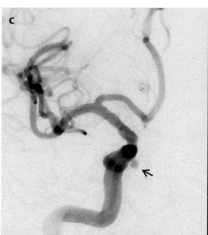
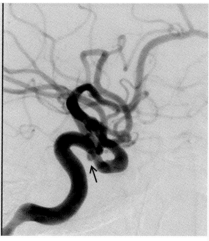
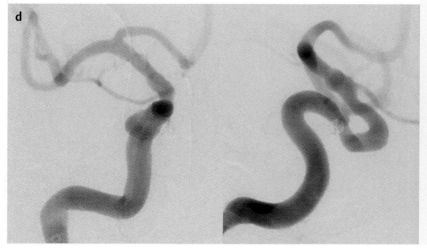

Fig. 6.13 (*continued*) (**c**, *arrow*). Given her previous contralateral infarct, a diminutive anterior communicating artery, treatment with flow diversion and coil embolization was elected over vessel sacrifice for hemostasis. An Echelon microcatheter was jailed in the aneurysm by deploying a 4.75 × 18 mm Pipeline Flex device across the neck. After placement of a single 3 mm × 6 cm platinum coil, there was no residual filling of the aneurysm (**d**). Patient experienced no further epistaxis and had no neurological complications.

6.8 Extracranial Disease

Extracranial vascular injuries resulting in dissection or pseudoaneurysm, as well as spontaneous dissections, have been successfully treated with flow diversion. In certain instances of carotid dissections (failure of medical therapy, severe flow limitation or clinical symptoms, and location at the high cervical region or skull base), flow diversion offers some advantages. The tortuosity of the skull base and high cervical region make placement of a traditional carotid stent technically challenging due to their rigidity. Additionally, the large cell design of intracranial self-expanding stents (Neuroform, Enterprise) may not provide sufficient flow diversion to occlude pseudoaneurysms. Brzezicki et al[31] reported 13 dissections (spontaneous and traumatic) treated with Pipeline flow diversion with a 91% near-complete revascularization rate. Half of the pseudoaneurysms were immediately obliterated after device placement. At follow-up, 75% of pseudoaneurysms had healed. Additionally, there are several reported cases of using flow diversion for the treatment of iatrogenic pseudoaneurysms of the vertebral artery.[32,33]

6.9 Conclusion

While the initial experience with flow diversion, in general, and the PED, in particular, was in aneurysms that met the initial U.S. FDA indications, the popularity of this treatment strategy has led to the expansion of its indications in routine clinical use. With continued meticulous testing and reporting of study results, it is highly likely that subsequent generations of flow diverters will have an expanded indication list to mirror the current practice.

References

[1] Kallmes DF, Hanel R, Lopes D, et al. International retrospective study of the pipeline embolization device: a multicenter aneurysm treatment study. AJNR Am J Neuroradiol. 2015; 36(1):108–115

[2] Ferns SP, Sprengers ME, van Rooij WJ, et al. Coiling of intracranial aneurysms: a systematic review on initial occlusion and reopening and retreatment rates. Stroke. 2009; 40(8):e523–e529

[3] Crobeddu E, Lanzino G, Kallmes DF, Cloft HJ. Review of 2 decades of aneurysm-recurrence literature, part 1: reducing recurrence after endovascular coiling. AJNR Am J Neuroradiol. 2013; 34(2):266–270

[4] Murayama Y, Nien YL, Duckwiler G, et al. Guglielmi detachable coil embolization of cerebral aneurysms: 11 years' experience. J Neurosurg. 2003; 98 (5):959–966

[5] Raymond J, Darsaut TE. An approach to recurrent aneurysms following endovascular coiling. J Neurointerv Surg. 2011; 3(4):314–318

[6] Daou B, Starke RM, Chalouhi N, et al. The use of the Pipeline Embolization Device in the management of recurrent previously coiled cerebral aneurysms. Neurosurgery. 2015; 77(5):692–697, 697

[7] Heiferman DM, Billingsley JT, Kasliwal MK, et al. Use of flow-diverting stents as salvage treatment following failed stent-assisted embolization of intracranial aneurysms. J Neurointerv Surg. 2016; 8(7):692–695

[8] Daou B, Starke RM, Chalouhi N, et al. Pipeline Embolization Device in the treatment of recurrent previously stented cerebral aneurysms. AJNR Am J Neuroradiol. 2016; 37(5):849–855

[9] Lin N, Brouillard AM, Keigher KM, et al. Utilization of Pipeline embolization device for treatment of ruptured intracranial aneurysms: US multicenter experience. J Neurointerv Surg. 2015; 7(11):808–815

[10] Cruz JP, O'Kelly C, Kelly M, et al. Pipeline embolization device in aneurysmal subarachnoid hemorrhage. AJNR Am J Neuroradiol. 2013; 34(2):271–276

[11] Munich SA, Tan LA, Keigher KM, Chen M, Moftakhar R, Lopes DK. The Pipeline Embolization Device for the treatment of posterior circulation fusiform aneurysms: lessons learned at a single institution. J Neurosurg. 2014; 121 (5):1077–1084

[12] Mazur MD, Kilburg C, Wang V, Taussky P. Pipeline embolization device for the treatment of vertebral artery aneurysms: the fate of covered branch vessels. J Neurointerv Surg. 2016; 8(10):1041–1047

[13] Siddiqui AH, Abla AA, Kan P, et al. Panacea or problem: flow diverters in the treatment of symptomatic large or giant fusiform vertebrobasilar aneurysms. J Neurosurg. 2012; 116(6):1258–1266

[14] Albuquerque FC, Park MS, Abla AA, Crowley RW, Ducruet AF, McDougall CG. A reappraisal of the Pipeline embolization device for the treatment of posterior circulation aneurysms. J Neurointerv Surg. 2015; 7(9):641–645

[15] Natarajan SK, Lin N, Sonig A, et al. The safety of Pipeline flow diversion in fusiform vertebrobasilar aneurysms: a consecutive case series with longer-term follow-up from a single US center. J Neurosurg. 2016; 125(1):111–119

[16] Phillips TJ, Wenderoth JD, Phatouros CC, et al. Safety of the pipeline embolization device in treatment of posterior circulation aneurysms. AJNR Am J Neuroradiol. 2012; 33(7):1225–1231

[17] Durst CR, Hixson HR, Schmitt P, Gingras JM, Crowley RW. Endovascular treatment of a fusiform aneurysm at the M3-M4 junction of the middle cerebral artery using the Pipeline Embolization Device. World Neurosurg. 2016; 86:511.e1–511.e4

[18] Lin N, Lanzino G, Lopes DK, et al. Treatment of distal anterior circulation aneurysms with the Pipeline Embolization Device: a US multicenter experience. Neurosurgery. 2016; 79(1):14–22

[19] Rouchaud A, Brinjikji W, Cloft HJ, Kallmes DF. Endovascular treatment of ruptured blister-like aneurysms: a systematic review and meta-analysis with focus on deconstructive versus reconstructive and flow-diverter treatments. AJNR Am J Neuroradiol. 2015; 36(12):2331–2339

[20] Linfante I, Mayich M, Sonig A, Fujimoto J, Siddiqui A, Dabus G. Flow diversion with Pipeline Embolic Device as treatment of subarachnoid hemorrhage secondary to blister aneurysms: dual-center experience and review of the literature. J Neurointerv Surg. 2017; 9(1):29–33

[21] Chalouhi N, Zanaty M, Tjoumakaris S, et al. Treatment of blister-like aneurysms with the pipeline embolization device. Neurosurgery. 2014; 74 (5):527–532, discussion 532

[22] Çinar C, Oran İ, Bozkaya H, Ozgiray E. Endovascular treatment of ruptured blister-like aneurysms with special reference to the flow-diverting strategy. Neuroradiology. 2013; 55(4):441–447

[23] Mazur MD, Taussky P, MacDonald JD, Park MS. Rerupture of a blister aneurysm after treatment with a single flow-diverting stent. Neurosurgery. 2016; 79(5):E634–E638

[24] Amuluru K, Al-Mufti F, Gandhi CD, Prestigiacomo CJ, Singh IP. Direct carotid-cavernous fistula: a complication of, and treatment with, flow diversion. Interv Neuroradiol. 2016; 22(5):569–576

[25] Pradeep N, Nottingham R, Kam A, Gandhi D, Razack N. Treatment of post-traumatic carotid-cavernous fistulas using pipeline embolization device assistance. BMJ Case Rep. 2015; 2015

[26] Nossek E, Zumofen D, Nelson E, et al. Use of Pipeline Embolization Devices for treatment of a direct carotid-cavernous fistula. Acta Neurochir (Wien). 2015; 157(7):1125–1129, discussion 1130

[27] Sylvester PT, Moran CJ, Derdeyn CP, et al. Endovascular management of internal carotid artery injuries secondary to endonasal surgery: case series and review of the literature. J Neurosurg. 2016; 125(5):1256–1276

[28] Navarro R, Brown BL, Beier A, Ranalli N, Aldana P, Hanel RA. Flow diversion for complex intracranial aneurysms in young children. J Neurosurg Pediatr. 2015; 15(3):276–281

[29] Vargas SA, Diaz C, Herrera DA, Dublin AB. Intracranial aneurysms in children: the role of stenting and flow diversion. J Neuroimaging. 2016; 26(1):41–45

[30] Ashok Vachhani J, Michael Nickele C, Elijovich L, Klimo P, Arthur AS. Flow diversion for treatment of growing A2 aneurysm in a child: case report and review of flow diversion for intracranial aneurysms in pediatric patients. World Neurosurg. 2016; 96:607.e13–607.e17

[31] Brzezicki G, Rivet DJ, Reavey-Cantwell J. Pipeline Embolization Device for treatment of high cervical and skull base carotid artery dissections: clinical case series. J Neurointerv Surg. 2016; 8(7):722–728

[32] Dolati P, Eichberg DG, Thomas A, Ogilvy CS. Application of Pipeline Embolization Device for iatrogenic pseudoaneurysms of the extracranial vertebral artery: a case report and systematic review of the literature. Cureus. 2015; 7(10):e356

[33] Ambekar S, Sharma M, Smith D, Cuellar H. Successful treatment of iatrogenic vertebral pseudoaneurysm using pipeline embolization device. Case Rep Vasc Med. 2014; 2014:341748

7 FLOW DIVERSION IN RUPTURED ANEURYSMS

ARTHUR WANG and MICHAEL F. STIEFEL

Abstract

Flow diversion is an established method for treating complex aneurysms not amenable to conventional endovascular or microsurgical techniques. Its utility is often limited to unruptured aneurysms because of the need for dual-antiplatelet therapy postintervention. There exist only a handful of case reports describing the use of flow diverters in the setting of subarachnoid hemorrhage. We discuss the use of flow diversion for ruptured aneurysms and its associated complications, the management of antiplatelet therapy, and the long-term durability in aneurysm occlusion.

Keywords: flow diversion, ruptured aneurysm, subarachnoid hemorrhage, Pipeline Embolization Device

7.1 Introduction

Flow diversion has been successfully applied to the treatment of large, wide-necked aneurysms; dissecting aneurysms; and small blood blister aneurysms whose morphology is not amenable to conventional endosaccular aneurysm occlusion.[1,2,3] Although the Pipeline Embolization Device (PED; Covidien, Irvine, CA) is the only flow-diverting stent approved for use by the U.S. Food and Drug Administration, other commercially available flow diverters include the SILK device (Balt Extrusion, Montmorency, France), Flow Redirection Endoluminal Device (FRED; MicroVention, Tustin, CA), Surpass (Stryker, Kalamazoo, MI), and p64 (Phenox, Bochum, Germany). These stents are self-expandable, endoluminal devices that disrupt pulsatile blood flow within an aneurysm. By altering the physiologic blood flow, these devices lead to thrombosis of the aneurysm and parent vessel reconstruction.[3,4]

The application of flow diversion in the setting of acute subarachnoid hemorrhage (SAH) is controversial because of three major limitations: requirement of dual-antiplatelet therapy, delayed aneurysm occlusion, and the potential for additional invasive procedures (ventriculostomy, ventriculoperitoneal shunt, decompressive craniectomy, tracheostomy, etc.). As a result, their use has only been described in a few small case series centered on ruptured dissecting aneurysms and ruptured blood blister aneurysms.[1,3,5,6] Additionally, variations in practice regimens in the selection of antiplatelet drugs, their dosing, and duration of therapy add another level of complexity to flow diversion treatment of ruptured aneurysms.[7]

7.2 Patient Selection

The decision to use flow diverters in the setting of acute SAH should be centered on the anatomy of the aneurysm, the condition of the patient, and the comfort level of the neurointerventionalist with flow diverters.

Flow-diverting stents can be considered in cases of morphologically challenging aneurysms such as small blister-type aneurysms, fragile walled dissecting aneurysms, and large wide-necked aneurysms.[1,3,5,6,8,9,10,11,12,13] In these select cases, endoluminal therapy with flow diverters can lead to improved neck and parent vessel reconstruction without the added risk of manipulating the aneurysm sac in the immediate postrupture period.

The clinical grade and condition of the patient need to be taken into account because these will determine the potential need for further surgical intervention. Favorable patients include those with low Hunt-Hess and Fisher's grades who do not have hydrocephalus and those who present days after the initial rupture.[5,14] Patients who present in poor clinical condition generally require additional intracranial procedures such as external ventricular drains (EVDs), ventriculoperitoneal shunts/lumboperitoneal shunts (VPS/LPS), as well as feeding tubes and tracheostomies. These patients are at risk for EVD- or VPS-related tract hemorrhages after initiation of antiplatelet therapy.[5,15,16] Additionally, these patients are at a higher risk of symptomatic vasospasm that could potentially necessitate treatments for ischemic strokes.[14] In these high-risk patients, flow diversion may not be ideal because of the need to discontinue and reverse the effects of the antiplatelet agents for surgical interventions while placing the patient at risk for in-stent thrombosis in the immediate postsurgical period.

7.3 Antiplatelet Therapy Management

Evidence regarding antiplatelet therapy during flow diversion is largely based on the cardiac literature and data from stent-assisted coiling of ruptured aneurysms.[17,18,19,20,21] The common practice is to maintain patients on both aspirin and clopidogrel following stent placement. In the setting of SAH, physicians may modify and vary their regimens after evaluating the risk–benefit profile of potential hemorrhagic and thromboembolic complications associated with antiplatelet medications in the immediate aneurysm postrupture period. As a result, there are heterogeneous practice patterns with antiplatelet medications, their dosing, and duration of use in the setting of ruptured aneurysms.[7]

Pretreatment. Reports on stent-assisted coil embolization using the Neuroform (Boston Scientific, Fremont, CA) and Enterprise (Codman & Shurtleff Inc, Raynham, MA) stents suggest that antiplatelet medications can be initiated in the acute and subacute period of aneurysm rupture with acceptable complication rates.[10,13,22,23,24] Interventional cardiology studies have shown that a 600-mg loading dose of clopidogrel inhibits platelet aggregation by 55 to 59% within 4 hours of administration and results in platelet inhibition for up to 48 hours.[25] The most common pretreatment regimen in the setting of acute SAH has evolved to aspirin 325 or 650 mg and clopidogrel 600 mg.[5,7,8,12,14] Patients are usually loaded with both antiplatelet agents at least 24 to 72 hours before intervention.[1,8,12]

Posttreatment. The appropriate duration of antiplatelets remains controversial. Early withdrawal of antiplatelet medications has been associated with late in-stent PED thrombosis and delayed thromboembolic events.[17,26] At the same time, prolonged dual-antiplatelet use theoretically delays aneurysm thrombosis and exclusion from the circulation. From the literature, the most common practice in the setting of a ruptured aneurysm is to continue the patient on both aspirin and clopidogrel for 6 months postoperatively. The most common doses reported in the literature is clopidogrel 75 mg daily and either aspirin 81 or 325 mg.[5,8,12,13,14,27] The decision to discontinue clopidogrel is usually at the discretion of the neurointerventionalists and results of 6-month follow-up angiography.[14] Some reports of delayed thromboembolic events argue for prolonged use of longer than 1 year of dual-antiplatelet therapy.[26,28,29] The reported rate of delayed thromboembolic events after Neuroform stent-assisted coiling is 4.6 to 8.8%.[26,30,31,32] This risk needs to be weighed with the risk of delayed aneurysm rupture when the aneurysm is not fully excluded from the circulation.[33]

7.4 Delayed Aneurysm Occlusion/Angiographic Outcomes

Unlike coil embolization, flow diversion may not lead to immediate aneurysm occlusion but rather gradual aneurysm thrombosis over days to weeks.[5,34] One case series using the PED to treat three ruptured blister aneurysms demonstrated complete aneurysm occlusion immediately in one case and at 6 weeks of angiographic follow-up on two additional cases.[5] However, there are no large series that document immediate angiographic cure of ruptured aneurysms with the use of flow diverters. In the case of a ruptured aneurysm, the risk of re-rupture remains and could be exacerbated while the patient is maintained on dual-antiplatelet therapy. Furthermore, this risk may be increased if the patient requires hypertensive therapy for clinically symptomatic vasospasm. Although studies show that there is no added risk of rupture with unruptured aneurysms during the treatment of cerebral vasospasm, the effect on an unsecured ruptured aneurysm with dual-antiplatelet therapy remains unknown.[20,35]

Several case series investigating the use of flow-diverting stents in unruptured aneurysms report a 95% occlusion rate at 6 to 18 months of follow-up.[2,29,36,37] There are limited data on aneurysm

occlusion rates with flow diverters in the setting of SAH because of the risk of complications with antiplatelet therapy. Nevertheless, there are several moderate-sized case series investigating the utility of flow diversion in the treatment of ruptured blister aneurysms, dissecting, and giant wide-necked aneurysms (▶ Table 7.1). A U.S. multicenter investigation utilizing the PED for treatment of 26 ruptured intracranial aneurysms reported a 70% complete occlusion rate at 6 months.[12] A similar Canadian multicenter investigation using the PED to treat 20 ruptured aneurysms found complete occlusion rates of 75 and 94% at 6 and 12 months, respectively.[14] Another case series of 11 patients with SAH treated with the PED found a complete occlusion rate of 73% at 6 months.[38] Finally, a case series of 23 patients with dissecting aneurysms reported an occlusion rate of 69.5% at 6 months.[1]

In aneurysms amenable to the placement of coils, coil embolization and flow diversion may be more suitable than using a flow diverter as a stand-alone construct. The placement of coils may afford additional protection to the dome of the aneurysm and may also provide a more thrombotic microenvironment than flow diversion alone.

7.5 Complications/Risk of Additional Procedures

Although flow diversion is a feasible option for select ruptured aneurysms, there are many potential pitfalls. The complications associated with flow diversion in the setting of ruptured aneurysms are directly related to the risks associated with initiation of antiplatelet agents. The risks/benefits profile of hemorrhagic versus thromboembolic complications should be weighed before starting antiplatelet therapy. These complications can be categorized into early/periprocedural (< 30 days) and delayed.

7.5.1 Aneurysm Re-rupture

In contrast to coil embolization, flow diversion does not lead to immediate aneurysm occlusion. The fibrin-platelet plug that forms at the rupture site does not completely protect the dome of the ruptured aneurysm and there remains a potential risk of

Table 7.1 Summary of several case series applying flow diversion to the treatment of ruptured intracranial aneurysms

Study	No. of patients/Ruptured aneurysms	Flow diverter	% of complete angiographic occlusion at 6 mo
Aydin et al[4]	11/Blister	SILK[a]	82
Chalouhi et al[14]	20/Dissecting, Saccular	PED[b]	80
Cruz et al[8]	23/Blister, Dissecting, Giant, Saccular	PED	75
de Barros Faria et al[1]	23/Dissecting	PED	70
Lin et al[12]	26/Blister, Dissecting, Fusiform, Saccular	PED	78
McAuliffe and Wenderoth[38]	11/Fusiform, Saccular	PED	73
Yoon et al[3]	11/Blister	PED	88

[a]SILK (Balt Extrusion, Montmorency, France).
[b]Pipeline Embolization Device (Covidien, Irvine, CA).

rehemorrhage even after the flow diverter is placed.[27] Moreover, with systemic dual-antiplatelet therapy, aneurysmal re-rupture can be devastating. Furthermore, antiplatelet agents will potentially delay platelet aggregation in the ruptured aneurysm and may theoretically prolong the latency interval before complete aneurysm occlusion.[4,39] The aneurysm re-rupture rate reported in the literature after PED placement ranges between 3.8 and 18.2%.[1,12,14,38]

Data from stent-assisted coil embolization using the Neuroform and Enterprise stents have shown that antiplatelet therapy can be started in the acute setting following SAH with acceptable complication rates.[34] To reduce the risk of re-rupture, some neurointerventionalists choose to treat the aneurysm in a staged approach by first coiling the aneurysm rupture site and then placing the flow-diverting stent once the patient is cleared for antiplatelet therapy and further intracranial procedures.[13,14,40] Depending on the characteristics of the aneurysm, some may choose to "jail" the microcatheter and perform a flow-diverter-assisted coil embolization to protect the dome of the aneurysm with the coils and allow for parent vessel reconstruction.[8,14]

7.5.2 EVD-Associated Hemorrhage

Patients treated with stent-assisted coiling who require an EVD have a higher risk of hemorrhagic complications during the management of their hydrocephalus. Studies report that these patients have a higher hemorrhage rate than those not on dual-antiplatelet therapy. Patients on antiplatelet medications have a 32% rate of radiographic hemorrhage and an 8% rate of symptomatic hemorrhage associated with the EVD, compared to a 15% rate of radiographic and a 1% rate of symptomatic hemorrhage in those without stenting and concomitant dual-antiplatelet therapy.[15,39,41,42] To minimize this risk, an EVD is generally placed prior to the intervention to avoid reversal of the antiplatelet agents.[3,5,6,14]

7.5.3 Ventriculoperitoneal Shunt–Associated Hemorrhages

The literature reports up to a 33% risk of catheter-related hemorrhage in patients undergoing VPS placement while on antiplatelet therapy following stent-assisted coil embolization of ruptured brain aneurysms.[16] In preparation for an intracranial procedure, one of the antiplatelet agents, generally clopidogrel, is stopped 24 hours before surgery and platelets are administered preoperatively.[27] To further minimize the risk of ventricular tract hemorrhage, the ventricular catheter is soft passed without the metal stylet.[5,27,43] Still some physicians advocate for first placing a VPS before treating the aneurysm to avoid the risk of antiplatelets entirely.[14]

7.5.4 Extracranial Hemorrhages

Following SAH, patients often require tracheostomies and gastrostomies. In addition, these patients are at risk for stress-related gastric ulcers. One study described a 10% risk of extracranial hemorrhages after stent-assisted coil embolization of ruptured aneurysms, including groin hematomas, retroperitoneal hematomas, and gastrointestinal bleeds.[41]

7.5.5 Spontaneous Intracranial Hemorrhage

There exists a limited number of case reports highlighting the risk of spontaneous distal ipsilateral and contralateral hemorrhages after placement of a flow diverter and concomitant use of antiplatelet therapy.[8,43,44,45,46,47] This complication occurs in 2 to 4% of cases and is thought to occur secondary to loss of cerebral autoregulation, embolized foreign bodies, and hemorrhagic conversion of ischemic lesions.[44,45]

7.5.6 In-Stent Thrombosis/Thromboembolic Events

Flow-diverting stents are more thrombogenic than conventional devices because of their greater metal surface area. In-stent thrombosis and thromboembolic events become legitimate concerns in these patients. In the setting of SAH, the risk of rehemorrhage after starting antiplatelet therapy must be weighed against the risk of in-stent thrombosis from withholding antiplatelet therapy. To this end, neurointerventionalists often modify and vary their antiplatelet regimens in the hopes of mitigating the risk of hemorrhagic complications. As a result, the reported rate of in-stent thrombosis in ruptured aneurysms varies widely between 2 and 18.8% depending on the chosen regimen.[12,22,37,43,48,49]

7.6 Conclusion

Treatment of ruptured aneurysms with flow diverters has been shown to have high occlusion rates, favorable outcomes, and an acceptable complication rate in several case series. An understanding of the aneurysm morphology as well as careful patient selection should guide physicians in their decision to use flow diverters in SAH. Physicians placing these devices should also weigh the risks and benefits of antiplatelet therapy and understand the complications associated with these medications in the immediate period following aneurysm rupture. As of yet, there is still no consensus on a standard antiplatelet regimen or duration of therapy.

References

[1] de Barros Faria M, Castro RN, Lundquist J, et al. The role of the pipeline embolization device for the treatment of dissecting intracranial aneurysms. AJNR Am J Neuroradiol. 2011; 32(11):2192–2195

[2] Nelson PK, Lylyk P, Szikora I, Wetzel SG, Wanke I, Fiorella D. The pipeline embolization device for the intracranial treatment of aneurysms trial. AJNR Am J Neuroradiol. 2011; 32(1):34–40

[3] Yoon JW, Siddiqui AH, Dumont TM, et al. Endovascular Neurosurgery Research Group. Feasibility and safety of pipeline embolization device in patients with ruptured carotid blister aneurysms. Neurosurgery. 2014; 75 (4):419–429, discussion 429

[4] Aydin K, Arat A, Sencer S, et al. Treatment of ruptured blood blister-like aneurysms with flow diverter SILK stents. J Neurointerv Surg. 2015; 7(3):202–209

[5] Hu YC, Chugh C, Mehta H, Stiefel MF. Early angiographic occlusion of ruptured blister aneurysms of the internal carotid artery using the Pipeline Embolization Device as a primary treatment option. J Neurointerv Surg. 2014; 6 (10):740–743

[6] Nerva JD, Morton RP, Levitt MR, et al. Pipeline Embolization Device as primary treatment for blister aneurysms and iatrogenic pseudoaneurysms of the internal carotid artery. J Neurointerv Surg. 2015; 7(3):210–216

[7] Faught RWF, Satti SR, Hurst RW, Pukenas BA, Smith MJ. Heterogeneous practice patterns regarding antiplatelet medications for neuroendovascular stenting in the USA: a multicenter survey. J Neurointerv Surg. 2014; 6(10):774–779

[8] Cruz JP, O'Kelly C, Kelly M, et al. Pipeline embolization device in aneurysmal subarachnoid hemorrhage. AJNR Am J Neuroradiol. 2013; 34(2):271–276

[9] Fiorella D, Lylyk P, Szikora I, et al. Curative cerebrovascular reconstruction with the Pipeline embolization device: the emergence of definitive endovascular therapy for intracranial aneurysms. J Neurointerv Surg. 2009; 1(1):56–65

[10] Kulcsár Z, Wetzel SG, Augsburger L, Gruber A, Wanke I, Rüfenacht DA. Effect of flow diversion treatment on very small ruptured aneurysms. Neurosurgery. 2010; 67(3):789–793

[11] Leung GK, Tsang AC, Lui WM. Pipeline embolization device for intracranial aneurysm: a systematic review. Clin Neuroradiol. 2012; 22(4):295–303

[12] Lin N, Brouillard AM, Keigher KM, et al. Utilization of Pipeline embolization device for treatment of ruptured intracranial aneurysms: US multicenter experience. J Neurointerv Surg. 2015; 7(11):808–815

[13] Taylor RA, Callison RC, Martin CO, Hayakawa M, Chaloupka JC. Acutely ruptured intracranial saccular aneurysms treated with stent assisted coiling: complications and outcomes in 42 consecutive patients. J Neurointerv Surg. 2010; 2(1):23–30

[14] Chalouhi N, Zanaty M, Whiting A, et al. Treatment of ruptured intracranial aneurysms with the pipeline embolization device. Neurosurgery. 2015; 76 (2):165–172, discussion 172

[15] Kung DK, Policeni BA, Capuano AW, et al. Risk of ventriculostomy-related hemorrhage in patients with acutely ruptured aneurysms treated using stent-assisted coiling. J Neurosurg. 2011; 114(4):1021–1027

[16] Mahaney KB, Chalouhi N, Viljoen S, et al. Risk of hemorrhagic complication associated with ventriculoperitoneal shunt placement in aneurysmal subarachnoid hemorrhage patients on dual antiplatelet therapy. J Neurosurg. 2013; 119(4):937–942

[17] Fargen KM, Hoh BL, Welch BG, et al. Long-term results of enterprise stent-assisted coiling of cerebral aneurysms. Neurosurgery. 2012; 71(2):239–244, discussion 244

[18] Gurbel PA, DiChiara J, Tantry US. Antiplatelet therapy after implantation of drug-eluting stents: duration, resistance, alternatives, and management of surgical patients. Am J Cardiol. 2007; 100 8B:18M–25M

[19] Mehta SR, Yusuf S, Peters RJ, et al. Clopidogrel in Unstable angina to prevent Recurrent Events trial (CURE) Investigators. Effects of pretreatment with clopidogrel and aspirin followed by long-term therapy in patients undergoing percutaneous coronary intervention: the PCI-CURE study. Lancet. 2001; 358 (9281):527–533

[20] Platz J, Güresir E, Vatter H, et al. Unsecured intracranial aneurysms and induced hypertension in cerebral vasospasm: is induced hypertension safe? Neurocrit Care. 2011; 14(2):168–175

[21] Steinhubl SR, Berger PB, Mann JT, III, et al. CREDO Investigators. Clopidogrel for the Reduction of Events During Observation. Early and sustained dual oral antiplatelet therapy following percutaneous coronary intervention: a randomized controlled trial. JAMA. 2002; 288(19):2411–2420

[22] Akpek S, Arat A, Morsi H, Klucznick RP, Strother CM, Mawad ME. Self-expandable stent-assisted coiling of wide-necked intracranial aneurysms: a single-center experience. AJNR Am J Neuroradiol. 2005; 26(5):1223–1231

[23] Fiorella D, Albuquerque FC, Deshmukh VR, et al. Endovascular reconstruction with the Neuroform stent as monotherapy for the treatment of uncoilable intradural pseudoaneurysms. Neurosurgery. 2006; 59(2):291–300, discussion 291–300

[24] Meckel S, Singh TP, Undrén P, et al. Endovascular treatment using predominantly stent-assisted coil embolization and antiplatelet and anticoagulation management of ruptured blood blister-like aneurysms. AJNR Am J Neuroradiol. 2011; 32(4):764–771

[25] Müller I, Seyfarth M, Rüdiger S, et al. Effect of a high loading dose of clopidogrel on platelet function in patients undergoing coronary stent placement. Heart. 2001; 85(1):92–93

[26] Fiorella D, Hsu D, Woo HH, Tarr RW, Nelson PK. Very late thrombosis of a pipeline embolization device construct: case report. Neurosurgery. 2010; 67 (3) Suppl Operative:E313–E314, discussion E314

[27] Amenta PS, Dalyai RT, Kung D, et al. Stent-assisted coiling of wide-necked aneurysms in the setting of acute subarachnoid hemorrhage: experience in 65 patients. Neurosurgery. 2012; 70(6):1415–1429, discussion 1429

[28] Klisch J, Turk A, Turner R, Woo HH, Fiorella D. Very late thrombosis of flow-diverting constructs after the treatment of large fusiform posterior circulation aneurysms. AJNR Am J Neuroradiol. 2011; 32(4):627–632

[29] Szikora I, Berentei Z, Kulcsar Z, et al. Treatment of intracranial aneurysms by functional reconstruction of the parent artery: the Budapest experience with the pipeline embolization device. AJNR Am J Neuroradiol. 2010; 31(6):1139–1147

[30] Fiorella D, Albuquerque FC, Woo H, Rasmussen PA, Masaryk TJ, McDougall CG. Neuroform stent assisted aneurysm treatment: evolving treatment strategies, complications and results of long term follow-up. J Neurointerv Surg. 2010; 2(1):16–22

[31] Yahia AM, Gordon V, Whapham J, Malek A, Steel J, Fessler RD. Complications of Neuroform stent in endovascular treatment of intracranial aneurysms. Neurocrit Care. 2008; 8(1):19–30

[32] Yahia AM, Latorre J, Gordon V, Whapham J, Malek A, Fessler RD. Thromboembolic events associated with Neuroform stent in endovascular treatment of intracranial aneurysms. J Neuroimaging. 2010; 20(2):113–117

[33] Cebral JR, Mut F, Raschi M, et al. Aneurysm rupture following treatment with flow-diverting stents: computational hemodynamics analysis of treatment. AJNR Am J Neuroradiol. 2011; 32(1):27–33

[34] Martin AR, Cruz JP, Matouk CC, Spears J, Marotta TR. The pipeline flow-diverting stent for exclusion of ruptured intracranial aneurysms with difficult morphologies. Neurosurgery. 2012; 70(1) Suppl Operative:21–28, discussion 28

[35] Hoh BL, Carter BS, Ogilvy CS. Risk of hemorrhage from unsecured, unruptured aneurysms during and after hypertensive hypervolemic therapy. Neurosurgery. 2002; 50(6):1207–1211, discussion 1211–1212

[36] Colby GP, Lin LM, Gomez JF, et al. Immediate procedural outcomes in 35 consecutive pipeline embolization cases: a single-center, single-user experience. J Neurointerv Surg. 2013; 5(3):237–246

[37] Lylyk P, Miranda C, Ceratto R, et al. Curative endovascular reconstruction of cerebral aneurysms with the pipeline embolization device: the Buenos Aires experience. Neurosurgery. 2009; 64(4):632–642, discussion 642–643, quiz N6

[38] McAuliffe W, Wenderoth JD. Immediate and midterm results following treatment of recently ruptured intracranial aneurysms with the Pipeline embolization device. AJNR Am J Neuroradiol. 2012; 33(3):487–493

[39] Peschillo S, Caporlingua A, Cannizzaro D, et al. Flow diverter stent treatment for ruptured basilar trunk perforator aneurysms. J Neurointerv Surg. 2016; 8 (2):190–196

[40] Dornbos D, Pilla, i P, Sauvageau E. Flow diverter assisted coil embolization of a very small ruptured ophthalmic artery aneurysm. J NeuroIntervent Surg. 2016; 8(e1):e2–e4

[41] Jankowitz B, Thomas AJ, Vora N, et al. Risk of hemorrhage in combined neuroform stenting and coil embolization of acutely ruptured intracranial aneurysms. Interv Neuroradiol. 2008; 14(4):385–396

[42] Tumialán LM, Zhang YJ, Cawley CM, Dion JE, Tong FC, Barrow DL. Intracranial hemorrhage associated with stent-assisted coil embolization of cerebral aneurysms: a cautionary report. J Neurosurg. 2008; 108(6):1122–1129

[43] Chitale R, Chalouhi N, Theofanis T, et al. Treatment of ruptured intracranial aneurysms: comparison of stenting and balloon remodeling. Neurosurgery. 2013; 72(6):953–959

[44] Brinjikji W, Murad MH, Lanzino G, Cloft HJ, Kallmes DF. Endovascular treatment of intracranial aneurysms with flow diverters: a meta-analysis. Stroke. 2013; 44(2):442–447

[45] Hu YC, Deshmukh VR, Albuquerque FC, et al. Histopathological assessment of fatal ipsilateral intraparenchymal hemorrhages after the treatment of supraclinoid aneurysms with the Pipeline Embolization Device. J Neurosurg. 2014; 120(2):365–374

[46] Park SI, Kim BM, Kim DI, et al. Clinical and angiographic follow-up of stent-only therapy for acute intracranial vertebrobasilar dissecting aneurysms. AJNR Am J Neuroradiol. 2009; 30(7):1351–1356

[47] Velat GJ, Fargen KM, Lawson MF, Hoh BL, Fiorella D, Mocco J. Delayed intraparenchymal hemorrhage following pipeline embolization device treatment for a giant recanalized ophthalmic aneurysm. J Neurointerv Surg. 2012; 4(5):e24

[48] Katsaridis V, Papagiannaki C, Violaris C. Embolization of acutely ruptured and unruptured wide-necked cerebral aneurysms using the neuroform2 stent without pretreatment with antiplatelets: a single center experience. AJNR Am J Neuroradiol. 2006; 27(5):1123–1128

[49] Tähtinen OI, Vanninen RL, Manninen HI, et al. Wide-necked intracranial aneurysms: treatment with stent-assisted coil embolization during acute (<72 hours) subarachnoid hemorrhage–experience in 61 consecutive patients. Radiology. 2009; 253(1):199–208

8 PHARMACOLOGY FOR FLOW DIVERSION

AMIN NIMA AGHAEBRAHIM and ANDREW F. DUCRUET

Abstract

Flow-diverting devices are being used more commonly for the treatment of intracranial aneurysms. Owing to their high metal surface area, antiplatelet agents are essential to prevent potential catastrophic consequences of thromboembolism. This chapter reviews the various antiplatelet medications currently available and discuss issues specific to the application of antiplatelet and anticoagulant medications in the setting of flow diversion.

Keywords: antiplatelet, aspirin, clopidogrel resistance, dual antiplatelet, flow-diverting devices, glycoprotein IIb/IIIa inhibitors, platelet function testing, prasugrel, ticagrelor, ticlopidine

8.1 Introduction

Endovascular treatment of complex and wide-neck aneurysms remains challenging, with the degree of complexity often related to size (very large or giant) and aneurysm morphology (dysplastic or fusiform). The recent introduction of flow-diverting devices represents a considerable advance in the treatment of these aneurysms. Multiple studies have supported the safety and efficacy of flow diversion.[1,2] One study showed complete aneurysm occlusion at 180 days in 93% of patients who were treated with Pipeline Embolization Device (PED).[3] The concept of flow diversion is based on reconstruction of the diseased parent artery rather than occlusion of the saccular portion of the aneurysm. Currently, the PED (Covidien/ev3) is the only flow diverter that has been cleared by the U.S. Food and Drug Administration. Other products such as the Silk (Balt Extrusion, Montmorency, France), the Surpass (Stryker), and the FRED (MicroVention) flow-diverting devices remain under investigation.

To prevent potential catastrophic consequences of neurosurgical thromboembolism after intracranial stenting procedures, the need for a safe and efficacious antiplatelet regimen is particularly important. The use of aspirin and clopidogrel has been shown to exhibit an optimal safety and efficacy profile.[4,5,6] However, about one-third of patients appear to be nonresponders to clopidogrel and alternative antiplatelets are now being used for this group of patients.[7,8,9,10]

8.2 Antiplatelet Medications

Platelets provide the initial hemostatic plug at sites of vascular injury and also participate in pathological thrombosis leading to myocardial infarction, stroke, and peripheral vascular thrombosis. They are also believed to be the main cause of in-stent thrombosis. Antiplatelet agents act by inhibiting discrete mechanisms. Thus, in combination, their effects are additive or even synergistic.[11]

Aspirin inhibits thromboxane A2 (TxA2) synthesis by irreversibly acetylating cyclooxygenase-1 (COX-1). Ticlopidine, clopidogrel, and prasugrel irreversibly block P2Y12, a key ADP

receptor on the platelet surface. Cangrelor and ticagrelor are reversible inhibitors of P2Y12. Abciximab, eptifibatide, and tirofiban inhibit the final common pathway of platelet aggregation by blocking fibrinogen and von Willebrand factor (vWF) from binding to activated glycoprotein (GP) IIb/IIIa. SCH530348 and E5555 inhibit thrombin-mediated platelet activation by targeting protease-activated receptor-1 (PAR-1), the major thrombin receptor on platelets.[11]

8.3 Dual-Antiplatelet Therapy

Typically, dual-antiplatelet therapy with aspirin and clopidogrel is instituted prior to placement of an intracranial stent due to concern for potential thrombus formation.[4,5,6] The risk of thrombosis is likely magnified by the high metal surface area of flow-diverting devices, which generally exhibit 30 to 35% of total metal surface area. The preventative strategy of dual-antiplatelet therapy with aspirin and an ADP receptor antagonist has been shown in multiple studies to reduce thromboembolic rates in neurointerventional patients and is commonly used in both coronary and carotid artery stenting.[12] However, increasing reports of clopidogrel resistance along with stent thrombosis in certain cases has prompted many physicians to use alternative antiplatelet medications and to routinely use platelet function testing.[13,14,15,16,17]

8.4 Aspirin (ASA)

Aspirin blocks production of TxA2 by inhibiting COX-1. Because platelets do not produce new proteins, the action of aspirin on platelet COX-1 is permanent, lasting for the life of the platelet (7–10 days). Complete inactivation of platelet COX-1 is achieved with a daily aspirin dose of 75 mg and numerous trials indicate that aspirin, when used as an antithrombotic drug, is maximally effective at doses of 50 to 320 mg/day.[18] Higher doses do not improve efficacy; moreover, they potentially are less efficacious because of inhibition of prostacyclin production, which can be largely spared by using lower doses of aspirin.[11] Therefore, 325 mg/day is typically used for flow-diverting devices and other intracranial stents.

8.5 Clopidogrel (Plavix)

Clopidogrel is an irreversible inhibitor of platelet P2Y12 receptors. Clopidogrel is a prodrug with a relatively slow onset of action. The usual dose is 75 mg/day with or without an initial loading dose of 300 or 600 mg. The loading dose can be detected in blood within 2 hours with peak effect of 6 hours, whereas the maintenance dose typically is detected by the second day of treatment, with peak effect of 5 to 7 days. Platelet aggregation and bleeding time gradually return to baseline after about 5 days after discontinuation.[11]

8.5.1 Clopidogrel Resistance

It has been shown that patients who suffer stent thrombosis exhibit high posttreatment platelet reactivity despite the dual-antiplatelet treatment, suggesting that nonresponsiveness to clopidogrel may be the main cause of the thrombotic event.[13,14,15,16,17] Prabhakaran and colleagues found that aspirin resistance is relatively uncommon, whereas clopidogrel resistance can occur in as high as half of patients undergoing cerebrovascular stent placement.[19] Clopidogrel is a prodrug, which must be metabolized in the liver to produce an active metabolite via CYP2C19 enzyme. Therefore, clopidogrel may not be effective in patients with genetic mutations of the CYP2C19.[20] Currently, there is no standardized definition for clopidogrel resistance. Furthermore, poor response to clopidogrel may be related to noncompliance, inadequate dosing or absorption, body mass index, genetic polymorphisms of cytochrome P450 3A4 and the P2Y12 receptor, and increased platelet activity related to an acute thrombotic event.[21,22,23,24] Significant association has been shown between older age and percentage platelet inhibition possibly due to age-related decreases in drug absorption or in the activity of cytochrome P450 3A4, which is essential in the conversion of clopidogrel to its active form.[19] In addition, drug–drug interactions could also impair clopidogrel hepatic metabolism.[25,26] Specifically, the concurrent use with drugs known to inhibit CYP2C19 such as proton pump inhibitors may reduce levels of active metabolite and subsequently reduce clinical efficacy.[27]

8.6 Ticlopidine

Similar to clopidogrel, ticlopidine permanently inhibits the P2Y12 receptor by forming a disulfide bridge between the thiol on the drug and a free cysteine residue in the extracellular region of the receptor, and thus has a prolonged effect. Maximal inhibition of platelet aggregation is not seen until 8 to 11 days after starting therapy and the usual dose is 250 mg twice a day. Loading dose of 500 mg is sometimes given to achieve a more rapid onset of action. This drug, however, is associated with severe neutropenia which occurred in 2.4% of patients with stroke during premarketing clinical trials. Therefore, it is no longer available in the united States.[11]

8.7 Prasugrel (Effient)

Prasugrel is a third-generation thienopyridine. It has a faster onset of action and more completely converts to its active form, but has been associated with 30% increase in the relative risk of bleeding when compared with clopidogrel.[28] In addition to the faster onset of action, it produces greater and more predictable inhibition of ADP-induced platelet aggregation. Virtually all of the absorbed prasugrel undergoes activation; on the contrary, only 15% of absorbed clopidogrel undergoes metabolic activation, with the remainder inactivated by esterases. Prasugrel binds irreversibly to the P2Y12 receptor and therefore also has a prolonged effect (typically 5 days) after discontinuation.[11]

Prasugrel has been compared with clopidogrel in patients with acute coronary syndromes undergoing a coronary intervention and has been shown to significantly decrease risk of cardiovascular death, myocardial infarction, and stroke in addition to lowering the incidence of stent thrombosis. However, it demonstrated higher rates of fatal and life-threatening bleeds. Because of this risk, the use of this drug for coronary interventions is contraindicated in patients with a history of cerebrovascular disease. In contrast to clopidogrel, CYP2C19 polymorphisms appear to be less important determinants of the activation of prasugrel; therefore, prasugrel may be a reasonable alternative to clopidogrel in patients with the loss-of-function CYP2C19 allele.[28]

Although there is limited published evidence to support its use in cerebrovascular procedures, there have been several reports of successful treatment with prasugrel.[29] The typical loading dose is 60 mg with a 5- to 10-mg daily maintenance dose, depending on age or weight (▶ Table 8.1). Current medication labeling recommends a dose reduction from 10 to 5 mg daily in patients weighing less than 60 kg or who are older than 75 years.

8.8 Ticagrelor (Brilinta)

Ticagrelor is an orally active, reversible inhibitor of P2Y12. It has more rapid onset and offset of action than clopidogrel and must be given twice daily. It has been compared with clopidogrel in patients with acute coronary syndromes[30] and has been

Table 8.1 Oral antiplatelet agents

Feature	Aspirin	Clopidogrel	Prasugrel	Ticagrelor
Commercial name		Plavix	Effient	Brilinta
Description	Inhibits production of thromboxane A2 by inhibiting COX-1	Inhibits ADP-induced platelet–fibrinogen interaction	Inhibits ADP-induced platelet–fibrinogen interaction	Inhibits ADP-induced platelet–fibrinogen interaction
Loading dose	325 mg	300–600 mg	60 mg	180 mg
Maintenance dose	50–325 mg/day	75 mg	5–10 mg daily	90 mg twice daily
Onset of action	1 h	Loading: 2 h Maintenance: 2 d	Loading dose: < 30 min	Loading dose: 30 min
Peak effect	1–2 h non–enteric-coated, 3–4 h enteric-coated	Loading: 6 h Maintenance: 5–7 d	30 min, 1.5 h with high-fat/ high-calorie meal	2 h
Duration of action	Life time of the platelets (~10 d)	5 ds	5–9 d	3 d

shown to reduce cardiovascular death, myocardial infarction, and stroke at 1 year. Rates of major bleeding were similar. Unlike clopidogrel, ticagrelor does not require hepatic activation and is primarily metabolized via the CYP34A enzyme. Thus, this drug can be advantageous in patients with genetic mutations of the CYP2C19 enzyme. Although reports are limited, ticagrelor has been shown to be safe in nonresponders to clopidogrel undergoing neuroendovascular procedures.[31] Loading dose is 180 mg with maintenance of 90 mg twice daily.

8.9 Glycoprotein IIb/IIIa Inhibitors

Glycoprotein IIb/IIIa is a platelet-surface integrin which is inactive on resting platelets but undergoes a conformational transformation when platelets are activated by platelet agonists such as thrombin, collagen, or TxA2. This transformation endows glycoprotein IIb/IIIa with the capacity to serve as a receptor for fibrinogen and vWF, which anchor platelets to foreign surfaces and to each other, thereby mediating aggregation. Inhibition of binding to this receptor blocks platelet aggregation. Three agents are approved for use currently (▶ Table 8.2). These drugs are all administered intravenously. Abciximab is the Fab fragment of a humanized monoclonal antibody directed against the αIIbβ3 receptor. The unbound antibody is cleared from the circulation within 30 minutes, but the antibody remains bound to the receptor and inhibits platelet aggregation for 18 to 24 hours after infusion is stopped. The duration of action of Eptifibatide, on the other hand, is relatively short, and platelet aggregation is restored within 6 to 12 hours after cessation of infusion.[11] Among cardiac patients, the addition of glycoprotein IIb/IIIa inhibitors has been shown to enhance the antiplatelet effect of clopidogrel alone.[32]

The major side effect of these agents is bleeding. The frequency of major hemorrhage in clinical trials varies from 1 to 10% depending on the intensity of anticoagulation with heparin. Additionally, thrombocytopenia with a platelet count less than 50,000 occurs in about 2% of patients.

8.10 Heparinization

Although data supporting a particular heparinization threshold is lacking, flow diversion procedures are typically performed under full heparinization, with an activated clotting time (ACT) goal of more than 250 seconds.

8.11 Institution and Duration of Dual-Antiplatelet Treatment

In general, dual-antiplatelet agents are administered beginning a minimum of 7 to 10 days prior to the planned procedure. For lesions with a relatively short segment of aneurysmal involvement separating normal vascular segments, as in a typical saccular aneurysm, patients remain on dual-antiplatelet therapy for 3 to 6 months. If angiography demonstrates complete aneurysmal occlusion at the end of that time interval, patients can be transitioned to antiplatelet monotherapy. For more complex aneurysms where multidevice constructs are used to bridge a substantial circumferential aneurysmal segment, such as in fusiform aneurysms, patients may be treated with dual-antiplatelet therapy for up to 1 year and then transitioned to monotherapy at the discretion of the neurointerventionalist. If an aneurysm remains patent, dual-antiplatelet therapy can be extended, as this suggests that endothelialization is not complete. One rationale for prolonged dual-antiplatelet therapy is due to the observation of the very late thrombosis of flow-diverting constructs 1 year or longer after initial treatment.[33]

8.12 Platelet Function Testing

Platelet function testing is often performed in preparation for flow diversion, although concrete guidelines have yet to be established. Point-of-care testing is available to evaluate responsiveness to both aspirin and clopidogrel. Although a lack of response to aspirin is rarely observed, nonresponse to clopidogrel is more frequently observed.[19] Many practitioners rely on testing to identify over- and under-responders to clopidogrel.

At our center, we use the VerifyNow PRU Test which is a whole blood test used in the laboratory or point-of-care setting to measure the level of platelet P2Y12 receptor blockade. Substances known to specifically block the P2Y12 receptor include the thienopyridine class of drugs, including clopidogrel,

Table 8.2 Intravenous antiplatelet agents

Feature	Abciximab (ReoPro)	Eptifibatide (Integrilin)	Tirofiban (Aggrastat)
Description	Fab fragment of humanized mouse monoclonal antibody	Cyclical KGD-containing heptapeptide	Nonpeptidic RGD-mimetic
Specific for GPIIb/IIIa	No	Yes	Yes
Plasma $t_{1/2}$	Short (min)	Long (2.5 h)	Long (2.0 h)
Platelet-bound $t_{1/2}$	Long (d)	Short (s)	Short (s)
Renal clearance	No	Yes	Yes
Dose	0.25-mg/kg bolus followed by 0.125 μg/kg/min for 12 h	180 μg/kg followed by 2 μg/kg/min for up to 96 h	0.4 μg/kg/min for 30 min, and then continued at 0.1 mg/kg/min for 12–24 h, 0.4 μg/kg/min for 30 min, and then continued at 0.1 mg/kg/min for 12–24 h

prasugrel, and ticagrelor. The test is based on the ability of activated platelets to bind fibrinogen. Fibrinogen-coated microparticles aggregate in whole blood in proportion to the number of expressed platelet GP IIb/IIIa. The rate of microbead aggregation is more rapid and reproducible if platelets are activated; therefore, the reagent adenosine-5-diphosphate (ADP/PGE1) is incorporated into the test channel to induce platelet activation without fibrin formation. The reagent is formulated to specifically measure P2Y12-mediated platelet aggregation. Light transmittance increases as activated platelets bind and aggregate fibrinogen-coated beads. This instrument measures this change in optical signal and reports results in P2Y12 reaction units (PRU). A PRU greater than 194 means there is no evidence of drug effect. If the result is less than 194, this suggests that there is a drug effect, with the lower PRU value signifying a higher level of platelet inhibition. For patients found to be clopidogrel hyperresponders, generally with PRU less than 60, a reduction in dose to 75 mg every other day is often used. On the other hand, for patients with Plavix nonresponsiveness, PRU greater than 194, an alternative ADP antagonist, such as prasugrel, can be used. Alternatively, percent reduction PRU from baseline can be used to identify nonresponders as shown in the formula below. PRU inhibition greater than 30% from baseline is considered to be an adequate drug response.[34,35]

$$\% \text{ Reduction} = \frac{(\text{Baseline PRU} - \text{Post PRU}) \times 100}{\text{Baseline PRU}}$$

Similarly, a VerifyNow Aspirin test can also be used to qualitatively test the detection of platelet dysfunction due to aspirin ingestion in citrated whole blood or the point-of-care or laboratory setting. The results are reported in aspirin reaction units (ARU). Results greater than 550 means there is no drug effect and results less than 550 means there is a drug effect. However, as aspirin resistance is less common compared to clopidogrel resistance, this test is not performed as routinely.[19]

Alternatively, there remain many neurointerventionalists who do not routinely evaluate platelet function testing.[36] Future evaluation and rigorous comparisons would be helpful to establish the efficacy of this practice, as well as to determine appropriate cutoffs.

Flow diversion for acutely ruptured intracranial aneurysms has been reported.[37] Management of antiplatelet agents in this setting is crucial to minimize the risk of both thromboembolic and hemorrhagic complications. Experience in this setting is limited, and guidelines are not established. The safest route to minimize procedure-related hemorrhagic complications may be to delay aneurysm treatment for patients with hydrocephalus until after the removal of the ventriculostomy or placement of a ventriculoperitoneal shunt. However, this exposes the patient to the potentially greater risks of re-rupture of an unsecured aneurysm. In cases where acute treatment of a ruptured aneurysm with flow diversion is necessary, placement of an EVD prior to the flow diversion procedure is strongly recommended for patients with symptomatic hydrocephalus.

Pretreatment loading with dual-antiplatelet agents is recommended, even in the setting of acute SAH. There have been minimal reports of re-bleeding prior to flow diversion in this setting.[37] In centers that measure antiplatelet responsiveness, it is critical to achieve an effective antiplatelet effect before placing a flow diverter. Most commonly, this will involve loading

clopidogrel/aspirin at a minimum on the day before the planned treatment. In some cases, the flow diverter can be placed using a GPIIb/IIIa infusion to bridge while clopidogrel is loaded following a procedure, as in unplanned cases for which flow diversion is emergently required. The use of prasugrel or ticagrelor may avoid the issue of antiplatelet agent nonresponsiveness, and the reversible and short half-life of ticagrelor makes it potentially attractive for use in this setting.

8.13 Conclusion

The introduction of flow-diverting devices has changed the face of the treatment of intracranial aneurysms. The extent of metal coverage afforded by these devices makes it imperative to optimize antiplatelet regimens to minimize complications. In general, dual-antiplatelet medication with aspirin and Plavix is recommended for a minimum of 3 to 6 months. Platelet function testing can be used to identify nonresponders, and alternative medications are emerging. Further work is necessary to determine the role of platelet function testing and the optimal antiplatelet function thresholds.

References

[1] Kallmes DF, Ding YH, Dai D, Kadirvel R, Lewis DA, Cloft HJ. A second-generation, endoluminal, flow-disrupting device for treatment of saccular aneurysms. AJNR Am J Neuroradiol. 2009; 30(6):1153–1158

[2] Kallmes DF, Ding YH, Dai D, Kadirvel R, Lewis DA, Cloft HJ. A new endoluminal, flow-disrupting device for treatment of saccular aneurysms. Stroke. 2007; 38(8):2346–2352

[3] Nelson PK, Lylyk P, Szikora I, Wetzel SG, Wanke I, Fiorella D. The pipeline embolization device for the intracranial treatment of aneurysms trial. AJNR Am J Neuroradiol. 2011; 32(1):34–40

[4] Heer T, Juenger C, Gitt AK, et al. Acute Coronary Syndromes (ACOS) Registry Investigators. Efficacy and safety of optimized antithrombotic therapy with aspirin, clopidogrel and enoxaparin in patients with non-ST segment elevation acute coronary syndromes in clinical practice. J Thromb Thrombolysis. 2009; 28(3):325–332

[5] Bowry AD, Brookhart MA, Choudhry NK. Meta-analysis of the efficacy and safety of clopidogrel plus aspirin as compared to antiplatelet monotherapy for the prevention of vascular events. Am J Cardiol. 2008; 101(7):960–966

[6] Cooke GE, Goldschmidt-Clermont PJ. The safety and efficacy of aspirin and clopidogrel as a combination treatment in patients with coronary heart disease. Expert Opin Drug Saf. 2006; 5(6):815–826

[7] Cuisset T, Quilici J, Cohen W, et al. Usefulness of high clopidogrel maintenance dose according to CYP2C19 genotypes in clopidogrel low responders undergoing coronary stenting for non ST elevation acute coronary syndrome. Am J Cardiol. 2011; 108(6):760–765

[8] Srinivas NR. Genetic CYP2C19 polymorphism dependent non-responders to clopidogrel therapy–does structural design, dosing and induction strategies have a role to play? Eur J Drug Metab Pharmacokinet. 2009; 34(3–4):147–150

[9] Gurbel PA, Bliden KP. Interpretation of platelet inhibition by clopidogrel and the effect of non-responders. J Thromb Haemost. 2003; 1(6):1318–1319

[10] Müller I, Besta F, Schulz C, Massberg S, Schönig A, Gawaz M. Prevalence of clopidogrel non-responders among patients with stable angina pectoris scheduled for elective coronary stent placement. Thromb Haemost. 2003; 89 (5):783–787

[11] Brunton L, Chabner BA, Knollmann BC. Goodman & Gilman's The Pharmacological Basis of Therapeutics. 12th ed. McGraw-Hill; 2011

[12] Kang HS, Kwon BJ, Kim JE, Han MH. Preinterventional clopidogrel response variability for coil embolization of intracranial aneurysms: clinical implications. AJNR Am J Neuroradiol. 2010; 31(7):1206–1210

[13] Matetzky S, Shenkman B, Guetta V, et al. Clopidogrel resistance is associated with increased risk of recurrent atherothrombotic events in patients with acute myocardial infarction. Circulation. 2004; 109(25):3171–3175

[14] Gurbel PA, Bliden KP, Samara W, et al. Clopidogrel effect on platelet reactivity in patients with stent thrombosis: results of the CREST Study. J Am Coll Cardiol. 2005; 46(10):1827–1832

[15] Gurbel PA, Bliden KP, Guyer K, et al. Platelet reactivity in patients and recurrent events post-stenting: results of the PREPARE POST-STENTING Study. J Am Coll Cardiol. 2005; 46(10):1820–1826

[16] Ajzenberg G, Aubry P, Huisse MG, et al. Enhanced shear-induced platelet aggregation in patients who experienced stent thrombosis. J Am Coll Cardiol. 2005; 45:1653–1656

[17] Cuisset T, Frere C, Quilici J, et al. High post-treatment platelet reactivity identified low-responders to dual antiplatelet therapy at increased risk of recurrent cardiovascular events after stenting for acute coronary syndrome. J Thromb Haemost. 2006; 4(3):542–549

[18] Collaboration AT, Antithrombotic Trialists' Collaboration. Collaborative meta-analysis of randomised trials of antiplatelet therapy for prevention of death, myocardial infarction, and stroke in high risk patients. BMJ. 2002; 324 (7329):71–86

[19] Prabhakaran S, Wells KR, Lee VH, Flaherty CA, Lopes DK. Prevalence and risk factors for aspirin and clopidogrel resistance in cerebrovascular stenting. AJNR Am J Neuroradiol. 2008; 29(2):281–285

[20] Cattaneo M. Ticagrelor versus clopidogrel in acute coronary syndromes. N Engl J Med. 2009; 361(24):2386–, author reply 2387–2388

[21] Feher G, Koltai K, Alkonyi B, et al. Clopidogrel resistance: role of body mass and concomitant medications. Int J Cardiol. 2007; 120(2):188–192

[22] Lau WC, Gurbel PA, Watkins PB, et al. Contribution of hepatic cytochrome P450 3A4 metabolic activity to the phenomenon of clopidogrel resistance. Circulation. 2004; 109(2):166–171

[23] Taubert D, Kastrati A, Harlfinger S, et al. Pharmacokinetics of clopidogrel after administration of a high loading dose. Thromb Haemost. 2004; 92 (2):311–316

[24] Soffer D, Moussa I, Harjai KJ, et al. Impact of angina class on inhibition of platelet aggregation following clopidogrel loading in patients undergoing coronary intervention: do we need more aggressive dosing regimens in unstable angina? Catheter Cardiovasc Interv. 2003; 59(1):21–25

[25] Neubauer H, Günesdogan B, Hanefeld C, Spiecker M, Mügge A. Lipophilic statins interfere with the inhibitory effects of clopidogrel on platelet function–a flow cytometry study. Eur Heart J. 2003; 24(19):1744–1749

[26] Serebruany VL, Midei MG, Malinin AI, et al. Absence of interaction between atorvastatin or other statins and clopidogrel: results from the interaction study. Arch Intern Med. 2004; 164(18):2051–2057

[27] Ho PM, Maddox TM, Wang L, et al. Risk of adverse outcomes associated with concomitant use of clopidogrel and proton pump inhibitors following acute coronary syndrome. JAMA. 2009; 301(9):937–944

[28] Wiviott SD, Braunwald E, McCabe CH, et al. TRITON-TIMI 38 Investigators. Prasugrel versus clopidogrel in patients with acute coronary syndromes. N Engl J Med. 2007; 357(20):2001–2015

[29] Jones GM, Twilla JD, Hoit DA, Arthur AS. Prevention of stent thrombosis with reduced dose of prasugrel in two patients undergoing treatment of cerebral aneurysms with pipeline embolisation devices. BMJ Case Rep. 2012; 2012: bcr2012010482

[30] Wallentin L, Becker RC, Budaj A, et al. PLATO Investigators. Ticagrelor versus clopidogrel in patients with acute coronary syndromes. N Engl J Med. 2009; 361(11):1045–1057

[31] Hanel RA, Taussky P, Dixon T, et al. Safety and efficacy of ticagrelor for neuroendovascular procedures. A single center initial experience. J Neurointerv Surg. 2014; 6(4):320–322

[32] Gurbel PA, Bliden KP, Zaman KA, Yoho JA, Hayes KM, Tantry US. Clopidogrel loading with eptifibatide to arrest the reactivity of platelets: results of the Clopidogrel Loading With Eptifibatide to Arrest the Reactivity of Platelets (CLEAR PLATELETS) study. Circulation. 2005; 111(9):1153–1159

[33] Fiorella D, Hsu D, Woo HH, Tarr RW, Nelson PK. Very late thrombosis of a pipeline embolization device construct: case report. Neurosurgery. 2010; 67 (3) Suppl Operative:E313–E314, discussion E314

[34] Malinin A, Pokov A, Spergling M, et al. Monitoring platelet inhibition after clopidogrel with the VerifyNow-P2Y12(R) rapid analyzer: the VERIfy Thrombosis risk ASsessment (VERITAS) study. Thromb Res. 2007; 119(3):277–284

[35] Serebruany VL, Steinhubl SR, Berger PB, Malinin AI, Bhatt DL, Topol EJ. Variability in platelet responsiveness to clopidogrel among 544 individuals. J Am Coll Cardiol. 2005; 45(2):246–251

[36] Lin L-M, Colby GP, Kim JE, Huang J, Tamargo RJ, Coon AL. Immediate and follow-up results for 44 consecutive cases of small (<10 mm) internal carotid artery aneurysms treated with the pipeline embolization device. Surg Neurol Int. 2013; 4:114

[37] Kulcsár Z, Wetzel SG, Augsburger L, Gruber A, Wanke I, Rüfenacht DA. Effect of flow diversion treatment on very small ruptured aneurysms. Neurosurgery. 2010; 67(3):789–793

9 OVERVIEW OF CURRENT FLOW-DIVERTING DEVICES

PEDRO AGUILAR-SALINAS, BARTLEY MITCHELL, DOUGLAS GONSALES, RICARDO A. HANEL, and ERIC SAUVAGEAU

Abstract

The treatment of intracranial aneurysms has impressively evolved over the past 20 years along with the development of less invasive techniques. However, large or giant wide-necked aneurysms remain a challenging and complex pathology to treat by traditional microsurgery or endovascular embolization due to the high rate of recanalization. Therefore, flow-diverting technology has been acknowledged as playing a central role in treating those complex aneurysms. Although the flow-diverting devices have been recently introduced to the endovascular armamentarium, multiple types are already available. All of them have the same mechanism of action but vary slightly in stent design and deployment technique. The Pipeline Embolization Device (PED; Covidien/Medtronic, Irvine, CA), the Silk flow diverter (SILK; Balt Extrusion, Montmorency, France), the Surpass flow diverter (SURPASS; Stryker Neurovascular, Fremont, CA), and the Flow Redirection Endoluminal Device (FRED; MicroVention, Tustin, CA) are discussed in this chapter. The PED is the most widely used stent and the only Food and Drug Administration (FDA)-approved device for clinical use in the United States. The SILK stent was the first flow diverter available. Both stents have 48 braided strands as a mesh design and may require telescoping devices to increase the metal surface coverage. The SURPASS has single-layer mesh that maintains a constant porosity across all sizes available, thus potentially reducing the need of telescoping stents. Conversely, the FRED has a unique double-layer mesh design. It consists of a low-porosity inner mesh and a high-porosity outer stent. The dual-layer system offers an improved scaffolding effect as well as full-stent length fluoroscopic visualization.

Keywords: endovascular, flow diverter, Flow Redirection Endoluminal Device, intracranial aneurysm, Pipeline Embolization Device, Silk flow diverter, Surpass flow diverter

9.1 Introduction

The method of treating intracranial aneurysms has impressively evolved over the past 20 years along with the advance of technology and less invasive techniques. Currently, neuroendovascular intervention is considered an effective and safe option after the long-term results of groundbreaking studies were published.[1,2] However, the occlusion rates of aneurysms with complex morphology are far from definitive when treated only with coiling or stent-assisted embolization.[3,4,5,6] Flow-diverting devices play a critical role in the neuroendovascular armamentarium with their higher rates of aneurysm occlusion over time, independent of lesion morphology.[7,8,9,10] These devices work by modifying the blood-flow dynamics through the parent artery, as well as by inducing physiological and biological events to facilitate aneurysm occlusion without endovascular intervention.[10,11] Although this technology has recently been introduced, the development of competing flow-diverting devices has rapidly increased with a growing body of literature to support their efficacy. The aim of this chapter is to provide an overview of the currently available flow-diverting devices. The technique and nuances of each flow diverter will be discussed in detail in the following sections.

9.2 Flow-Diverting Devices

Several features such as the pore density, porosity, metal coverage of the aneurysm neck, and deployment procedure contribute to determine the effectiveness of a flow diverter. However, experimental models suggest that low porosity and high-pore density are the main factors in decreasing the blood flow into the aneurysm with an optimal range between 60 and 76%.[12,13,14] Although the principle of action is the same, the currently available flow diverters vary slightly in the aforementioned properties. The following devices will be discussed: the Pipeline Embolization Device (PED; Covidien/Medtronic, Irvine, CA), the Silk flow diverter (SILK; Balt Extrusion, Montmorency, France), the Surpass flow diverter (SURPASS; Stryker Neurovascular, Fremont, CA), and the Flow Redirection Endoluminal Device (FRED; MicroVention, Tustin, CA). ▶ Table 9.1 summarizes the main characteristics of the four types of flow-diverting devices.

Table 9.1 Summary of the main properties of the flow diverters

Flow diverter	FDA/CE mark	Mesh design	Surface coverage (%)	Diameter and lengths (mm)
PED	FDA/CE mark	48 braided strands of 75% cobalt-chromium/25% platinum-tungsten	30–35	D: 2.5–5 L: 10–35
SILK	CE mark	48 braided nitinol strands and platinum filaments	30–35	D: 2–5 L: 15–40
SURPASS	CE mark	Cobalt-chromium and platinum wires	30	D: 2–5 L: 12–50
FRED	CE mark	Dual-layer design: low-porosity inner mesh (48 nitinol wires) and high-porosity outer mesh (16 nitinol wires)	30	D: 3–5.5 L: 7–56[a]

Abbreviations: CE, Conformité Européenne; D, diameter; FDA, Food and Drug Administration; FRED, Flow Redirection Endoluminal Device; L, length; PED, Pipeline Embolization Device; SILK, Silk flow diverter; SURPASS, Surpass flow diverter.
[a]Work lengths (dual-layer segment).

9.2.1 Pipeline Embolization Device

The PED is the only Food and Drug Administration (FDA)-approved flow diverter in the United States and the most widely used worldwide. The first generation received the European CE mark approval in June 2008 and became available in the United States in April 2011 after the Pipeline for Uncoilable and Failed Aneurysms (PUFS) trial.[8] The PED is a self-expanding stent, cylindrically shaped, composed of 48 braided strands in a standard pattern, and made of 75% chromium-cobalt and 25% platinum-tungsten alloy microfilaments. The cell sizes range from 0.02 to 0.05 mm. Its porosity consists of 65 to 75% and when deployed properly, it affords 30 to 35% coverage of the arterial wall surface. It is available in lengths from 10 to 35 mm and in diameters from 2.5 to 5.0 mm. However, when expanded, the device may reach 0.25 mm in diameter larger than stated.[11,15]

The second generation of this stent is known as the Pipeline Flex Embolization Device (PED Flex). It obtained the CE mark in March 2014 and the FDA approval in February 2015. This new generation keeps the same stent design, material, and configuration of the previous generation but has a new delivery system that makes it almost completely resheathable.[16,17]

9.2.2 Silk Flow Diverter

The SILK device received the European CE mark approval in 2008 and was the first flow-diverting device available in the neuroendovascular field, but it is not available for clinical use in the United States. This is a self-expanding stent designed as a closed-cell mesh cylinder composed of 48 interwoven nitinol strands and 4 platinum microfilaments with flared ends. Its porosity is of 45 to 60%, resulting in a metal surface coverage of approximately 35%. It is available in several diameters from 2 to 5 mm and lengths from 15 to 40 mm. In addition, stents may be placed to vessels from 0.5 mm smaller or up to 0.25 mm larger than the labeled diameter. A new generation has been released, Silk+, designed with a lower porosity, higher radial force, and eight platinum markers.[18,19]

9.2.3 Surpass Flow Diverter

The SURPASS device has been used in Europe after CE mark approval in 2010. It is currently undergoing evaluation under an investigational device exemption in the United States in the SCENT trial, a single arm study to examine its efficacy and safety.[20] This is a self-expanding braided tubular stent with a porosity of 70% and a pore density ranging from 21 to 32 pores/mm^2 with a metal surface coverage of 30%. It is available in diameters from 2.0 to 5.0 mm and in lengths from 12 to 50 mm. Its design keeps the porosity relatively constant (70%) while the wire struts increase across all diameters, the 2-mm stent has 48 wires, the 3- and 4-mm stents have 72 wires, and the 5-mm stent has 96 wires. In addition, the braid angle avoids changes of pore density in curved arterial segments and 12 platinum wires integrated in the mesh improve the radiopacity.[13,21,22,23]

9.2.4 Flow Redirection Endoluminal Device

The FRED device has a unique dual-layer design made of a nickel-titanium alloy. It is only CE mark approved and currently under evaluation in the United States through a clinical trial.[24] It consists of a low-porosity inner mesh (48 nitinol wires) and a high-porosity outer stent (16 nitinol wires). Its stent-within-a-stent design is limited to the midsection of the device to cover the neck of the aneurysm. Two helical markers attach both layers across the total length of the inner mesh. The dual layer covers 80% of the device length; this is known as the working length. Its integrated dual-layer system enhances radial force, provides full-stent length fluoroscopic visualization, and may offer an improved scaffolding effect. Each end of the stent is flared and marked by four radiopaque tips. It is available in fully expanded diameters from 3.5 to 5.5 mm and various working lengths from 7 to 48 mm.[25,26]

9.3 Technical Specifications and Indications

The placement of any current flow diverter follows a similar endovascular protocol. Owing to the high metal surface of these devices associated with thrombogenic risk, patients should be started on dual-antiplatelet therapy with aspirin (100–325 mg/day) and a thienopyridine derivative (clopidogrel 75 mg/day) typically 5 to 7 days prior to the procedure. However, the antiplatelet regimen should be decided on a case-by-case basis. Interventions can be performed under general anesthesia. Optimal views of the proximal and distal landing zones within the parent artery are paramount and should be determined from the working angle angiogram and three-dimensional reconstructions. Thus, stents are deployed through their appropriate microcatheter and wall apposition is confirmed under fluoroscopy. After the procedure, dual-antiplatelet therapy is maintained for 6 months followed by aspirin alone indefinitely. ▸ Table 9.2 compares the technical specifications and indications of the flow diverters.

9.3.1 Pipeline Embolization Device

This device is only cleared to treat adults (> 22 years) with large or giant, wide-necked, intracranial aneurysms from the petrous to the superior hypophyseal segments of the internal carotid artery (ICA). However, it is a Premarket Approval (PMA) device and it may be used off-label by physicians in the United States. The PED is mounted on a 0.016-inch stainless steel pusher wire and compressed inside an introducer sheath. It is deployed through a 0.027-inch microcatheter (3F) such as the Marksman (Covidien/Medtronic), Headway 27 (MicroVention Inc., Tustin, CA), and Excelsior XT-27 (Stryker Neurovascular). The PED Flex has a different delivery system in comparison with the PED classic. The distal capture coil has been removed and substituted by two protective sleeves of polytetrafluoroethylene. These protective sleeves allow the device to be released instantly, eliminating the need to torque the delivery wire. This new system allows the device to be re-sheathed until deployed over 90% and facilitates a more controlled and precise

Table 9.2 Comparison of technical specifications and indications of flow-diverting devices

Flow diverter	Guide catheter	Delivery microcatheter (inches)	Specials features and considerations	Indication
PED	6F	0.027	Longitudinal shortening after deployment (50–60%). Resheathing and repositioning are possible only with the PED Flex Telescoping stent is permissible	Patients aged ≥ 22 with large or giant, wide-necked aneurysms in the ICA from the petrous to the superior hypophyseal segment
SILK	6F	0.021 (Vasco + 21) 0.027 (Vasco + 27)	Longitudinal shortening after deployment (50–60%). It may be retrieved and/or repositioned up to its 90% deployment length Telescoping stent is permissible	Large or giant, wide-necked aneurysms. Adjuvant coiling is recommended for giant aneurysms
SURPASS	6F	Surpass delivery catheter, 0.057	Longitudinal shortening after deployment (≈ 35%). Constant porosity and high-pore density across stent diameters may reduce the need of telescoping devices	Large or giant, wide-necked aneurysms
FRED	6F	0.027	Longitudinal shortening after deployment (60%) Recapturing is possible up to 50% deployment length	Large or giant, wide-necked aneurysms

Abbreviations: ICA, internal carotid artery; FRED, Flow Redirection Endoluminal Device; PED, Pipeline Embolization Device; SILK, Silk flow diverter; SURPASS, Surpass flow diverter.

placement. When the stent is deployed, it expands radially and shortens longitudinally (up to 50–60%). Additionally, its design allows telescoping multiple devices within each other to increase the metal surface coverage or the length of the reconstructed vessel. If this is done, smaller devices should be deployed first in order for larger stents to expand within the smaller ones.[27,28]

9.3.2 Silk Flow Diverter

The SILK stent is indicated to treat large, giant, fusiform and wide-necked aneurysms. However, the manufacturer highly recommends adjuvant coiling for giant aneurysms. This stent is loaded on a stainless delivery wire that has a 9-mm distal radiopaque tip. The stent is deployed through a 0.021-inch microcatheter (2.4F) known as Vasco + 21 (Balt, Montmorency, France) when using diameters from 2.0 to 4.5 mm. For stent diameters 5.0 and 5.5 mm, a 0.027-inch microcatheter is required (Vasco + 27, Balt, Montmorency, France). The overall deployment technique consists of microcatheter retraction while holding the delivery wire stable. This tension is paramount to maintain the stent system in the correct place. A slight push on the stent might be necessary to accomplish proper stent opening. This device may be retrieved and repositioned up to 90% deployment.[19,29]

9.3.3 Surpass Flow Diverter

The SURPASS is indicated to treat large or giant, wide-necked aneurysms. This stent is loaded on its own delivery microcatheter. This system is composed of an inner (the pusher) and an outer catheter (the delivery catheter). The distal outer diameter of the delivery system measures 3.9F and the proximal segment measures 3.7F. The system (inner catheter) may be navigated through any 0.014-inch microwire and the positioning of the device may be done by either the exchange or direct technique. Once the system is accurately placed, the pusher is slowly advanced while the outer catheter is held stable or retracted to release tension and maintain a proper position. The design of the device allows a precise deployment, keeps the porosity constant (70%), and maintains a high-pore density across all diameters, which may reduce the need of telescoping devices.[21,22,30]

9.3.4 Flow Redirection Endoluminal Device

The FRED has been designed to treat large or giant aneurysms with wide necks. The device may be delivered by a 0.027-inch microcatheter. The stent is attached to a delivery microwire with a radiopaque distal tip and a proximal marker. The distal radiopaque marker should be placed approximately 7 mm past the aneurysm neck to ensure that the double layer will adequately cover it. The deployment technique is through the pull–push method. The device may be recaptured up to 50% deployment of its total length.[25,26,31]

9.4 Conclusion

Flow-diverting technology continues to rapidly evolve with the development of new-generation devices. This is the result of continued innovation in device design and a desire to simplify device deployment. At the time of this writing, the most abundant clinical data involve the PED and SILK devices, which have demonstrated safety and efficacy in a number of studies.[7,32] Although the data on other available stents are more limited, their mesh design, deployment technique, and clinical results offer considerable promise.

Flow-diverting devices have expanded the treatment options for intracranial aneurysms, specifically targeting complex lesions. Additionally, because of a better understanding of blood-flow disruption, these devices are constantly improving. Long-term clinical data are still limited and results from ongoing trials will elucidate the safety and effectiveness of the new-generation devices.

References

[1] Spetzler RF, McDougall CG, Zabramski JM, et al. The Barrow Ruptured Aneurysm Trial: 6-year results. J Neurosurg. 2015; 123(3):609–617

[2] Molyneux AJ, Birks J, Clarke A, Sneade M, Kerr RS. The durability of endovascular coiling versus neurosurgical clipping of ruptured cerebral aneurysms: 18 year follow-up of the UK cohort of the International Subarachnoid Aneurysm Trial (ISAT). Lancet. 2015; 385(9969):691–697

[3] King B, Vaziri S, Singla A, Fargen KM, Mocco J. Clinical and angiographic outcomes after stent-assisted coiling of cerebral aneurysms with Enterprise and Neuroform stents: a comparative analysis of the literature. J Neurointerv Surg. 2015; 7(12):905–909

[4] Moret J, Cognard C, Weill A, Castaings L, Rey A. The "remodelling technique" in the treatment of wide neck intracranial aneurysms. Angiographic results and clinical follow-up in 56 cases. Interv Neuroradiol. 1997; 3(1):21–35

[5] White PM, Lewis SC, Gholkar A, et al. HELPS trial collaborators. Hydrogel-coated coils versus bare platinum coils for the endovascular treatment of intracranial aneurysms (HELPS): a randomised controlled trial. Lancet. 2011; 377(9778):1655–1662

[6] Ferns SP, Sprengers ME, van Rooij WJ, et al. Coiling of intracranial aneurysms: a systematic review on initial occlusion and reopening and retreatment rates. Stroke. 2009; 40(8):e523–e529

[7] Kallmes DF, Hanel R, Lopes D, et al. International retrospective study of the pipeline embolization device: a multicenter aneurysm treatment study. AJNR Am J Neuroradiol. 2015; 36(1):108–115

[8] Becske T, Kallmes DF, Saatci I, et al. Pipeline for uncoilable or failed aneurysms: results from a multicenter clinical trial. Radiology. 2013; 267(3):858–868

[9] Gross BA, Frerichs KU. Stent usage in the treatment of intracranial aneurysms: past, present and future. J Neurol Neurosurg Psychiatry. 2013; 84 (3):244–253

[10] Lylyk P, Miranda C, Ceratto R, et al. Curative endovascular reconstruction of cerebral aneurysms with the pipeline embolization device: the Buenos Aires experience. Neurosurgery. 2009; 64(4):632–642, discussion 642–643, quiz N6

[11] Fiorella D, Lylyk P, Szikora I, et al. Curative cerebrovascular reconstruction with the Pipeline embolization device: the emergence of definitive endovascular therapy for intracranial aneurysms. J Neurointerv Surg. 2009; 1 (1):56–65

[12] Aurboonyawat T, Blanc R, Schmidt P, et al. An in vitro study of silk stent morphology. Neuroradiology. 2011; 53(9):659–667

[13] Sadasivan C, Cesar L, Seong J, et al. An original flow diversion device for the treatment of intracranial aneurysms: evaluation in the rabbit elastase-induced model. Stroke. 2009; 40(3):952–958

[14] Wakhloo AK, Tio FO, Lieber BB, Schellhammer F, Graf M, Hopkins LN. Self-expanding nitinol stents in canine vertebral arteries: hemodynamics and tissue response. AJNR Am J Neuroradiol. 1995; 16(5):1043–1051

[15] Nelson PK, Lylyk P, Szikora I, Wetzel SG, Wanke I, Fiorella D. The pipeline embolization device for the intracranial treatment of aneurysms trial. AJNR Am J Neuroradiol. 2011; 32(1):34–40

[16] Duckworth EA, Nickele C, Hoit D, Belayev A, Moran CJ, Arthur AS. The first North American use of the Pipeline Flex flow diverter. BMJ Case Rep. 2015 Jan 30; 2015. DOI: doi:10.1136/bcr-2014-011548

[17] Colby GP, Lin LM, Caplan JM, et al. Immediate procedural outcomes in 44 consecutive Pipeline Flex cases: the first North American single-center series. J Neurointerv Surg. 2016; 8(7):702–709

[18] Maimon S, Gonen L, Nossek E, Strauss I, Levite R, Ram Z. Treatment of intracranial aneurysms with the SILK flow diverter: 2 years' experience with 28 patients at a single center. Acta Neurochir (Wien). 2012; 154(6):979–987

[19] Alghamdi F, Morais R, Scillia P, Lubicz B. The Silk flow-diverter stent for endovascular treatment of intracranial aneurysms. Expert Rev Med Devices. 2015; 12(6):753–762

[20] Stryker N. The Surpass Intracranial Aneurysm Embolization System Pivotal Trial to Treat Large or Giant Wide Neck Aneurysms (SCENT Trial). In: ClinicalTrials.gov. Bethesda, MD: National Library of Medicine (US). 2012 [cited January 8, 2016]. Available at: https://clinicaltrials.gov/ct2/show/NCT01716117; NLM Identifier: NCT01716117

[21] De Vries J, Boogaarts J, Van Norden A, Wakhloo AK. New generation of Flow Diverter (surpass) for unruptured intracranial aneurysms: a prospective single-center study in 37 patients. Stroke. 2013; 44(6):1567–1577

[22] Wakhloo AK, Lylyk P, de Vries J, et al. Surpass Study Group. Surpass flow diverter in the treatment of intracranial aneurysms: a prospective multicenter study. AJNR Am J Neuroradiol. 2015; 36(1):98–107

[23] Seong J, Wakhloo AK, Lieber BB. In vitro evaluation of flow diverters in an elastase-induced saccular aneurysm model in rabbit. J Biomech Eng. 2007; 129(6):863–872

[24] Microvention-Terumo, Inc. Pivotal Study of the FRED Stent System in the Treatment of Intracranial Aneurysms. In: ClinicalTrials.gov. Bethesda, MD: National Library of Medicine (US). 2013 [cited January 8, 2016]. Available at: https://clinicaltrials.gov/ct2/show/NCT01801007; NLM Identifier: NCT01801007

[25] Möhlenbruch MA, Herweh C, Jestaedt L, et al. The FRED flow-diverter stent for intracranial aneurysms: clinical study to assess safety and efficacy. AJNR Am J Neuroradiol. 2015; 36(6):1155–1161

[26] Kocer N, Islak C, Kizilkilic O, Kocak B, Saglam M, Tureci E. Flow Re-direction Endoluminal Device in treatment of cerebral aneurysms: initial experience with short-term follow-up results. J Neurosurg. 2014; 120(5):1158–1171

[27] Pereira VM, Kelly M, Vega P, et al. New Pipeline Flex device: initial experience and technical nuances. J Neurointerv Surg. 2015; 7(12):920–925

[28] Martínez-Galdámez M, Gil A, Caniego JL, et al. Preliminary experience with the Pipeline Flex Embolization Device: technical note. J Neurointerv Surg. 2015; 7(10):748–751

[29] Lubicz B, Collignon L, Raphaeli G, et al. Flow-diverter stent for the endovascular treatment of intracranial aneurysms: a prospective study in 29 patients with 34 aneurysms. Stroke. 2010; 41(10):2247–2253

[30] Colby GP, Lin LM, Caplan JM, et al. Flow diversion of large internal carotid artery aneurysms with the surpass device: impressions and technical nuance from the initial North American experience. J Neurointerv Surg. 2016; 8 (3):279–286

[31] Poncyljusz W, Sagan L, Safranow K, Rać M. Initial experience with implantation of novel dual layer flow-diverter device FRED. Wideochir Inne Tech Malo Inwazyjne. 2013; 8(3):258–264

[32] Briganti F, Leone G, Marseglia M, et al. Endovascular treatment of cerebral aneurysms using flow-diverter devices: a systematic review. Neuroradiol J. 2015; 28(4):365–375

10 TECHNIQUES AND NUANCES OF PIPELINE DEPLOYMENT

EDISON P. VALLE-GILER, RYAN HEBERT, MICHAEL J. LANG, STAVRAPOLA I. TJOUMAKARIS, PASCAL JABBOUR, and ROBERT H. ROSENWASSER

Abstract

Flow diversion is an important tool for treatment of cerebral aneurysms, particularly with the Pipeline Embolization Device (PED). Complications are avoided by appropriate preoperative management, vessel imaging, and understanding of device deployment nuances. We recommend obtaining 3D rotational and high-magnification 2D angiography to accurately determine measurements of the aneurysm neck, as well as inflow and outflow parent vessel diameters. The PED is sized to the inflow vessel diameter. A triaxial setup is used with a long sheath, intermediate catheter and 0.027" delivery catheter. This improves support during loading and unloading of the PED system necessary for precise control of PED expansion and deployment. The "push-pull" technique maximizes metal coverage of the stent over the aneurysm neck and improves apposition to the parent vessel wall, though at the expense of foreshortening of up to 50% of nominal length. Procedural nuances can avoid the most common causes of device failure, such as incomplete expansion in highly tortuous vessels, incomplete device detachment from pusher wire, and endoleak. We recommend use of a single PED device, even if stasis is not immediately apparent, except in complex cases such as long fusiform dilatation, very wide-necked giant aneurysms, or significant inflow-outflow diameter mismatch. Second-generation Flex devices have a modified delivery platform. A second device can be deployed in a telescoping manner, but requires maintaining distal access following deployment of the initial stent. Giant aneurysms are treated with low coil mass embolization via a jailed microcatheter to prevent delayed rupture due thrombus remodeling and resulting inflammatory changes.

Keywords: endoleak, flow diversion, giant aneurysm, inflow-outflow mismatch, Pipeline Embolization Device, technique

10.1 Introduction

Flow diversion has been a major breakthrough in the neurovascular field, allowing the treatment of very challenging aneurysms.[1,2,3] From all the flow diverters (FDs), the Pipeline Embolization Device (PED, Medtronic, Inc.) has been the most popular worldwide since its initial approval in 2011.[1]

The popularity of the PED relies on its efficacy to treat aneurysms when compared to conventional coiling (> 80 vs. 66% aneurysm obliteration rates, respectively). It has also shown that it is an effective treatment, with minimal, if any, aneurysm recurrence rates.[2,3,4,5,6,7,8,9,10]

The PED is approved to use only for the endovascular treatment of adults (22 years of age or older) with large or giant, wide-neck intracranial aneurysms in the internal carotid artery, from the petrous to the superior hypophyseal segment.

In an attempt to widen the PED indications, the Prospective Study on Embolization of Intracranial Aneurysms with Pipeline Embolization Device (PREMIER) trial is evaluating the use of PED in all anterior or posterior aneurysms with a wide neck.

Although still off-label, the PED is used for the treatment of fusiform aneurysms and remnants of previously treated aneurysms. It is also a very good treatment option for very small and blister aneurysms located at curved vessels, where the use of intrasaccular treatments would increase the risk of aneurysm rupture.[4]

Contraindications to PED are patients with active bacterial infection and those in whom dual-antiplatelet therapy is contraindicated or cannot be done.

10.2 Pipeline Properties

The Pipeline is a highly flexible, in stretch and compression, braided stent with high metal coverage (low porosity) that has flow diversion properties.[1,2,3,11,12] The device is composed of 48 braided strands of cobalt chromium (75%) and platinum tungsten (25%). The individual strands measure between 28 and 33 μm.[2] The PED is available with nominal diameters of 2.5 to 5 mm, with 0.25-mm increments in size. The length of the devices ranges from 10 to 35 mm, in 2-mm increments for the 10- to 20-mm lengths, and 5-mm increments for the 25- to 35-mm lengths.[4]

When expanded to nominal diameter, the construct provides approximately 30 to 35% metal surface area coverage, with an average pore size of 0.02 to 0.05 mm^2 and a radial force of 2.0 mN/mm (3.0 mm vessel diameter).[2,4]

The low porosity reduces the hemodynamic exchange between the aneurysm and parent artery, promoting thrombosis within the aneurysm. It also provides scaffolding for neointimal growth over the aneurysm neck, which creates a more durable treatment of aneurysms.[2,6] The stages of aneurysm transition have been described as follows[2,13]:

- Mechanical-anatomical change, after flow diversion of the primary vector of blood flow once the device is deployed.
- Physiological change, after several days to weeks, when the blood staggering within the aneurysm goes through thrombosis.
- Biological, after months, when the device goes through endothelialization and thrombus resorption. There is a permanent biological seal across the diseased parent artery, while preserving physiological flow in the parent vessel and adjacent branches.

10.3 Preoperative Antiplatelet Therapy

In the following paragraphs, we describe our protocol for management of dual-antiplatelet therapy for patients undergoing flow diversion. Patients undergoing PED placement receive 75 mg/day of clopidogrel and 81 mg/day of aspirin 10 days prior to the intervention. Platelet function is tested using P2Y12 assay (VerifyNow; Accumetrics, San Diego, CA). A baseline test is obtained upon scheduling the case, and a "day-of-procedure" test is checked to calculate the percentage of platelet inhibition.

Patients who have platelet inhibition between 30 and 90% are cleared for the procedure. Patients with inhibition less than 30% are reloaded and the assay is rechecked. Patients who are poor responders to clopidogrel are then switched to prasugrel (40 mg loading dose, followed by a 5-mg daily maintenance dose). Patients with inhibition more than 90% are admitted to the hospital, their procedure is canceled, and clopidogrel is held until the platelet inhibition level falls to less than 90%.[9] Dual-antiplatelet therapy is continued for 6 months after the procedure, and then the patients stay on 81 mg/day of aspirin for life.

10.4 Intraoperative Measures

It is our preference to perform the procedures under general endotracheal anesthesia and continuous neurophysiological monitoring, including electroencephalography, somatosensory-evoked potentials, and brain stem auditory-evoked potentials. There are some centers that have shown that doing the procedure under conscious sedation may be equally safe.[14]

As soon as fluoroscopic confirmation of good groin access is achieved, an intravenous bolus of 100 U/kg of heparin is given. Activated clotting time (ACT) is checked at baseline and every 30 minutes thereafter to aim for a goal of double to triple the baseline value. Heparin is discontinued, but not reversed, at the end of the procedure.

To select the correct PED size, we recommend having a three-dimensional rotational angiography as well as high-magnification fluoroscopic runs (anteroposterior and lateral views) for parent vessel and aneurysm measurements. Parent vessel inflow and outflow diameters as well as length of coverage are measured in all the views. To achieve best flow diversion and braid wall apposition, the rule is to match the size of the nominal PED diameter relative to the diameters of the proximal landing zone and parent vessel at the aneurysmal neck (inflow diameter).[4,12] A good wall apposition of the PED requires an equal or very close diameter of the target vessel.

Other factors to consider when choosing the correct size of the pipeline are as follows:
- Foreshortening of approximately 50% and possible device shift during deployment must be kept in mind when choosing the length of the device.
- During delivery, the device may expand to its maximum size, which is approximately 0.25 mm larger than the nominal diameter.
- In case of giant aneurysms, where there could be a significant mismatch in the inflow and outflow parent vessel diameters, creating a multiple device construct may be necessary to achieve good wall apposition and maximize flow diversion.

Implantation of an undersized device may result in poor wall apposition, with the potential risk of an endoleak phenomenon and lack of vessel endothelialization in the future. It can also lead to migration of the device with potential aneurysm rupture.[15] Implantation of an oversized device increases the braid porosity due to an incomplete compaction of the strands, leading to lack of flow diversion and aneurysm obliteration failure.[4,12]

10.5 Deployment Technique

We recommend using a triaxial system (long sheath, intermediate catheter, and a standard 0.027-inch internal diameter delivery catheter). Generally, an 8F femoral sheath, a 6F shuttle sheath (Cook Medical, Bloomington, IN), a 0.058-inch Navien catheter (Medtronic, Inc.), and a 0.027-inch Marksman microcatheter (Medtronic, Inc.) are used.

Once the appropriately sized PED has been selected, the introducer sheath is partially inserted into the rotating hemostatic valve at the catheter hub and sealed. Confirm back flush of saline at the proximal end of the introducer sheath and advance the introducer sheath until it is fully engaged in the hub. Push the PED until you see the fluoro-safe marker on the delivery wire, then start fluoroscopy.

The triaxial system is used to maximize support during forward loading of the system, thus facilitating the initial expansion of the PED and its conformation to the parent vessel while avoiding kickback.[16] The long sheath is generally brought up to the carotid bulb; the intermediate catheter is brought up to the petrous ICA; and under high-magnification fluoroscopic roadmap control, the delivery microcatheter and a Synchro II guidewire (Stryker Neurovascular, Fremont, CA) are manipulated to pass the neck of the aneurysm. Creating a generous "J" on the guidewire is generally enough to pass the aneurysm neck. The distal tip of the Marksman catheter needs to be a minimum of 20 mm past the aneurysm.

A straight vessel segment (generally M1 or M2) is chosen to bring the PED and push the distal part of the braid out of the delivery microcatheter. It is important, before deployment, to reduce the load in the system by slowly pulling back the Marksman microcatheter and the delivery wire together. Once completely unloaded, and in the desired deployment position within the parent vessel, a combination of a "push and pull" technique is used to deliver the PED (push the delivery wire while pulling the delivery catheter).[17]

The "art" of the PED deployment comes to play by understanding that the metal coverage area of the device can be increased or decreased by loading or unsheathing the braid while deploying it. Forward wire pushing will increase the metal coverage area to a point, before starting to compress the device. Unsheathing the PED will decrease metal coverage area and eventually will stretch the braid. It is important to keep in mind that a higher metal coverage area is directly correlated with early obliteration of the aneurysm[18] (▸ Fig. 10.1).

Once the PED had been deployed, the distal coil needs to be pulled inside the Marksman (Medtronic, Inc.), so that it does not get caught in the braid when being removed. To complete this step, rail the microcatheter over the delivery wire. Care must be taken to minimize bumping of the proximal end of the device with the microcatheter, thus potentially pushing the device into the aneurysm. Once the Marksman (Medtronic, Inc.) tip had passed through the PED braid, retract the delivery coil into the microcatheter tip. If the delivery coil cannot be retracted into the microcatheter, advance the Marksman to a straight vessel segment (generally M1) and try to retract the wire again. If this maneuver does not work, pull the delivery wire until the distal coil gets snugged together with the delivery catheter, and remove them simultaneously, paying attention not to move the PED braid from its original position.

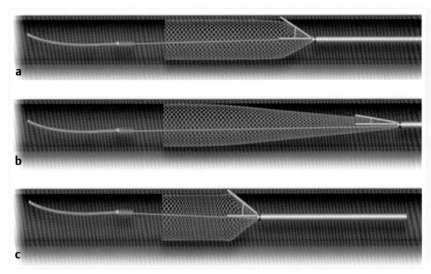

Fig. 10.1 (a) Appropriate amount of forward push on the delivery wire. **(b)** Stretching of the braid due to too much unsheathing of the delivery catheter. **(c)** Too much forward push on the delivery wire and possible compression of the braid. (Reproduced with permission of Medtronic, Inc.)

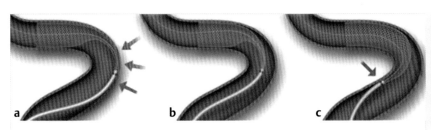

Fig. 10.2 Center-and-push technique. When the braid does not expand because it is leaning against the convexity of the curvature **(a)**, unload the system by pulling both microcatheter and delivery wire together **(b)**. In that way, a new vector of deployment is created **(c)**. This is the so-called center-and-push technique. (Reproduced with permission of Medtronic, Inc.)

It is important to recognize possible deployment failures.

- When bringing the PED up to the distal tip of the delivery catheter, ***if the delivery forces start to increase too much***, stop pushing the wire before causing damage to the microcatheter (sometimes the Marksman can accordion). At this point, try to straighten the system by pulling the microcatheter and delivery wire together to create a different vector of deployment. This concept, called "unloading" is especially important when trying to deploy the PED in vessel curvatures.

- When working in *tortuous anatomy and the PED does not expand after unloading the system and pushing and torquing* the delivery wire, bring the Navien catheter (Medtronic, Inc.) intracranially for more support. The Navien is advanced over the Marksman (Medtronic, Inc.) to the unopened part of the PED. The PED is then fully unsheathed within the Navien catheter. At this point, the PED deployment is a combination of unsheathing from the Navien and pushing on the Marksman (Navien functions as the Marksman, and Marksman functions as pusher/delivery wire).[19]

- If, while deploying the PED against the convexity of a curve, the *PED does not expand*, get a new vector of deployment. It is important to "unload" the system until the system achieves a new vector of deployment, along the concavity of the curve. At this point, push more wire to continue the deployment; this is the so-called center-and-push technique[16] (▶ Fig. 10.2).

- If, after deployment, there is *inadequate vessel wall apposition (endoleak),* create a generous "J" on the Synchro II guidewire

(Stryker Neurovascular, Fremont, CA) and pass it through the PED several times to push the device against the vessel wall. Another option, although not very frequently used in our practice, is to use a hyperglide balloon (Medtronic, Inc) to assure device-wall apposition. Ballooning may be associated with mechanical vessel injury that predisposes to intimal hyperplasia and in-stent stenosis.[4,20]

The number of devices that are optimal to achieve flow diversion is still a matter of discussion. Complete intra-aneurysmal stasis during initial embolization is not required for ultimate aneurysm thrombosis and should not be the end point of the procedure.[4,11,20] We prefer to use a single PED, reserving multiple device placement only for those aneurysms that remain unchanged or do not sufficiently decrease in size at the 6-month follow-up.[15,21] Less than 24% of patients in our series required more than one PED.[9] Placement of multiple devices in a single setting increases the length of the procedure and the number of complications.[20]

Multiple device constructs during the first treatment setting are reserved for complex cases with suboptimal aneurysm neck coverage, long fusiform aneurysms, very wide neck aneurysms, reconstruction of a dilated long vessel, and ruptured aneurysms in which immediate occlusion is needed. We also consider multiple PED placements when there is a dramatic mismatch between the inflow and outflow parent vessel diameter, choosing the first device based on the outflow parent vessel diameter, and the second device based on the inflow parent vessel diameter. Using multiple PEDs may increase the device stability, increase the metal coverage area, and prevent PED migration into the aneurysm.[4,15,20]

When creating a multiple device construct, it is very important not to lose distal access past the aneurysm. Once the first device is deployed, the Marksman (Medtronic, Inc.) is railed over the delivery wire to a straight vessel segment to capture the distal coil and remove the pusher wire. The goal would be to deliver and "telescope" the second PED within the already deployed PED. The distal coil is pushed out of the delivery catheter at a straight vessel segment, so the second device is at the tip of the microcatheter, ready to be delivered. At this point, the entire system is unloaded and pulled to the desired landing zone within the already deployed PED. An initial "push" is necessary to deliver the second device, then a combination of pushing the delivery wire and pulling (unsheathing) the Marksman (Medtronic, Inc) is necessary for deployment. When telescoping devices, it is very important to avoid "dragging" the second device because it can create damage to the strands of the already deployed PED.

In case of giant aneurysms, it is our approach to do low coil mass embolization and use steroids to prevent delayed aneurysm rupture and attenuate the effects of intra-aneurysmal thrombosis, worsening mass effect, and neurological deficits.[21,22] After positioning the Marksman microcatheter (Medtronic, Inc) distal to the aneurysm neck, we navigate a second microcatheter, parallel to the Navien, into the aneurysm sac to deploy coils via the "jailing" technique. After deployment of the PED, the aneurysm is coiled, without achieving high coil packing density and without occluding the aneurysm neck covered by the PED.[22] Subtotal aneurysm packing reduces the need to coil across the aneurysm neck, thus reducing the risk of coils protruding into the parent vessel subjacent to the PED.[22]

Finding the parent vessel outflow in giant aneurysms can be challenging. Sometimes, it requires creating a Marksman "loop" within the aneurysm before the outflow is found. These circumstances would require straightening the delivery catheter before PED deployment, which most of the times can be achieved by unloading the system. Seldom, the Marksman cannot be straightened without losing outflow access. In these cases, after positioning the Marksman catheter in a straight M1 segment, a second Marksman catheter is brought up parallel to the Navien catheter (Medtronic, Inc.). A Solitaire stent (Medtronic, Inc.) is partially deployed to "jail" the Marksman (Medtronic, Inc.) carrying the PED and create a distal anchor point. At this point, the looped Marksman can be reduced safely, without losing outflow access.[23]

10.6 Classic versus Flex

There are two kinds of devices available on the market, the Pipeline Classic and the Pipeline Flex. The device itself is the same with changes only to the delivery system (▸ Fig. 10.3).

10.6.1 Pipeline Classic-Specific Deployment Properties

A radiopaque 15-mm platinum tip extends beyond the end of the PED. The PED is pushed approximately 5 mm distal to the Marksman, or until the portion of the device outside of the microcatheter takes a pillow case/cigar shape. If the landing zone is optimal, a torque device is attached to the delivery wire to "push and torque" the wire in order to detach the distal braid from the capture coil. Following distal detachment, the push-and-pull technique is used to ensure adequate opening of the stent.[16,17]

Once the PED is entirely deployed, the Marksman is driven up, over the delivery wire to recapture the coil and remove the delivery system together, without moving or damaging the deployed device.[16]

Possible Pipeline Classic deployment failures need to be recognized:

- If, after pushing the distal device out of the Marksman (Medtronic, Inc), the **device forms the cigar shape but does not open (is not released from the capture coil)**, unload/decrease the tension of the system by pulling both the Marksman and delivery wire together. Then, with the help of a torque device, spin the torque clockwise up to three times while pushing the delivery wire to "push the device out" of the delivery coil. By pushing and turning the delivery wire, the capture coil separates from the device, allowing full expansion.
- If **recapturing of the distal coil is not possible**, the delivery wire is pulled until resistance is felt (distal capture coil snugged against Marksman), so the entire system can be pulled together through the PED without pulling or damaging the already deployed device.[16]

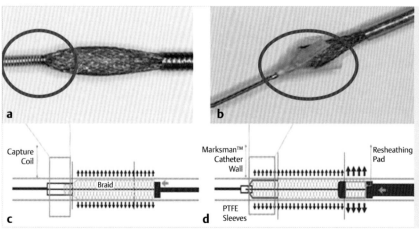

Fig. 10.3 Schematic and magnified views of the Classic and Flex pipeline models. The PED in the Classic model is held distally by the capture coil (**a,c**). The capture coil (*red circle*, **a**) explains why pushing and turning (up to three clockwise turns) the delivery wire would dislodge the PED from the capture coil and let the braid blossom. The PED in the Flex model is held proximally by the resheathing pad (**d**). Distally, the PED remains constrained by two 3-mm PTFE sleeves (**b**). This new design explains the easy initial expansion of the PED once it is pushed 5 mm out of the Marksman delivery catheter. (Reproduced with permission of Medtronic, Inc.)

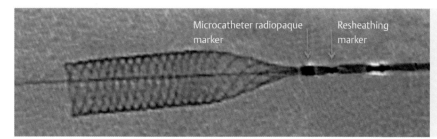

Microcatheter radiopaque marker

Resheathing marker

Fig. 10.4 Resheathing marker in the Pipeline Flex. There is a radiopaque marker that shows the point of "no return" when trying to resheath the braid. (Reproduced with permission of Medtronic, Inc.)

10.6.2 Pipeline Flex-Specific Deployment Properties

The 15-mm radiopaque platinum tip coil is 30% softer and allows 55-degree angle turns (compared with 25-degree angle from the Classic), facilitating deployment in tortuous anatomy.

The capture platinum coil was replaced by PTFE (polytetrafluoroethylene; Teflon-Dupont Co.) sleeves. The device remains constrained until the PTFE sleeves are 5 mm outside of the microcatheter. No torquing is required for initial deployment, which provides better distal landing zone accuracy (▶ Fig. 10.3).

The Pipeline Flex has a resheathing pad that holds the device proximally, and allows resheathing up to two times. The device has a proximal marker that defines the point of "no return" (▶ Fig. 10.4).

The delivery wire is slightly bigger, but more flexible, making it easier to navigate through tortuous anatomy.

Once the system is positioned in the desired deployment location, an initial push (at least 5 mm) in the delivery wire brings the PED out of the Marksman, separates the PTFE sleeves, and lets the device fully expand. At this point, the technique of deployment is the same "push-and-pull" technique as in the Classic system. If resheathing is needed, remove any energy from the system, apply forward pressure in the Marksman, and pull the delivery wire at the same time.

To remove the distal coil, rail the Marksman over the delivery wire without dislodging the already deployed device. Then, find a straight vessel segment distal to the device and retract the distal coil into the microcatheter tip. A slight resistance will be felt, before the delivery wire retracts into the Marksman (PTFE sleeves retracting into the Marksman).

It is important to recognize potential delivery failures in the Pipeline Flex system:

- If the **braid does not expand** upon initial pushing on the delivery wire, it could be because the PTFE sleeves did not separate from the braid. In this case, resheath the braid, so the Marksman can push the PTFE sleeves forward and let the braid expand (▶ Fig. 10.5). This "re-sheathing before final deployment" technique is especially helpful when facing tortuous anatomy and precise deployment is needed. Once the PTFE sleeves are separated from the braid, there is less kick back upon initial deployment, allowing better control while deploying the device in the desired location.

10.7 Avoidance of Complication

Complications during Pipeline placement range from groin-related issues to worsening cranial neuropathy and ischemic/

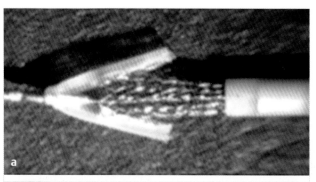

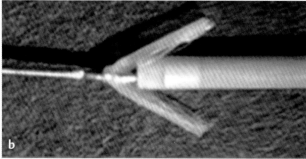

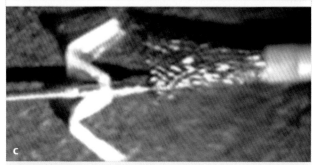

Fig. 10.5 Distal braid opening. If the PTFE sleeves do not separate from the braid (and are pinned against the vessel wall), preventing it from expanding **(a)**, resheath the distal braid to push the PTFE sleeves forward **(b)**. At this point, the PTFE sleeves would let the braid expand freely **(c)**. (Reproduced with permission of Medtronic, Inc.)

hemorrhagic stroke. They occur in 5.6% of the patients according to major pipeline trials,[3,6,21] and they are more frequent (almost twice as common) when treating vessels of the posterior circulation in comparison to the anterior circulation.[5]

We suggest the following strategies to avoid complications:

- Heparinize the patient only after the groin angiography confirms good access. This maneuver minimizes groin complications related to bleeding and retroperitoneal hematomas.

- Minimize the time of the procedure as much as possible. Using one pipeline provides similar aneurysm obliteration rates but lower complication rates than using multiple device constructs.[3,20]
- Use three-dimensional, as well as two-dimensional, high-magnification angiography views for vessel measurement and selection of the correct PED size. Device migration usually occurs when there is mismatch in the inflow and outflow vessel diameter, and the PED diameter is not correctly chosen. Migration can be associated with hemorrhagic or thromboembolic events.[15]
- Do not lose distal access through the pipeline until good deployment is confirmed. When trying to recapture the distal coil, the PED device can rarely be pushed by the Marksman into the aneurysm. In this situation, it is very important not to lose the distal delivery wire, to use it to rail the Marksman up past the PED. If the delivery microcatheter does not pass through the proximal end of the PED (microcatheter colliding with the proximal braids of the PED), push the delivery wire up to an M2 or M3 segment. At this point, slowly unload the system to create a new vector on the delivery wire for navigation of the Marksman through the PED.
- We routinely prescribe a 2-week dexamethasone taper starting at 8 mg every 6 hours to all patients with giant aneurysms. This regimen may provide symptomatic relief of headaches and decrease the incidence of cranial neuropathies.[16]

10.8 Postoperative Course and Follow-up

The groin access sheath is generally removed and closed immediately after the procedure. Patients who are not candidates for a vascular closure device have manual pressure applied after sheath removal. On these patients, we wait until the partial thromboplastin time or ACT has gone back to baseline before the sheath is removed. Patients are admitted to the intensive care unit for neurological checks and groin evaluations for 24 hours.

If there are no complications, the patients are discharged on postoperative day 1. They receive a prescription for clopidogrel (75 mg/day) and aspirin (81 mg/day) until they come back for follow-up angiography and MRI in 6 months.

References

[1] Nelson PK, Lylyk P, Szikora I, Wetzel SG, Wanke I, Fiorella D. The pipeline embolization device for the intracranial treatment of aneurysms trial. AJNR Am J Neuroradiol. 2011; 32(1):34–40

[2] Fiorella D, Lylyk P, Szikora I, et al. Curative cerebrovascular reconstruction with the Pipeline embolization device: the emergence of definitive endovascular therapy for intracranial aneurysms. J Neurointerv Surg. 2009; 1(1):56–65

[3] Lylyk P, Miranda C, Ceratto R, et al. Curative endovascular reconstruction of cerebral aneurysms with the pipeline embolization device: the Buenos Aires experience. Neurosurgery. 2009; 64(4):632–642, discussion 642–643, quiz N6

[4] Fischer S, Vajda Z, Aguilar Perez M, et al. Pipeline embolization device (PED) for neurovascular reconstruction: initial experience in the treatment of 101 intracranial aneurysms and dissections. Neuroradiology. 2012; 54(4):369–382

[5] Kallmes DF, Hanel R, Lopes D, et al. International retrospective study of the pipeline embolization device: a multicenter aneurysm treatment study. AJNR Am J Neuroradiol. 2015; 36(1):108–115

[6] Becske T, Kallmes DF, Saatci I, et al. Pipeline for uncoilable or failed aneurysms: results from a multicenter clinical trial. Radiology. 2013; 267(3):858–868

[7] Briganti F, Leone G, Marseglia M, et al. Endovascular treatment of cerebral aneurysms using flow-diverter devices: a systematic review. Neuroradiol J. 2015; 28(4):365–375

[8] Molyneux AJ, Kerr RS, Yu LM, et al. International Subarachnoid Aneurysm Trial (ISAT) Collaborative Group. International subarachnoid aneurysm trial (ISAT) of neurosurgical clipping versus endovascular coiling in 2143 patients with ruptured intracranial aneurysms: a randomised comparison of effects on survival, dependency, seizures, rebleeding, subgroups, and aneurysm occlusion. Lancet. 2005; 366(9488):809–817

[9] Chalouhi N, Tjoumakaris S, Starke RM, et al. Comparison of flow diversion and coiling in large unruptured intracranial saccular aneurysms. Stroke. 2013; 44(8):2150–2154

[10] Raymond J, Guilbert F, Weill A, et al. Long-term angiographic recurrences after selective endovascular treatment of aneurysms with detachable coils. Stroke. 2003; 34(6):1398–1403

[11] Shapiro M, Raz E, Becske T, Nelson PK. Building multidevice pipeline constructs of favorable metal coverage: a practical guide. AJNR Am J Neuroradiol. 2014; 35(8):1556–1561

[12] Shapiro M, Raz E, Becske T, Nelson PK. Variable porosity of the pipeline embolization device in straight and curved vessels: a guide for optimal deployment strategy. AJNR Am J Neuroradiol. 2014; 35(4):727–733

[13] D'Urso PI, Lanzino G, Cloft HJ, Kallmes DF. Flow diversion for intracranial aneurysms: a review. Stroke. 2011; 42(8):2363–2368

[14] Rangel-Castilla L, Cress MC, Munich SA, et al. Feasibility, safety, and periprocedural complications of pipeline embolization for intracranial aneurysm treatment under conscious sedation: University at Buffalo Neurosurgery Experience. Neurosurgery. 2015; 11 Suppl 3:426–430

[15] Chalouhi N, Satti SR, Tjoumakaris S, et al. Delayed migration of a pipeline embolization device. Neurosurgery. 2013; 72(2) Suppl Operative:ons229–ons234, discussion ons234

[16] Chitale R, Gonzalez LF, Randazzo C, et al. Single center experience with pipeline stent: feasibility, technique, and complications. Neurosurgery. 2012; 71(3):679–691, discussion 691

[17] Ma D, Xiang J, Choi H, et al. Enhanced aneurysmal flow diversion using a dynamic push-pull technique: an experimental and modeling study. AJNR Am J Neuroradiol. 2014; 35(9):1779–1785

[18] Jou LD, Chintalapani G, Mawad ME. Metal coverage ratio of pipeline embolization device for treatment of unruptured aneurysms: reality check. Interv Neuroradiol. 2016; 22(1):42–48

[19] Lin LM, Colby GP, Jiang B, et al. Intra-DIC (distal intracranial catheter) deployment of the Pipeline embolization device: a novel rescue strategy for failed device expansion. J Neurointerv Surg. 2016; 8(8):840–846

[20] Chalouhi N, Tjoumakaris S, Phillips JL, et al. A single pipeline embolization device is sufficient for treatment of intracranial aneurysms. AJNR Am J Neuroradiol. 2014; 35(8):1562–1566

[21] Jabbour P, Chalouhi N, Tjoumakaris S, et al. The Pipeline Embolization Device: learning curve and predictors of complications and aneurysm obliteration. Neurosurgery. 2013; 73(1):113–120, discussion 120

[22] Nossek E, Chalif DJ, Chakraborty S, Lombardo K, Black KS, Setton A. Concurrent use of the Pipeline Embolization Device and coils for intracranial aneurysms: technique, safety, and efficacy. J Neurosurg. 2015; 122(4):904–911

[23] Clarençon F, Wyse G, Fanning N, et al. Solitaire FR stent as an adjunctive tool for pipeline stent deployment in the treatment of giant intracranial aneurysms. Neurosurgery. 2013; 72(2) Suppl Operative:onsE241–E244, discussion E244

11 TECHNIQUE AND NUANCES OF SILK DEPLOYMENT (BALT EXTRUSION)

OR COHEN-INBAR, JASON M. DAVIES, YAAQOV AMSALEM, and ELAD I. LEVY

Abstract

The Silk flow diverter (SFD; Balt Extrusion, Montmorency, France) is a first-generation endovascular flow diversion stent for minimally invasive treatment of intracranial aneurysms. SFD stents can be effective devices for the treatment of unruptured aneurysms with complex anatomy in which primary coiling, coiling in conjunction with conventional stents, and clipping may be problematic. These devices have been shown to induce complete angiographic occlusion along with a patent parent artery in more than 80% of patients at 1 year after treatment. Disappearance or shrinkage of the aneurysm sac was reported in more than 80% of aneurysms. Proper SFD deployment and rigorous monitoring of the antiplatelet therapy are mandatory components of treatment to limit ischemic complications. A risk of delayed aneurysm bleeding after SFD treatment does exist (ranging from 0 to 5%), highlighting the need for a better understanding of related pathophysiology. We herein review proper periprocedural management and stenting techniques.

Keywords: nitinol, obliteration, progressive aneurysm obliteration, self-expandable stents, Silk flow diverter stents

11.1 Introduction

Our understanding of intracranial vascular pathologies and interactions with therapeutic devices ha**s** been rapidly coevolving over the past decade. Computational and experimental models have demonstrated the importance of angioarchitectural and hemodynamic factors on the formation and eventual rupture of intracranial aneurysms (IAs), and this knowledge has in turn informed device design in important ways. Intrasaccular occlusion of aneurysms has long been practiced for aneurysmal lesions, but the geometrical constraints of the technique left certain lesions, such as wide-necked, giant, and fusiform aneurysms, without suitable endovascular options. To address these lesions, technology and technique have pushed the boundary, with progression from balloon-assisted coiling to stent-assisted coiling. Studies of these techniques yielded intriguing insights into mechanisms of action: although stents were initially intended to simply isolate a coil mass from the parent artery, evidence suggested a secondary effect whereby blood flow was redirected, changing the hemodynamic factors that propagated aneurysmal growth.[1,2] Standalone stents, whose primary purpose was modification of flow, were hypothesized, developed, proven in animal models, and subsequently shown efficacious in humans.[3]

Flow-diverting stents (FDSs) are a paradigm shift in our approach to the treatment of IAs. Flow diverters have the basic form of other intracranial intraluminal stents, but with tighter meshes this additional metal coverage serves to divert blood flow from the aneurysm sac toward the downstream artery. This intraluminal reconstruction results in flow reduction outside of the vessel lumen.[4] Over time, this alteration of inflow and outflow jets at the parent artery–aneurysm sac interface induces aneurysm thrombosis.[5,6] FDSs further function through a secondary mechanism: neointimal overgrowth. The dense mesh of the stent wall serves as a scaffold for ingrowth of cells that ultimately covers the stent, reconstructing the parent artery wall and eliminating the aneurysm–parent vessel interface. Neointimal overgrowth, being a latent process, has been shown to spare the origin of branching perforators, likely through a demand mechanism.[7,8] In the short term, aneurysmal thrombosis may result in inflammation, perianeurysmal edema in surrounding brain parenchyma, and even transient neurological findings.[9] With time, however, the aneurysm dome tends to shrink and collapse around the device construct, ultimately eliminating local mass effect and related symptoms.[4,10]

Flow-diverting stents have been used in clinical practice since 2007 for IA configurations that were deemed poorly amenable to traditional coiling.[10,11,12] These include fusiform/dissecting IAs,[13] giant/large internal carotid artery IAs,[14,15] carotid-ophthalmic aneurysms,[16] as well as blisterlike aneurysms.[17] Fusiform IAs are typically circumferentially diseased vessels that are difficult to reconstruct with previous techniques, given that there is no good tissue to clip or sew to, and the fusiform segment often cannot be sacrificed or embolized without compromising parent vessel flow. FDSs smoothly reconstruct an endothelial-covered channel in continuation with the parent artery.[7] Blisterlike aneurysms are small, broad-based, shallow pseudoaneurysms commonly located at nonbranching sites; they are difficult to treat with conventional endovascular or microsurgical techniques.[17,18] As experience with flow diverters has increased, practitioners have come to appreciate that flow diversion techniques cause aneurysms to occlude over time, with occlusion rates demonstrated to increase as far as 6 to 12 months after deployment of an FDS.[11,12] This mechanism often seems to be better tolerated physiologically, as well.

We will devote the rest of this chapter to a discussion on the treatment of IAs with Silk flow diverters (SFDs; Balt Extrusion, Montmorency, France), reviewing the published literature and different technical nuances.

11.1.1 Nitinol Alloy

Most modern stents, including the Silk, are constructed using a shape-memory alloy called nitinol (nitinol is a tradename for *ni*ckel *ti*tanium *N*aval *O*rdnance *L*aboratory), first introduced as a material for stents in 2003.[19] Nitinol offers shape-memory effects particularly suited for self-expanding stents (SESs),[19,20,21] like the Silk, with a unique balance between the desirable features of both conventional stent materials and natural materials (hair, bone, tendon). The elastic deformation of conventional stent-forming metals is limited to approximately 1% strain, and stent elongation typically increases and decreases proportionally with the applied force. On the other hand, natural materials (like hair, tendon, and bone) can be elastically deformed, in some cases up to 10% strain in a nonlinear way (▶ Fig. 11.1).[22] Nitinol SESs do not require postdeployment heating, imparting a superelastic quality to the stent, thus being crush-recoverable.[19,20,21] After deployment, these stents exert a gentle chronic outward force and are generally more physiologically compatible than balloon-expandable stents. Despite the high nickel content of nitinol, its corrosion resistance and biocompatibility is equal to that of other implant materials.[19,20,21]

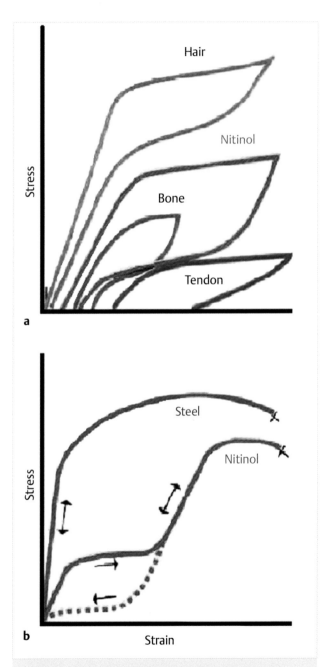

Fig. 11.1 Biomechanical compatibility of nitinol. **(a)** Deformation characteristics of nitinol and living tissues; **(b)** Schematic stress–strain diagram for nitinol and stainless steel. (Modified from Cohen-Inbar et al[21][http://www.SciRP.org/journal/ojmn].)

11.1.2 Silk Device Parameters

The SFD received Conformité Européenne (CE) mark approval in 2008. It is a closed-cell mesh cylinder composed of 48 braided 35-μm microfilament strands, 44 nitinol, and 4 platinum. This construct results in metal surface coverage ranging from 35 to 60% with a pore size of 110 to 250 μm², depending on the degree of compression/elongation of the stent at deployment.[23,24] The SFD has two flared ends with four sinusoidal radiopaque platinum markers running the length of the stent. The SFD is deployed from its delivery microcatheter (Vasco + 21, Balt Extrusion) through a combination of pushing the delivery wire and retrieving the microcatheter, which allows the operator to fine-tune placement of the stent. The delivery procedure is similar to that for other self-expanding intracranial stents; however, in contrast to others, the SFD allows resheathing and repositioning, even when as much as 90% of its length has been deployed.[20,21,22,23,24]

The SFD is available in a wide range of diameters (2–5.5 mm) and lengths (15–40 mm) for the treatment of aneurysms of different sizes and locations. The shapes, forms, and available sizes are presented in ▶ Fig. 11.2. The original Silk stent, although quite flexible, had a relatively lower radial force than other closed-cell stents, such as the Enterprise (Codman, Raynham, MA), that resulted in the potential for stent migration and even vessel occlusion in stenotic vessels. Adjunctive stenting with other stents with greater radial force was thus sometimes performed (discussed later).[25,26] The Silk Plus (Silk +) stent, characterized with 15% more radial force, addressed this point and negated the need for additional stents.

11.2 Reported Obliteration and Complication Rates—Literature Review

A literature review of SFD series is presented in ▶ Table 11.1.[4,14,17,24,26,27,28,29,30,31,32,33,34,35,36,37] Although the ultimate goals of treatment are to prevent hemorrhage and rupture-related morbidity and mortality as well as the alleviation of local aneurysm-related mass effect, these events are, fortunately, rarely encountered during the course of typical clinical follow-up. As a result, aneurysm obliteration and recanalization rates are typically employed as surrogates for aneurysm rupture rate/risk.[3] A review of the data presented in ▶ Table 11.1 shows that deployment failure was reported in approximately 3% of cases and deployment difficulty in an additional 11% of cases. Complete aneurysm obliteration was reported in 59 to 90.9% of cases, varying depending on the center, experience of the interventionists, and date of publication.[2,12,15,22,24,25,26,27,28,29,30,31,32,33,34,35] The series by Velioglu et al[36] featured the longest mean follow-up of 17.5±11.1 months (range: 2–48 months). These authors reported an 87.9% complete obliteration rate. No recanalization was reported. Among the studies reviewed, the mean acute periprocedural complication rate was 12.5% (95% confidence interval [CI]: 8.7–

	REFERENCE	VESSEL Ø (MM)	SILK+ LENGTH AT NOMINAL Ø (MM)	DELIVERY CATHETER	UNCONSTRAINED STENT	
					Ø (MM)	LENGTH (MM)
SILK+2,0	SILK2,0 x 15	1,50 to 2,25	15	VASCO+21 (2.4F)	2.5	7
	SILK2,0 x 20		20			9
SILK+2,5	SILK2,5 x 15	2,00 to 2,75	15	VASCO+21 (2.4F)	3.0	5
	SILK2,5 x 20		20			7
	SILK2,5 x 25		25			10
SILK+3,0	SILK3,0 x 15	2,50 to 3,25	15	VASCO+21 (2.4F)	3.5	6
	SILK3,0 x 20		20			8
	SILK3,0 x 25		25			10
	SILK3,0 x 30		30			12
SILK+3,5	SILK3,5 x 15	3,00 to 3,75	15	VASCO+21 (2.4F)	4.0	7
	SILK3,5 x 20		20			9
	SILK3,5 x 25		25			12
	SILK3,5 x 30		30			13
	SILK3,5 x 35		35			17
SILK+4,0	SILK4,0 x 15	3,50 to 4,25	15	VASCO+21 (2.4F)	4.5	8
	SILK4,0 x 20		20			11
	SILK4,0 x 25		25			14
	SILK4,0 x 30		30			17
	SILK4,0 x 35		35			21
	SILK4,0 x 40		40			23
SILK+4,5	SILK4,5 x 15	4,00 to 4,75	15	VASCO+21 (2.4F)	5.0	7
	SILK4,5 x 20		20			10
	SILK4,5 x 25		25			13
	SILK4,5 x 30		30			16
	SILK4,5 x 35		35			19
	SILK4,5 x 40		40			22
SILK+5,0	SILK5,0 x 25	4,50 to 5,25	25	VASCO+25 (3F)	5.5	13
	SILK5,0 x 30		30			15
	SILK5,0 x 40		40			21
SILK+5,5	SILK5,5 x 25	5,00 to 5,75	25	VASCO+25 (3F)	6.0	11
	SILK5,5 x 30		30			15
	SILK5,5 x 40		40			19

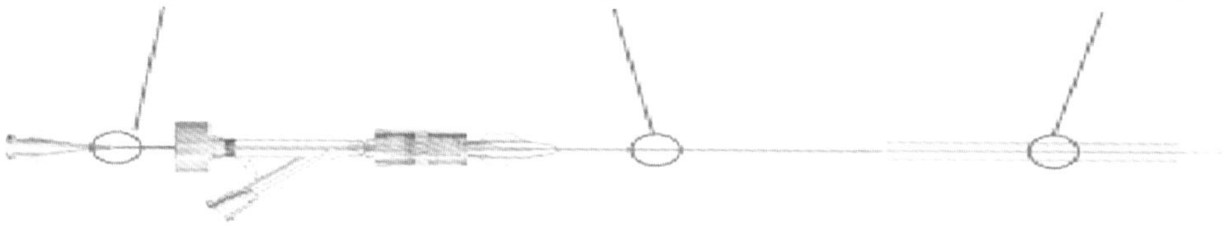

Pusher   Delivery catheter   Silk flow diverter

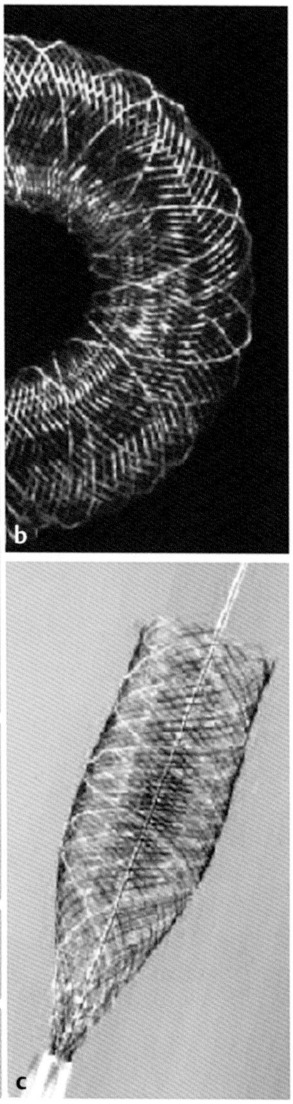

Fig. 11.2 Product manual and size options. **(a)** Catalog of diameters and length. **(b,c)** Images of the Silk stent. **(d)** The Silk flow diverter, which is made of cobalt-chromium alloy; also note the inner body that functions as a delivery wire.

16.3%), and the mean delayed complication rate was 9.9% (95% CI: 6.4–13.4%). Ischemic postprocedural complications included parent artery occlusion in 0 to 8% of cases and embolic events in 0 to 6% of cases. One series, devoted to basilar artery aneurysms treated with SFD, reported a 25% incidence of ischemic events.[29] In-stent stenosis was reported in 1 to 10% of cases, whereas intracranial hemorrhage was reported in 0 to 5% of cases. The overall neurological morbidity and mortality rates reported ranged from 0 to 6% and 0 to 4%, respectively.

11.3 Technical Note

11.3.1 Stent Size Selection

The Silk stent should be sized such that its diameter is the smallest compatible with the parent artery. A general rule of thumb is to choose a stent with a nominal diameter, less than 0.25 mm smaller than the diameter of the parent artery (refer to sections "Nitinol Alloy" and "Silk Device Parameters" for rationale). This enables it to be deployed to its

Table 11.1 Literature review of patients treated with Silk flow diversion

Authors (year)	Na	Nb	FUc time (range and/ or mean)	Previous coiling (%)	Deployment failure, no. (%)/difficulty, no. (%)	Aneurysm location (%) (A/ Pd)	Aneurysm size (%) (S/L/ Ge)	Obliteration in 12-mo FU (%)
Byrne et al[14] (2010)	70	70	4	14.3	3 (4.3)/15 (21.4)	A = 71.4 P = 28.6	S = 26, L = 53, G = 21	82.8
Kulcsár et al[29] (2010)	12	12	4	50	0 (0)/1 (8.3)	P = 100	NA	58.3
Lubicz et al[31] (2010)	29	34	6–18	0	3 (8.8)/NA	A = 83.9 P = 16.1	S = 54.8, L = 38.7, G = 6.5	69
Leonardi et al[30] (2011)	25	25	6–19	0	0 (0)/NA	A = 92 P = 8	S = 20, L = 40, G = 40	60
Berge et al[4] (2012)	65	77	12	33.8	1 (1.3)/9 (11.7)	A = 88.3 P = 11.7	S = 37.7, L = 39, G = 23.3	84.3
Briganti et al[27] (2012)	143	143	3–12	5.2	5 (3.5)/5 (3.5)	A = 89.2 P = 10.8	<5 mm: 10.8% 5–15 mm: 42.2% >15 mm: 46.9%	85
Maimon et al[26] (2012)	28	32	6–24	25	0 (0)/NA	A = 75 P = 25	S = 10.7, L = 71.4, G = 18.9	80
Pistocchi et al[33] (2012)	20	24	13	20.8	0 (0)/NA	A = 30	S = 96.7, L = 3.3, G = 0	78.9
Tähtinen et al[24] (2012)	24	24	7.5	16.7	1 (4.2)/7 (29.2)	A = 79.2 P = 20.8	NA	69.6
Velioglu et al[36] (2012)	76	87	17.5 ± 11.1 (2–48)	NA	0 (0)/18 (20.6)	A = 95.4 P = 4.6	S = 48.3, L = 33.3, G = 18.4	87.9
Wagner et al[37] (2012)	22	26	13.2	42.3	0 (0)/NA	A = 73 P = 26	S = 50, L = 46.2, G = 3.8	85.7
Shankar et al[34] (2013)	19	29	6–24	0	0 (0)/NA	A = 84.2 P = 15.8	S = 10.5, L = 89.5, G = 0	59
Buyukkaya et al[28] (2014)	32	34	12	11.7	0 (0)/5 (14.7)	A = 88.2 P = 11.8	NA	87.9
Aydin et al[17] (2015)	11	11	6	0	0 (0)/0 (0)	A = 81.8 P=18.2	S = 100, L = 0, G = 0	90.9
Slater et al[35] (2015)	14	14	6–24	0	0 (0)/NA	NA	NA	78.6

aNumber of patients.
bNumber of aneurysms treated.
cFollow-up, months.
dA, anterior circulation; P, posterior circulation.
eS, small, aneurysms < 10 mm; L, large, aneurysms 10–25 mm; G, giant, aneurysms > 25 mm. NA, data not available.

maximum diameter. Stent length should be a minimum of three times the vessel diameter plus the width of the aneurysm neck. This point is emphasized, considering the significant shortening that occurs upon deployment. The deployed SFD is usually no more than 50% of the length inside the deployment catheter. Another way to ensure sufficient length is to leave a minimum of 1 cm of the stent extending beyond each end of the aneurysm or at a minimum distance of 1.5 times the diameter of the artery. For cases in which the proximal and distal parent arterial diameters are disparate, the stent is sized to the larger parent vessel. Alternatively, consideration may be given to using a tapered stent or placing two stents, one appropriately sized for each parent vessel, and deploying the smaller stent first with subsequent overlapping with the larger stent.

11.3.2 Deployment Technique

It is important to obtain good catheter access close to the site of intended stent deployment. Absolute stability of the guide catheter and microcatheters and strict control with push–pull movements are required for stent deployment. This is achieved through the use of a triaxial system consisting of a long sheath, a supple intermediate distal access catheter, and a maneuverable delivery microcatheter. The triaxial system forms a *Tower of Power* to establish stability in the distal vasculature and ensure 1:1 maneuverability. This can be achieved by positioning a Fargo guide catheter (Balt Extrusion) or Neuron guide catheter (Penumbra, Inc., Alameda, CA) in the internal carotid artery or vertebral artery adjacent to the aneurysm. The distal access catheter is then positioned at the distal aspect of the carotid siphon or in the A1 segment of the anterior cerebral artery. This helps prevent recoil of the device that can occur during stent deployment. It may also prevent the premature or inappropriate release of the proximal aspect of the device at the level of the carotid terminus when the FDS is deployed to cover an A1 segment aneurysm.[38] A three-dimensional angiogram should be obtained once the guide catheter is in place to find the best working projection with optimal views of the proximal and distal landing zones within the parent artery.[3,38,39]

Microcatheter Access

The Silk stents are intended for use with the Vasco microcatheter (Balt Extrusion), as discussed. The Vasco + 21 is used for stents 2 to 4.5 mm in diameter; the Vasco + 25 is used for stents 5 to 5.5 mm in diameter. Under roadmap guidance, the Vasco microcatheter is advanced over a 0.14-inch wire to a position located 10 to 20 mm distal to the aneurysm and in a straight segment of the artery. The wire is gradually withdrawn to remove any slack in the microcatheter until it is completely removed.[3]

Insertion and Deployment

The introducer sheath-mounted stent is inserted into the rotating hemostatic valve or copilot device. Saline is used to irrigate the introducer sheath. Upon advancement of the introducer to the hub, the rotating hemostatic valve is tightened to prevent any back bleeding. The stent is positioned under roadmap guidance at the tip of the delivery wire, so as not to traumatize the vessel. The insertion technique involves deploying the distal tip of the delivery microcatheter to the aneurysm and then pushing the SFD to the tip of the delivery wire to which it is attached. When the deployment position is reached, the stent must be centered over the aneurysm because shortening occurs upon device deployment.[39]

Once the system is aligned with the aneurysm, the SFD is deployed by unsheathing the self-expanding Silk stent from the constraints of the microcatheter, while holding the delivery wire stable. This process involves a combination of pushing the delivery wire while simultaneously retrieving the microcatheter to allow the SFD to expand and to compensate for any resulting foreshortening. Often, there may be friction between the stent and the microcatheter requiring considerable force on the delivery wire to ensure its stability. The entire assembly is then gently nudged slightly forward as the stent unfolds to ensure good wall apposition.

Treatment with the SFD may require the deployment first of a Leo stent (Balt Extrusion) for support in cases of wide-necked or long-segment fusiform lesions.[23] The Leo is a finely braided, nitinol SES that can be used for stent-assisted coiling of wide-necked aneurysms.[20,21] The decision to use the Leo stent is made at the time of stenting if the operator determines that the Silk stent will need additional support scaffolding. There are no strict guidelines for when the Leo stent should and should not be used.

Releasing the Stent

As the last portion of the Silk stent begins to exit the microcatheter, the interventionist ensures that the stent is optimally positioned across the aneurysm neck, with no apparent kinks or twists. At this point, it is still possible to resheath and reposition the stent, if necessary. Consideration may be given to performing an angiogram through the guide catheter prior to final deployment of the stent, especially when the parent artery is smaller than 3 mm in diameter. At this stage, if the SFD occludes the parent artery, it still can be retrieved. When 90% of the stent has left the microcatheter, the stent must be fully deployed. Once deployed, the microcatheter is carefully advanced through the stent to capture the delivery wire. ▶ Fig. 11.3, ▶ Fig. 11.4, ▶ Fig. 11.5 demonstrate the placement of the SFD for IAs.

Silk Remodeling

Once deployed, a follow-up angiogram allows for careful inspection of the deployed stent, with attention paid to coverage and wall apposition. Several strategies, including balloon remodeling or deployment of additional stents, can be employed to manage stents that may not be optimally deployed. For balloon remodeling, a Hyperglide balloon (ev3 Neurovascular, Irvine, CA) or an Eclipse balloon (Cook Medical, Bloomington, IN) is advanced into the stent and gently inflated for angioplasty purposes. Care is taken not to overinflate the balloon to prevent stent prolapse into the aneurysm dome. Should the stent be twisted, resulting in compromised flow through the vessel, patency can be restored by deploying an appropriately sized Wingspan stent (Stryker, Kalamazoo, MI) within the lumen.

As discussed previously, the use of multiple Silk stents may be indicated when increased coverage across the aneurysm neck is necessary to slow down blood flow into the aneurysm, when treating a large aneurysm neck that requires more than one stent, or when there is a large size discrepancy between the parent vessels proximal and distal to the aneurysm.

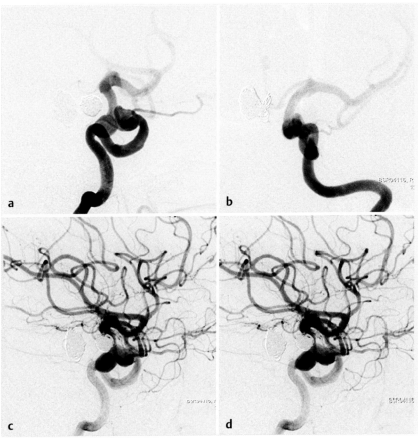

Fig. 11.3 Illustrative case. A 55-year-old woman presented with a massive subarachnoid hemorrhage (Hunt and Hess grade 4). A ruptured right posterior communicating artery aneurysm was treated with coils with a good radiological occlusion and clinical recovery. A right middle cerebral artery aneurysm was than electively treated with stent-assisted coiling and a good recovery. Two additional wide-necked aneurysms (**a–d**) were noted: an 8-mm paraophthalmic artery aneurysm and a 7-mm supraclinoid aneurysm (**a,b**). Angiogram, left lateral view (**c,d**). Angiogram, anteroposterior (AP) view.

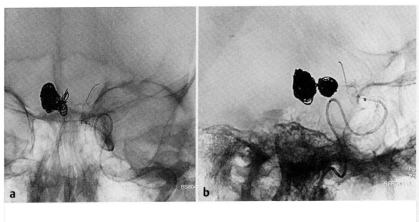

Fig. 11.4 Same patient as presented in ▶ Fig. 11.3, SFD stenting: The paraophthalmic artery aneurysm and the supraclinoid aneurysm demonstrated progressive growth and were treated 24 months later. Aspirin and clopidogrel were administered prestenting, as indicated (refer to text). (**a**) Anteroposterior view. The Vasco + 21 microcatheter (Balt Extrusion) is shown deploying the Silk stent (Balt Extrusion). A tapered 30-mm stent measuring 4 mm distally and 3 mm proximally was used due to significant difference in vessel sizes proximal and distal to the aneurysm neck. (**b**) Lateral view. The Vasco + 21 microcatheter is advanced through the stent to capture the delivery wire and assure proper wall apposition.

11.4 Postdeployment Treatment

Postprocedural headaches are common, as with other flow diverter devices, and are usually responsive to a short course of steroid therapy. As with other endovascular stents and devices, dual-antiplatelet therapy is mandatory prior to implantation of flow diverters. The current practice is to use a pretreatment regimen consisting of 300 to 600 mg of clopidogrel and 325 to 500 mg of aspirin before the stent placement procedure (8 days before the procedure), with 75 mg daily as the maintenance dose.[39]

Long-term dual-antiplatelet therapy (aspirin, 100–325 mg, with clopidogrel, 75 mg on a daily basis) is recommended. Aspirin is typically continued indefinitely, although clopidogrel may be stopped, depending on the angiographic and clinical results. The clopidogrel maintenance dose should continue for at least 3 months (preferably 6 months, more so if the communicating arteries originate from the aneurysmal sac covered by the Silk).[4,10,11,40] A follow-up angiogram should be performed 6 months after the procedure, and treatment is guided in accordance with the findings. If aneurysm thrombosis is seen at 6 months, the clopidogrel therapy may be discontinued.

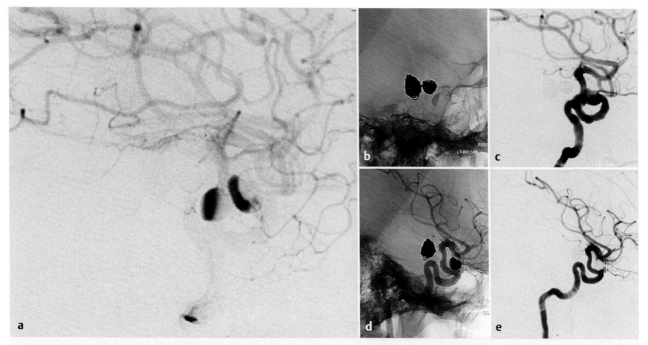

Fig. 11.5 Same patient as presented in ▶ Fig. 11.3. Outcome: **(a)** angiogram taken 5 minutes after Silk flow diverter deployment showing immediate blood stagnation within the aneurysm dome. **(b,c)** Three-month follow-up angiogram showing near-complete aneurysm obliteration. **(d,e)** 12-month follow-up angiogram, showing complete obliteration.

Thromboembolic complications, including in-stent thrombosis, have been reported to occur upon stopping clopidogrel, even in short-term follow-up reports of 3 months.[40] Patients with stenosis after flow-diverting device implantation seem to be at a higher risk of in-stent thrombosis upon discontinuation of clopidogrel.[41] If there is still flow in the aneurysm 6 months after device deployment, the dual-antiplatelet regimen should be continued for an additional 6 months, followed by a repeat angiogram. For cases in which there are signs of parent artery stenosis, dual-antiplatelet therapy should be continued indefinitely. The use of platelet aggregation assays or thromboelastography to measure medication resistance and drive decision making is controversial.[42,43] In addition, there are no data to guide the use of ticlopidine, cilostazol, or other antiplatelet medications in patients resistant to clopidogrel who undergo flow diverter implantation.

11.5 Report Limitations

The results, as reviewed in ▶ Table 11.1, are primarily from single-center studies, and as such may be skewed by both reporting and publication bias. Follow-up for most of these studies averaged less than 1 year and in many series, late follow-up was lost in a significant percentage of patients.[14] As such, the reported recanalization rates, as well as delayed complication rates, may be underestimated. When comparing the reported outcome parameters from different centers, we did not account for varying antiplatelet regimens and endovascular techniques, which may serve as an important consideration when pooling outcomes and complication rates. In addition, given that outcome parameters are largely self-assessed (clinical symptoms reported by patients and angiographic features reported by the operator), minimally symptomatic events may be discounted and occlusion rates inflated, further feeding the publication bias.

The development of a prospective multi-institutional registry, facilitating multicenter data analysis, formation of standards of care and guidelines, and third-party adjudication of outcomes, can address most of these limitations. Such an undertaking is currently embraced by the National Neurosurgery Quality and Outcomes Database (N²QOD), as well as subspecialty-specific registries. In the interim, these pooled results are better used for trends and for comparison among different stents, rather than to assess absolute pooled rates.

11.6 Conclusion

Unruptured aneurysms with complex anatomy can be safely and effectively treated with SFD. Based on reports in the literature, SFDs have been shown to induce complete angiographic occlusion with a patent parent artery in more than 80% of patients at 1 year after treatment, with disappearance or shrinkage of the aneurysm sac reported in more than 80% of aneurysms (▶ Table 11.1). Ischemic complications are among the most common SFD-related complications, and avoidance requires both precise device deployment and rigorous monitoring of the antiplatelet treatment. Further studies are required to elucidate longer-term rates of complete occlusion and complications.

References

[1] D'Urso PI, Lanzino G, Cloft HJ, Kallmes DF. Flow diversion for intracranial aneurysms: a review. Stroke. 2011; 42(8):2363–2368

[2] Lawson MF, Newman WC, Chi YY, Mocco JD, Hoh BL. Stent-associated flow remodeling causes further occlusion of incompletely coiled aneurysms. Neurosurgery. 2011; 69(3):598–603, discussion 603–604

[3] Gross BA, Frerichs KU. Stent usage in the treatment of intracranial aneurysms: past, present and future. J Neurol Neurosurg Psychiatry. 2013; 84 (3):244–253

[4] Berge J, Biondi A, Machi P, et al. Flow-diverter silk stent for the treatment of intracranial aneurysms: 1-year follow-up in a multicenter study. AJNR Am J Neuroradiol. 2012; 33(6):1150–1155

[5] Ionita CN, Natarajan SK, Wang W, et al. Evaluation of a second-generation self-expanding variable-porosity flow diverter in a rabbit elastase aneurysm model. AJNR Am J Neuroradiol. 2011; 32(8):1399–1407

[6] Sadasivan C, Cesar L, Seong J, et al. An original flow diversion device for the treatment of intracranial aneurysms: evaluation in the rabbit elastase-induced model. Stroke. 2009; 40(3):952–958

[7] Kallmes DF, Ding YH, Dai D, Kadirvel R, Lewis DA, Cloft HJ. A new endoluminal, flow-disrupting device for treatment of saccular aneurysms. Stroke. 2007; 38(8):2346–2352

[8] Yavuz K, Geyik S, Saatci I, Cekirge HS. Endovascular treatment of middle cerebral artery aneurysms with flow modification with the use of the pipeline embolization device. AJNR Am J Neuroradiol. 2014; 35(3):529–535

[9] Berge J, Tourdias T, Moreau JF, Barreau X, Dousset V. Perianeurysmal brain inflammation after flow-diversion treatment. AJNR Am J Neuroradiol. 2011; 32(10):1930–1934

[10] Szikora I, Berentei Z, Kulcsar Z, et al. Treatment of intracranial aneurysms by functional reconstruction of the parent artery: the Budapest experience with the pipeline embolization device. AJNR Am J Neuroradiol. 2010; 31(6):1139–1147

[11] Lylyk P, Miranda C, Ceratto R, et al. Curative endovascular reconstruction of cerebral aneurysms with the pipeline embolization device: the Buenos Aires experience. Neurosurgery. 2009; 64(4):632–642, discussion 642–643, quiz N6

[12] Nelson PK, Lylyk P, Szikora I, Wetzel SG, Wanke I, Fiorella D. The pipeline embolization device for the intracranial treatment of aneurysms trial. AJNR Am J Neuroradiol. 2011; 32(1):34–40

[13] Fischer S, Vajda Z, Aguilar Perez M, et al. Pipeline embolization device (PED) for neurovascular reconstruction: initial experience in the treatment of 101 intracranial aneurysms and dissections. Neuroradiology. 2012; 54(4):369–382

[14] Byrne JV, Beltechi R, Yarnold JA, Birks J, Kamran M. Early experience in the treatment of intra-cranial aneurysms by endovascular flow diversion: a multicentre prospective study. PLoS One. 2010; 5(9):e12492

[15] Saatci I, Yavuz K, Ozer C, Geyik S, Cekirge HS. Treatment of intracranial aneurysms using the pipeline flow-diverter embolization device: a single-center experience with long-term follow-up results. AJNR Am J Neuroradiol. 2012; 33(8):1436–1446

[16] Lanzino G, Crobeddu E, Cloft HJ, Hanel R, Kallmes DF. Efficacy and safety of flow diversion for paraclinoid aneurysms: a matched-pair analysis compared with standard endovascular approaches. AJNR Am J Neuroradiol. 2012; 33 (11):2158–2161

[17] Aydin K, Arat A, Sencer S, et al. Treatment of ruptured blood blister-like aneurysms with flow diverter SILK stents. J Neurointerv Surg. 2015; 7(3):202–209

[18] Abe M, Tabuchi K, Yokoyama H, Uchino A. Blood blisterlike aneurysms of the internal carotid artery. J Neurosurg. 1998; 89(3):419–424

[19] Stoeckel D, Pelton A, Duerig T. Self-expanding nitinol stents: material and design considerations. Eur Radiol. 2004; 14(2):292–301

[20] Cohen-Inbar O, Amsalem Y. Cerebral nitinol stenting in progressive stroke and in crescendo TIAs. J Neurol Surg A Cent Eur Neurosurg. 2015; 76(6):499–507

[21] Cohen-Inbar O, Amsalem Y, Soustiel JF. Nitinol stenting in post-traumatic pseudo-aneurysm of internal carotid artery. Open J Modern Neurosurg. 2012; 2:45–49

[22] Shabalovskaya SA. On the nature of the biocompatibility and on medical applications of NiTi shape memory and superelastic alloys. Biomed Mater Eng. 1996; 6(4):267–289

[23] Binning MJ, Natarajan SK, Bulsara KR, Siddiqui AH, Hopkins LN, Levy EI. SILK flow-diverting device for intracranial aneurysms. World Neurosurg. 2011; 76 (5):477.e1–477.e6

[24] Tähtinen OI, Manninen HI, Vanninen RL, et al. The silk flow-diverting stent in the endovascular treatment of complex intracranial aneurysms: technical aspects and midterm results in 24 consecutive patients. Neurosurgery. 2012; 70(3):617–623, discussion 623–624

[25] Kulcsár Z, Houdart E, Bonafé A, et al. Intra-aneurysmal thrombosis as a possible cause of delayed aneurysm rupture after flow-diversion treatment. AJNR Am J Neuroradiol. 2011; 32(1):20–25

[26] Maimon S, Gonen L, Nossek E, Strauss I, Levite R, Ram Z. Treatment of intracranial aneurysms with the SILK flow diverter: 2 years' experience with 28 patients at a single center. Acta Neurochir (Wien). 2012; 154(6):979–987

[27] Briganti F, Napoli M, Tortora F, et al. Italian multicenter experience with flow-diverter devices for intracranial unruptured aneurysm treatment with peri-procedural complications–a retrospective data analysis. Neuroradiology. 2012; 54(10):1145–1152

[28] Buyukkaya R, Kocaeli H, Yildirim N, Cebeci H, Erdogan C, Hakyemez B. Treatment of complex intracranial aneurysms using flow-diverting silk® stents. An analysis of 32 consecutive patients. Interv Neuroradiol. 2014; 20(6):729–735

[29] Kulcsár Z, Ernemann U, Wetzel SG, et al. High-profile flow diverter (silk) implantation in the basilar artery: efficacy in the treatment of aneurysms and the role of the perforators. Stroke. 2010; 41(8):1690–1696

[30] Leonardi M, Cirillo L, Toni F, et al. Treatment of intracranial aneurysms using flow-diverting silk stents (BALT): a single centre experience. Interv Neuroradiol. 2011; 17(3):306–315

[31] Lubicz B, Collignon L, Raphaeli G, et al. Flow-diverter stent for the endovascular treatment of intracranial aneurysms: a prospective study in 29 patients with 34 aneurysms. Stroke. 2010; 41(10):2247–2253

[32] Murthy SB, Shah S, Shastri A, Venkatasubba Rao CP, Bershad EM, Suarez JI. The SILK flow diverter in the treatment of intracranial aneurysms. J Clin Neurosci. 2014; 21(2):203–206

[33] Pistocchi S, Blanc R, Bartolini B, Piotin M. Flow diverters at and beyond the level of the circle of Willis for the treatment of intracranial aneurysms. Stroke. 2012; 43(4):1032–1038

[34] Shankar JJ, Vandorpe R, Pickett G, Maloney W. SILK flow diverter for treatment of intracranial aneurysms: initial experience and cost analysis. J Neurointerv Surg. 2013; 5 Suppl 3:iii11–iii15

[35] Slater LA, Soufan C, Holt M, Chong W. Effect of flow diversion with silk on aneurysm size: a single center experience. Interv Neuroradiol. 2015; 21 (1):12–18

[36] Velioglu M, Kizilkilic O, Selcuk H, et al. Early and midterm results of complex cerebral aneurysms treated with Silk stent. Neuroradiology. 2012; 54 (12):1355–1365

[37] Wagner A, Cortsen M, Hauerberg J, Romner B, Wagner MP. Treatment of intracranial aneurysms. Reconstruction of the parent artery with flow-diverting (Silk) stent. Neuroradiology. 2012; 54(7):709–718

[38] Clarençon F, Di Maria F, Gabrieli J, et al. Flow diverter stents for the treatment of anterior cerebral artery aneurysms: safety and effectiveness. Clin Neuroradiol. 2017; 27:51–56 [Epub 2015]

[39] Balt. Tips and tricks for optimal Silk placement (REV 1.3). Available at: silverekenmedicalny.mamutweb.com/TIPSNTRPDF.PDF; Accessed December 21, 2015

[40] Augsburger L, Farhat M, Reymond P, et al. Effect of flow diverter porosity on intraaneurysmal blood flow. Klin Neuroradiol. 2009; 19(3):204–214

[41] De Vries J, Boogaarts J, Van Norden A, Wakhloo AK. New generation of Flow Diverter (surpass) for unruptured intracranial aneurysms: a prospective single-center study in 37 patients. Stroke. 2013; 44(6):1567–1577

[42] Comin J, Kallmes DF. Platelet-function testing in patients undergoing neurovascular procedures: caught between a rock and a hard place. AJNR Am J Neuroradiol. 2013; 34(4):730–734

[43] Sambu N, Radhakrishnan A, Dent H, et al. Personalised antiplatelet therapy in stent thrombosis: observations from the Clopidogrel Resistance in Stent Thrombosis (CREST) registry. Heart. 2012; 98(9):706–711

12 TECHNIQUE AND NUANCES OF SURPASS STREAMLINE FLOW DIVERTER

AJAY K. WAKHLOO and BARUCH B. LIEBER

Abstract

Manufacturing of the Surpass flow diverter (FD) is based on scientific and biological concepts that were developed over the past three decades in endovascular treatment of brain aneurysms. The braided tubular chromium-cobalt implant is engineered to address regional flow conditions and fine-tune the needs of porosity and mesh density of the implant. Braid angle and introduction of larger number of wires provide biomechanical stability, consistent and reliable deployment, and prevent kinking and torque of the Surpass FD even under extreme conditions. Development of the Streamline delivery system addresses challenges inherent to the neurovascular system and allows for a torque-free, over-the-wire deployment of the device. The maintenance of continuous distal access allows for the recapture and redeployment of the device. In tortuous vasculature, the use of a triaxial access system is required.

Keywords: aneurysm flow dynamics, brain aneurysm, chromium-cobalt alloy, endothelialization, endovascular treatment, flow diverter, implants, stroke, Surpass FD

12.1 Introduction and Basic Concepts of Flow Diversion

The introduction of flow diverters (FDs) in the management of intracranial aneurysms (IAs) is truly a great example how accumulated knowledge in physiology, biomedical engineering, and clinical science was used to solve an important health problem. No other IA treatment has involved a more rigorous scientific effort and scrutiny than the concept of flow diversion. The final design of the Surpass FD (Stryker, Kalamazoo, MI), one of the flow diverters in clinical use, was based on a careful evaluation of the hydrodynamics involving the parent artery–aneurysm complex using *Computational Fluid Dynamics* (CFD), *Laser-Induced Fluorescence* (LIF), and *Particle Imaging Velocimetry* (PIV) studies, along with preclinical in vivo studies.[1,2,3,4,5] These studies showed that the reconstitution of the blood flow of the diseased segment to near-physiological condition was dependent on the FD design.

When properly engineered, the inflow from the parent artery into the aneurysm is reduced sufficiently to form a stable clot within the aneurysm pouch while maintaining the flow within covered side branches and perforators.[5] Various factors were critical in manufacturing Surpass, such as the choice of the metal alloy. Other parameters included the manufacturing modality used (i.e., laser cut, knitting, and braiding) that determines the flexibility and kink resistance of the product and the vessel wall apposition in tortuous intracranial arteries. Radial and crush force is pivotal to maintain sufficient outward force and mechanical stability during the cardiac cycle to prevent device migration. However, excessive radial forces may create undesired intimal response. The type of material used should

also withstand fatigue-related fractures and galvanic corrosion over time.

Given these challenges and its long history of use in the medical domain, the Surpass FD utilizes a cobalt-chromium alloy and fine-wire braiding to control the mesh size of the device. Cobalt-chromium is a well-known alloy for its excellent biocompatibility and fatigue properties, corrosion resistance, and mechanical strength.[6] Additionally, the use of chromium-cobalt braided FDs in the hemodynamically challenging, elastase-induced aneurysm model in rabbits was very favorable.[7,8,9] The Surpass FD resisted migration and fracture when placed close to the heart in the rabbit subclavian artery. This location is subjected to excessive motion during each cardiac cycle (heart rate on average of 180 beats/min) resulting in a biomechanical stress not encountered in the human cerebrovasculature.

12.2 Surpass FD Implant

CFD, as well as semi-quantitative LIF, followed by quantitative *PIV* methods were utilized to refine and optimize the properties of the Surpass FD. The goal was to optimize blood flow reduction into the aneurysm and increase the circulation time of blood within the aneurysm, while maintaining flow through side branches and perforators.[5] Two major parameters were found to be important for FDs to be hydrodynamically effective: (1) *porosity* and (2) *pore or mesh density* of the implant. The *in vivo* and *in vitro hemodynamic* studies indicated that there was a fine-tuning required to balance the *porosity* (metal free/metal area) and *pore* or *mesh density* (number of pores/mm^2) of the FD to optimize the effect on flow reduction.[2,3,4,5]

$$\text{porosity}(\%) = \frac{(\text{Total surface area} - \text{Metal surface area})}{\text{Total surface area}} \times 100$$

The FD creates a resistance to the flow at the aneurysm neck and subsequently decreases the hydrodynamic circulation and the peak and mean kinetic energy transfer from the parent artery into the aneurysm with each pulse cycle. The FD modifies the predominantly convective flow to a more diffusive form that eventually leads to aneurysm thrombosis and occlusion.[7,8,9] Before finalizing the Surpass FD, various samples were manufactured and tested for their hydrodynamic properties with follow-up testing in an in vivo rabbit elastase aneurysm model (▶ Fig. 12.1a, b).

The Surpass FD is braided out of cobalt-chromium alloy wires with small amounts of Nitinol (Ni-Ti) to form a tubular structure. The braid angle β (▶ Fig. 12.2) and the number of wires also help preserve the structural integrity of the device, the diamond cell shape, and mesh density, regardless of large variabilities in the arterial diameter over the length of the construct (▶ Fig. 12.2, ▶ Fig. 12.3). Consistent mesh density ensures a more even effect on flow reduction, preventing pockets of increased flow impingement zones within the aneurysm. Various lengths and diameters of the Surpass FD implants are available for the clinical use. Unlike other products, the device is

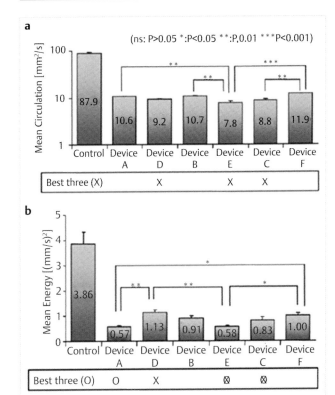

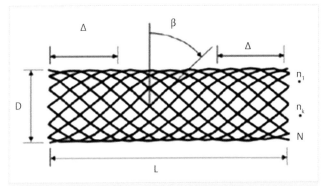

Fig. 12.2 Critical dimensions for manufacturing of Surpass flow diverter (simplified for illustrative purposes). L, implant length; Δ, proximal and distal landing zone for a stable placement; β, braid angle; n_1 to N, number of wires. (Reproduced with permission from Lieber and Sadasivan.[5])

Fig. 12.1 (a) Mean circulation time in a silicone aneurysm replica of the rabbit elastase model for various flow diverter (FD) implants as compared with control (reproduced with permission from Lieber and Sadasivan[5]). **(b)** Mean energy transfer in a silicone aneurysm replica of the rabbit elastase model for various FD implants as compared with control. (Reproduced with permission from Lieber and Sadasivan.[5])

manufactured in diameters of 1-mm increments. The number of wires for each device varies depending on the device diameter to maintain biomechanical stability and a consistent reduction in aneurysm inflow (up to 96 wires for the largest device diameter of 5.3 mm; ▶ Fig. 12.4, ▶ Fig. 12.5, ▶ Fig. 12.6). Additionally, the wire diameter used for braiding ranges, for currently available implants, from 25 to 32 μm. The diameter is limited by the alloy chosen and the risk of material fracture during fine-wire braiding. The mesh density of the device ranges from 21 to 32 pores/mm². Twelve platinum-tungsten wires are braided into the implant to aid visibility under X-ray fluoroscopy without interfering with the mesh density or the biomechanics of the device. As recently shown, this increased number of wires may result in an earlier and more complete endothelialization of the diseased vessel. Interestingly, among other cellular mechanisms, CD + 34 progenitor cells are involved in endothelialization.[10]

The percentage foreshortening of a Surpass FD varies, like for all braided implants, and depends on the device diameter and length, with approximately 38, 42, and 26% foreshortening—under nominal diameter—experienced for 3-, 4-, and 5-mm systems, respectively. However, unlike with other similar products, Surpass FD foreshortens significantly less due to the braid angle and larger number of wires. These features also prevent kinking and torquing of the FD and facilitate a more reliable and consistent device opening in tortuous vasculature.

Surpass FD has been determined to be *MR conditional at 3T* or less magnetic field strength according to the terminology specified in the American Society for Testing and Materials (ASTM) International, Designation: F2503; Standard Practice for Marking Medical Devices and Other Items for Safety in the Magnetic Resonance Environment. A patient can safely be scanned immediately after placement of Surpass FD under the following conditions: (1) static magnetic field of 3 Tesla or less; (2) maximum spatial gradient magnetic field of 720 Gauss/cm, a higher value for the spatial gradient magnetic field may apply if properly calculated; and (3) maximum MR system–reported, whole-body–averaged specific absorption rate (SAR) of 2 W/kg for 15 minutes of scanning (per pulse sequence).[11] In nonclinical testing, the FD produced an increase temperature of 6.0°C or less using an MR system–reported, whole-body–averaged SAR of 2 W/kg for 15 minutes (per pulse sequence) of scanning in a 3-Tesla MR system. Although MRI can be used, the image quality may suffer in the area adjacent to and within the center of the implant.

12.3 Streamline FD Delivery System

Each Surpass FD implant is packaged preloaded at the distal end of its delivery system consisting of a 0.04-inch ID delivery microcatheter. The delivery system consists of an outer and an inner system with the inner system consisting of a smaller microcatheter that functions as the FD pusher (▶ Fig. 12.7). The FD is constrained on the inner pusher 10 mm proximal to the tip of the delivery catheter. In addition to the pusher tip marker, there are two additional radiopaque markers, the distal marker of the outer microcatheter and the proximal pusher marker. Surpass FD is well visible in its constrained form under fluoroscopy on standard state-of-the-art angiography equipment. The pusher has a lumen that accommodates a standard 0.014-inch microwire, which can be controlled by the operator. The microwire permits continued distal access and adds stability to the delivery system during device deployment, particularly in large or giant, wide-neck or fusiform aneurysms.

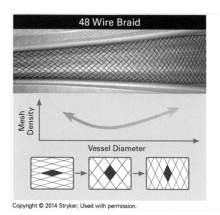

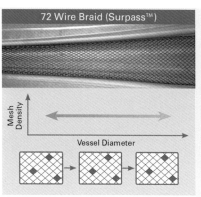

Fig. 12.3 Change of diamond cell shape as function of number of wires across tapering vessels. Consistent mesh density and subsequently an even flow diversion is achieved by increased number of wires. (Copyright ©2014 Stryker, reproduced with permission.)

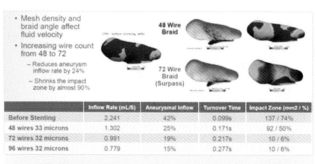

	Inflow Rate (mL/S)	Aneurysmal Inflow	Turnover Time	Impact Zone (mm2 / %)
Before Stenting	2.241	42%	0.099s	137 / 74%
48 wires 33 microns	1.302	25%	0.171s	92 / 50%
72 wires 32 microns	0.991	19%	0.217s	10 / 6%
96 wires 32 microns	0.779	15%	0.277s	10 / 6%

Fig. 12.4 Effect of Surpass flow diverter mesh density on aneurysm inflow and wall shear stress distribution in a human-specific paraophthalmic artery aneurysm using Computational Fluid Dynamics. (Images courtesy of G. De Santis and M. De Beule, FEOps, Ghent, Belgium.)

Over the past years, several changes have been made to the material and manufacturing of the Surpass delivery system, leading to reduction of the track force and improved navigability (▶ Fig. 12.8). The most recent generation, the *Streamline delivery system*, designed for larger internal carotid artery (ICA) aneurysms has an outer diameter (OD) distally of 3.7F (1.2 mm) and proximally of 3.9F (1.3 mm) for the 3-, 4-, and 5-mm systems with a working length of 135 cm. An additional 2-mm FD system, intended for aneurysms distal to the circle of Willis, was designed with a distal OD of 3.3F (1.1 mm) and a proximal OD of 3.7F (1.3 mm) with a working length of 150 cm. The Streamline delivery system also has a recapture feature indicated by a small marker on the proximal shaft of the delivery system (▶ Fig. 12.8c). The Surpass FD can be recaptured, repositioned, and redeployed, as long as there is a minimum gap between the microcatheter tip marker and the proximal pusher marker. This unique feature of the delivery system permits continuous distal wire access allowing for the safe recapture and repositioning both distally and proximally.

12.4 Surpass FD Streamline Preparation, Delivery, and Deployment

12.4.1 Sizing

It is mandatory to have accurate measurements of the parent vessel size both proximal and distal to the aneurysm neck to select the appropriate Surpass FD implant. Preferentially, the measurements should be conducted in at least two planes on a standard digital subtraction angiogram (DSA) after infusion of intra-arterial calcium antagonist, such as Verapamil or Nicardipine, into the target vessel to avoid poor wall FD apposition due to vasospasm. A Surpass FD should be selected at least 10 mm longer than the aneurysm neck to maintain a minimum of 5 mm on either side of the aneurysm neck and to allow the proximal and distal ends of the implant to land in a straight section of the vessel.[12,13] Depending on the diameter of the artery and taper of the vessel, the device may be longer than the indicated nominal diameter (▶ Fig. 12.9). These factors should be taken into account when selecting the proper size of the implant.

12.4.2 Preparation of the Implant/ Delivery System

1. After removal of the Surpass Streamline delivery system from packaging and inspection of the entire system for damage, the dispenser hoop should be flushed with sterilized heparinized normal saline (▶ Fig. 12.10).
2. Purge the Surpass FD outer microcatheter with sterile heparinized normal saline and attach to a continuous heparinized sterile normal saline drip.
3. Subsequently, purge the pusher with sterile heparinized normal saline and attach to a rotating hemostatic valve (RHV) with continuous heparinized sterile normal saline drip.

12.4.3 Direct Triaxial Access

1. Using standard access techniques based on patient anatomy, place a 70- to 90-cm-long guiding sheath, for example, a Shuttle 6F (Cook Medical, Bloomington, IN), a Neuron Max 8F delivery catheter (Penumbra, Alameda, CA), or a LS Infiniti guide catheter (Stryker Neurovascular, Kalamazoo, MI) within the distal common carotid artery or at the origin of the ICA.
2. After infusion of a calcium antagonist, completion of vessel and aneurysm measurements, and selection of the appropriate Surpass FD Streamline system, define work projections in at least two work planes.
3. Place a 115-cm-long intermediate catheter (IC) with an ID of no less than 0.053 inch either alone or over a microcatheter,

Surpass™ Flow Diverter Specifications	2mm	3mm	4mm	5mm
Maximum vessel diameter	2.5mm	3.5mm	4.4mm	5.3mm
Recommended minimum	2.0mm	2.5mm	3.4mm	4.3mm
Number of total wires	48	72	72	96
Wire diameter	25µm	32µm		
Number of marker wires	12			
Braided wire material	Cobalt chromium alloy			
Marker wire material	92% platinum 8% tungsten			
Mesh density (pores/mm²)	20-32			
Delivery System	2mm	3mm	4mm	5mm
Outer Diameter, distal/proximal	3.3F/3.7F (1.1mm/1.2mm)	3.7F/3.9F (1.2mm/1.3mm)		
Minimum recommended microcatheter ID	0.053in (1.447mm)			
Working length	150cm	135cm		

Copyright © 2014 Stryker; Used with permission.

Fig. 12.5 Surpass Streamline specifications for clinically available implants. (Copyright ©2014 Stryker, reproduced with permission.)

Length (mm)	Diameter: 2mm	Diameter: 3mm	Diameter: 4mm	Diameter: 5mm
12mm	✔			
15mm	✔	✔	✔	
20mm	✔	✔	✔	✔
25mm		✔	✔	✔
30mm			✔	✔
40mm			✔	✔
50mm			✔	✔

Copyright © 2014 Stryker; Used with permission.

Fig. 12.6 Available sizes for Surpass flow diverter. (Copyright ©2014 Stryker, reproduced with permission.)

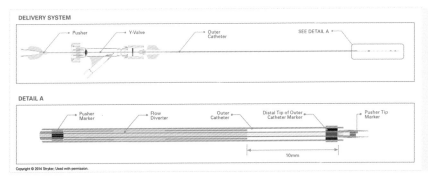

Fig. 12.7 Surpass flow diverter delivery system. Schematic illustration of various components including the outer and inner member of the system. (Copyright ©2014 Stryker, reproduced with permission.)

for example, XT-27 (Stryker Neurovascular) proximal to the aneurysm neck (▶ Fig. 12.11a). Infrequently, an IC placement distal to the aneurysm may be required. This should cautiously be executed to avoid aneurysm rupture.

4. Load the Surpass FD Streamline system on a 0.014-inch microwire (▶ Fig. 12.11b).
5. Under fluoroscopy and roadmap, advance the Surpass delivery system over the 0.014-inch microwire through the IC past the aneurysm.
6. For improved proximal support, the IC can also be navigated distally over the Streamline delivery system by using the "climbing" technique.[14] This may be advantageous especially

for the larger and longer systems that require higher track force.

7. After removal of the slack in the delivery and IC, the implant is deployed by a combination of initially unsheathing the outer microcatheter and exposing the Surpass FD, followed by loading the entire delivery system to ensure a proper vessel wall apposition. Pay attention during removal of the slack from the delivery system so that the IC does not climb up uncontrolled.
8. During deployment, maintain a load on the delivery system while pushing out the FD by activating the inner pusher. The axial load will translate into further deployment of the Surpass and sliding back of the outer microcatheter.

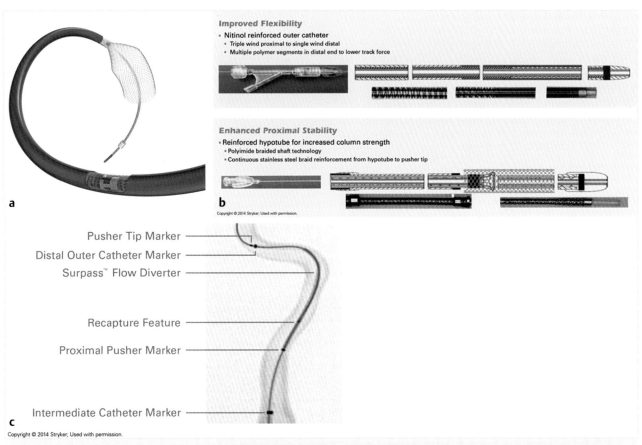

Fig. 12.8 (a) Surpass flow diverter (FD) Streamline delivery system. Schematic illustration of various components including the outer and inner member of the system (copyright ©2014 Stryker, used with permission). (b) Surpass FD Streamline delivery system. Schematic illustration of various components including the outer and inner member of the system (copyright ©2016 Stryker, used with permission). (c) Surpass FD Streamline delivery system. Radiograph depicts various components and marker bands of the delivery system including the recapture feature. (Copyright ©2016 Stryker, reproduced with permission.)

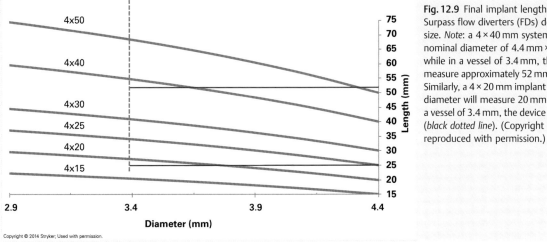

Fig. 12.9 Final implant length for various 4-mm Surpass flow diverters (FDs) dependent on vessel size. Note: a 4 × 40 mm system will measure at nominal diameter of 4.4 mm × 40 mm (blue line), while in a vessel of 3.4 mm, the same FD will measure approximately 52 mm (black dotted line). Similarly, a 4 × 20 mm implant at 4.4 mm nominal diameter will measure 20 mm (blue line), while in a vessel of 3.4 mm, the device will be 25 mm long (black dotted line). (Copyright ©2014 Stryker, reproduced with permission.)

9. In case the microcatheter does not slide back on its own, reduce the axial load by pulling slightly back on the entire delivery catheter.

10. Through the entire delivery procedure, the microwire should be stabilized to prevent loss of wire access or perforation.

11. If available, appropriate device expansion and deployment can be assessed with submillimeter thick cone-beam CT image features of the angiography unit.
12. If needed, balloon angioplasty of the implant should be performed for improved vessel wall apposition.
13. Follow-up DSA is performed immediately after deployment and at 10 minutes following deployment to confirm vessel wall apposition, patency of the parent vessels, and to rule out vasospasm, intraluminal thrombus, or dissections.

12.4.4 Exchange Triaxial Access

1. For large or giant aneurysms with complex inflow and outflow patterns or situations of extreme vessel tortuosity, crossing the aneurysm initially with a 0.017-inch microcatheter may be required followed by placement of a 0.014-inch exchange microwire.
2. Remove the microcatheter and carefully backload the Surpass delivery system onto the 0.014-inch microwire. Infrequently in more tortuous vasculature, the use of a more supportive 0.014-inch wire may be required.

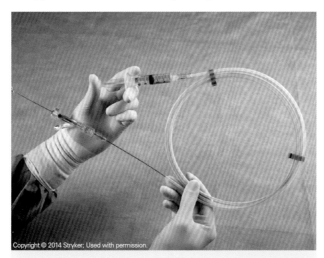

Copyright © 2014 Stryker; Used with permission.

Fig. 12.10 Preparation of the Surpass flow diverter Streamline Delivery System. (Copyright ©2014 Stryker, reproduced with permission.)

3. Under fluoroscopy, carefully advance the Surpass delivery system distal to the aneurysm over the microwire and through the IC. Ensure proper coverage of the aneurysm neck and unsheathe the outer microcatheter to release the Surpass FD.
4. Follow steps 7 to 13 of "Direct Triaxial Access."as described above.

12.4.5 Implant Deployment

1. Ensure proper device selection. Use of a single device is recommended.
2. Confirm the position of the constrained Surpass FD within the delivery microcatheter across the aneurysm neck. High frame-rate fluoroscopy (15–30 frames/second) or single radiographs, especially at the skull base may be helpful.
3. More distal IC placement will provide increased stability to the delivery system and facilitate accurate implant deployment.
4. The distal part of the Surpass FD must be at least 5 mm past the distal neck of the aneurysm (▶ Fig. 12.12a).
5. The distal and proximal landing zones should preferentially be located on a straight vessel segment to ensure adequate vessel wall apposition.
6. If the device lands in the anterior genu of the ICA leading to malapposition, a second telescoping device should be used to optimize wall apposition. Continuous wire access throughout the procedure facilitates easier placement of a second FD, as well as navigation of a balloon angioplasty catheter, if necessary.
7. Owing to the braid angle and number of wires (▶ Fig. 12.2), the Surpass implant and delivery system allows for precise placement of the distal part of the FD at the target site and consistent and reliable deployment without the risk of torque or kinking.
8. Once the target site is reached, loosen the RHV on the Surpass delivery system.
9. Begin deployment by retracting the outer microcatheter while holding forward tension on the inner pusher.
10. At least 10 mm of the Surpass FD must be exposed before the distal end begins to flare and appose the vessel wall.

Intermediate Catheters

System	ID (in)	Prox.OD (in)	Dist. OD (in)	Clearance w/ 6F Shuttle (.087)	Performance	Compatibility	CI Friendly
Surpass	-	0.053	-	-	-	-	-
Navien	0.058	0.070	0.070	0.017	**	****	****
5 Max/DDC	0.054	0.080	0.065	0.007	**	*	**
DAC™	0.057	0.068	0.068	0.019	*	**	**
Fargo	0.055	0.079	0.064	0.008	*	**	**

a Copyright © 2014 Stryker; Used with permission.

Guidewires

System	Diameter	Navigability	Support Level	Shape Retention	Tip Softness
Synchro™ Standard	0.014	****	***	*	*
Transend 300™ Floppy	0.014	***	***	*	***
Chikai	0.014	**	***	***	*
Traxcess	0.014 (.012 tip)	***	***	***	****

b Copyright © 2014 Stryker; Used with permission.

Fig. 12.11 (a) Most commonly used intermediate catheters with Surpass flow diverter (FD) Streamline delivery system. **(b)** Most commonly used microwires with Surpass FD Streamline delivery system. (Copyright ©2014 Stryker, reproduced with permission.)

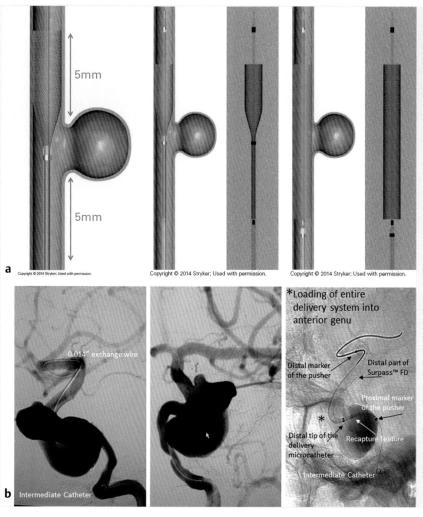

Fig. 12.12 (a) Schematic illustration of a proper positioning and deployment of a Surpass flow diverter (FD) by unsheathing only. (Copyright ©2014 Stryker, reproduced with permission.) **(b)** Illustrative case showing use of Surpass FD Streamline. (Images courtesy of Dr. Joost de Vries, Nijmegen, The Netherlands.)

Slow deployment will enhance precise placement and gradual opening of the FD.

11. A balanced combination of loading the entire delivery system after locking the RHV and pushing the inner pusher after loosening the RHV will result in desired wall apposition and allow precise deployment in the proximal landing zone. This loading and unloading maneuver requires a two-handed approach.

12. In less tortuous vasculature, an alternative technique for deploying the distal part of the Surpass FD may be employed. The microcatheter tip is positioned at the desired distal landing zone and the device is deployed using the inner pusher. However, in more tortous anatomy, this technique may fail due to high friction between the constrained FD and delivery microcatheter.

13. The Surpass FD is engineered to be recaptured and repositioned. A proximal marker indicates the capture area (▶ Fig. 12.8c). To recapture, reduce the slack on the delivery system. Then gently pull back on the pusher while maintaining slight forward force on the outer microcatheter. This will allow for a smooth recapture of the Surpass FD.

14. Once recaptured, the system can be repositioned both distally and proximally as long as the position of the microwire is maintained. According to the manufacturer's

recommendation, a partial deployment and recapture should not be exercised more than three times.

15. To prevent loss of distal access or perforation, the microwire should be monitored closely throughout delivery and deployment.

16. With excessive forward force, the Surpass FD can herniate across the neck of the aneurysm. This can be eliminated by locking the RHV and applying gentle retraction of the delivery system. This technique can be useful to fine-tune FD wall apposition at the neck.

17. For proper vessel wall apposition, maintain forward force on the delivery system especially when deploying around bends. This can be managed by keeping the delivery system on the outer curvature of the vessel, for example, the anterior and posterior ICA genu, during deployment.

18. After complete deployment, the RHV is locked and the delivery system is gently withdrawn. If the proximal part of the FD is not fully open, this maneuver will allow for consistent and reliable opening of the entire FD.

19. Subsequently, loosen the RHV and advance the pusher over the microwire into the FD. The microcatheter is then sleeved through the implant over the pusher, which is kept under tension.

20. The IC can now safely be navigated over the delivery system into the FD. Placement of the IC within the FD or distal to it enables improved wall apposition and allows for removal of the Surpass delivery catheter and the microwire while maintaining endoluminal access for a balloon microcatheter or an additional Surpass FD.

21. If the delivery catheter or the IC cannot be safely advanced into the FD, the microwire can be exchanged for an exchange length microwire through the inner pusher. The exchange microwire provides distal access for balloon catheter or a second Surpass FD.

22. Cine fluoroscopy with contrast injection through the long sheath or guide catheter is useful to assess Surpass FD under real-time, pulsatile conditions and evaluate vessel wall apposition.

12.4.6 Tips

1. Continuous heparinized saline drips are necessary to minimize friction between the outer delivery microcatheter and the Surpass FD and between the microwire and the inner pusher especially around tight bends.

2. Although use of a coaxial access system may suffice in straight craniocervical vasculature, routine implementation of a triaxial access system will enhance deliverability to ensure precise placement of Surpass FD.

3. To prevent perforation and dissection, keep the microwire and IC/guide catheter tip visible on the monitor.

4. Distal placement of an extra-support microwire may reduce track force and enable easier navigation of the Surpass FD delivery system.

5. Proper distal positioning of guide catheters and ICs may enable easier advancement of the delivery system.

6. Interchanging forward movements with the IC and FD delivery system may improve distal navigation.

7. Replace IC, microwire, and/or the Surpass FD delivery system if excessive friction is encountered.

8. Pulling the pusher inside the outer microcatheter may lock the FD inside the system and impede the delivery of the device.

9. Remove the slack from the IC and deliver system for an easier and more controlled deployment.

12.5 Summary

Manufacturing of the Surpass FD is based on scientific and biological concepts that were developed over the past three decades. The device was engineered to address regional flow conditions and fine-tune the needs of porosity and mesh density of the implant. Braid angle and introduction of larger number of wires provide biomechanical stability, consistent and reliable deployment, and prevent kinking and torque of the Surpass FD even under extreme conditions. Development of the Streamline delivery system addresses challenges inherent to the neurovascular system and allows for a torque-free, over-the-wire deployment of the device. The maintenance of continuous distal access allows for the recapture and redeployment of the device. In tortuous vasculature, a triaxial access system is required. Advancements in material sciences and microfabrication will propel future developments that will likely include further improvements of the implant, surface modifications of the implant, and the delivery system. Additionally, plans are ongoing for the development of a bifurcation FD for challenging locations such as the middle cerebral artery bifurcation and anterior communicating artery.

References

[1] Wakhloo AK, Lieber BB, Gounis M, Sandhu J. Flow dynamics in cerebral aneurysms. In: Le Roux PD, Winn HR, Newell DW, eds., Management of Cerebral Aneurysms. Philadelphia, PA: WB Saunders; 2003:99–120

[2] Aenis M, Stancampiano AP, Wakhloo AK, Lieber BB. Modeling of flow in a straight stented and nonstented side wall aneurysm model. J Biomech Eng. 1997; 119(2):206–212

[3] Lieber BB, Stancampiano AP, Wakhloo AK. Alteration of hemodynamics in aneurysm models by stenting: influence of stent porosity. Ann Biomed Eng. 1997; 25(3):460–469

[4] Lieber BB, Livescu V, Hopkins LN, Wakhloo AK. Particle image velocimetry assessment of stent design influence on intra-aneurysmal flow. Ann Biomed Eng. 2002; 30:768–777

[5] Lieber BB, Sadasivan C. Endoluminal scaffolds for vascular reconstruction and exclusion of aneurysms from the cerebral circulation. Stroke. 2010; 41(10) Suppl:S21–S25

[6] Marti A. Cobalt-base alloys used in bone surgery. Injury. 2000; 31 Suppl 4:18–21

[7] Lieber BB, Sadasivan C, Gounis MJ, Seong J, Miskolczi L, Wakhloo AK. Functional angiography. Crit Rev Biomed Eng. 2005; 33(1):1–102

[8] Sadasivan C, Cesar L, Seong J, Wakhloo AK, Lieber BB. Treatment of rabbit elastase-induced aneurysm models by flow diverters: development of quantifiable indexes of device performance using digital subtraction angiography. IEEE Trans Med Imaging. 2009; 28(7):1117–1125

[9] Sadasivan C, Cesar L, Seong J, et al. An original flow diversion device for the treatment of intracranial aneurysms: evaluation in the rabbit elastase-induced model. Stroke. 2009; 40(3):952–958

[10] Marosfoi M, Langan ET, Strittmatter L, et al. In situ tissue engineering: endothelial growth patterns as a function of flow diverter design. J Neurointerv Surg. 2016:neurintsurg-2016–012669 [Epub ahead of print]

[11] Karacozoff AM, Shellock FG, Wakhloo AK. A next-generation, flow-diverting implant used to treat brain aneurysms: in vitro evaluation of magnetic field interactions, heating and artifacts at 3-T. Magn Reson Imaging. 2013; 31 (1):145–149

[12] De Vries J, Boogaarts J, Van Norden A, Wakhloo AK. New generation of Flow Diverter (surpass) for unruptured intracranial aneurysms: a prospective single-center study in 37 patients. Stroke. 2013; 44(6):1567–1577

[13] Wakhloo AK, Lylyk P, de Vries J, et al. Surpass Study Group. Surpass flow diverter in the treatment of intracranial aneurysms: a prospective multicenter study. AJNR Am J Neuroradiol. 2015; 36(1):98–107

[14] Colby GP, Lin LM, Caplan JM, et al. Flow diversion of large internal carotid artery aneurysms with the surpass device: impressions and technical nuance from the initial North American experience. J Neurointerv Surg. 2016; 8 (3):279–286

13 TECHNIQUE AND NUANCES OF DEPLOYMENT OF THE FLOW RE-DIRECTION ENDOLUMINAL DEVICE

BRADLEY A. GROSS, FELIPE C. ALBUQUERQUE, KARAM MOON, and CAMERON G. McDOUGALL

Abstract

This chapter reviews the technique and nuances of Flow Re-direction Endoluminal Device (FRED; MicroVention, Inc., Tustin, CA) deployment. The device is composed of a high-porosity outer stent and a low-porosity inner mesh flow diverter. This dual-layer design allows for more reliable stent opening, better apposition to the parent vessel wall, easier deliverability, and improved preservation of flow in adjacent branch vessels. Deployment is facilitated by the visibility of two radiopaque helical strands along the inner mesh that help indicate stent opening. The results from four recent case series underscore the relative safety and potential efficacy of this novel device.

Keywords: aneurysm, endoluminal device, endovascular, flow diversion, flow diverter, flow redirection stent, FRED

13.1 Introduction

Flow diversion has revolutionized the treatment of challenging intracranial aneurysms for traditional microsurgical and endovascular approaches.[1,2,3,4] Complex wide-neck, fusiform/dissecting, blister, and giant aneurysms now have an expedient, endovascular treatment option that provides remarkable angiographic results.[4,5,6,7] In contrast to intracranial stents designed for stent-assisted coil embolization, flow-diverting stents are composed of a braided meshwork with a densely covered surface; this leads to intra-aneurysmal flow stasis and aneurysm thrombosis.[2,3,4]

The Flow Redirection Endoluminal Device (FRED; Micro-Vention Terumo Co., Tustin, CA) represents a potential technological advance in flow diversion with its dual-layer design. The device is composed of a high-porosity outer stent (16 nitinol wires) and a low-porosity inner mesh (48 nitinol wires) along its midsection (80% of the outer stent's length). The additional high-porosity outer stent may allow for a superior scaffolding effect with better outward stability of the stent in apposing the wall of the parent vessel. Furthermore, the 16 nitinol wires lining the outer stent wall potentially reduce friction within the delivery microcatheter, facilitating deployment compared to, for example, the Silk (Balt Extrusion, Montmorency, France) or Pipeline (Medtronic, Dublin, Ireland) flow diverters with 48 nitinol wires, or the Surpass flow diverters (Stryker Neurovascular, Fremont, CA) with 96 nitinol wires. The dual-stent design also provides additive radial force vectors, potentially improving the reliability of stent opening. An interwoven double helix of radiopaque tantalum strands attaches the outer stent and the inner mesh, facilitating visibility along the entire length of the dual layer.

In this chapter, we review the nuances of FRED deployment; a case of a large cavernous aneurysm is illustrated in ▶ Fig. 13.1 along with another case of FRED salvage after failed microsurgical clipping of a large ophthalmic aneurysm in ▶ Fig. 13.2.

13.2 Catheter/Microcatheter

Patients are pre-treated with 5 days of aspirin (325 mg daily) and clopidogrel (75 mg daily). We perform each procedure under general endotracheal anesthesia and via 6F access through the common femoral artery. Once access has been obtained, patients are systemically anticoagulated with heparin (initial bolus, 100 IU/kg) to an activated clotting time maintained between 200 and 300 seconds during the procedure. We prefer long sheaths; if feasible, based on parent vessel size and anatomy, we employ an 80-cm, 6F Flexor Shuttle (Cook Medical Inc., Bloomington, IN) for placement in either the cervical internal carotid artery (ICA) or the distal V2 segment of the vertebral artery. The target vessel is evaluated via biplane angiography and the aneurysm is carefully evaluated with various working angles after three-dimensional rotational angiographic images are obtained. Through the sheath, we often employ a 0.072-inch inner diameter, 105-cm Navien intermediate catheter (Medtronic) for placement in the petrous or cavernous ICA or the V4 segment (▶ Fig. 13.1b). Through the intermediate catheter, a Headway 27 microcatheter (0.027-inch inner diameter; Micro-Vention, Inc.) is advanced over a 0.014-inch microwire into position for FRED deployment (▶ Fig. 13.1b). Adequate distal positioning of at least 2 cm past the aneurysm is necessary before advancing the FRED into the system. Before advancing the FRED into the microcatheter, 5 to 10 mm of it should be unsheathed into a water bath and agitated to break off any potential air bubbles. The device should then be resheathed while still in the water bath and then passed into the microcatheter.

13.3 Device Markers and Sizing

Two radiopaque tantalum strands attach the inner and outer layers of the FRED and mark the full length of its dual-layer component (▶ Fig. 13.1c). In addition, each flared end of the stent is marked by four radiopaque dots (▶ Fig. 13.1c).

FRED diameters range from 3.5 to 5.5 mm in 0.5-mm increments and are recommended for vessel diameters ranging from 2.5 to 5.5 mm with working lengths spanning 7 to 48 mm (total length spans: 13–55 mm). From working angle views, the parent vessel should be measured proximal to, at, and distal to the aneurysm. An optimal stent diameter should be chosen for the maximal (typically proximal) parent artery diameter to mitigate the risk of an endovascular leak (▶ Fig. 13.1). Kocer et al observed anecdotally that the stent may expand an additional 0.3 mm over the stated nominal diameter.[8] The stent should be sized as close as possible to the maximal parent artery diameter to facilitate maximal coverage and avoid oversizing.

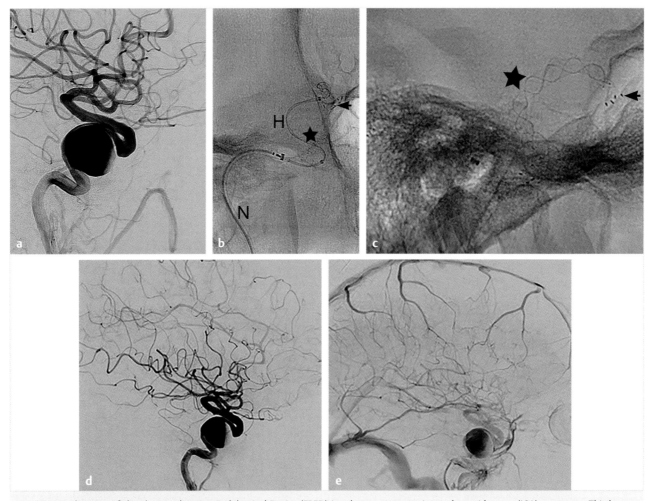

Fig. 13.1 Deployment of the Flow Re-direction Endoluminal Device (FRED) in a large, cavernous internal carotid artery (ICA) aneurysm. This large cavernous ICA aneurysm had a neck width of 12 mm (**a,** lateral projection). The maximal diameter of the proximal parent artery was 4 mm. Thus, a 4-mm FRED with a working length of 26 mm (total length, 32 mm) was selected. This lateral native image demonstrates the Navien intermediate catheter (N) in the mid-petrous segment, the Headway 27 microcatheter (H), the compressed helical working length of the FRED in the microcatheter (*star*), and the distal radiopaque dots (*arrow*) during initial deployment **(b)**. After deployment, this native image demonstrates a well-opened FRED stent spanning the aneurysm **(c)**. The tantalum wires (*star*) have an interwoven helical appearance with consistent spacing between each helical turn, suggesting the stent has opened well. These wires mark the inner mesh (working length). The outer stent lies between these wires and the terminal, flared out radiopaque markers (*arrow*). Postdeployment angiography demonstrates contrast stagnation in the aneurysm dome **(d)** into the venous phase **(e)**. (Used with permission from Barrow Neurological Institute, Phoenix, AZ.)

13.4 Deployment

The device is attached to a delivery microwire with a radiopaque distal tip and proximal marker. The device may be resheathed and repositioned so long as no more than 50% of the stent has been unsheathed (published but anecdotal evidence of up to 85%).[8]

The device is advanced into the microcatheter until the tip of the delivery system is visualized at the microcatheter tip. The microcatheter and FRED are then slowly withdrawn as a unit until the inner mesh is at its desired location. The device is then slowly deployed by withdrawal of the microcatheter with a steady forward pressure on the delivery microwire (pull–push). Careful scrutiny of the stent opening throughout a slow, meticulous deployment is crucial; if the stent does not open well initially, it should be recaptured. The helical markers can facilitate

this assessment because they should appear separately in a helical fashion; if they appear in parallel, this suggests the stent has not opened. This is a particularly important nuance for deploying the FRED around curves such as the carotid siphon. In addition, the radiopaque tantalum wires that denote the inner mesh should span the neck of the aneurysm for maximal effect of the FRED. Once the delivery microcatheter is fully withdrawn over the delivery microwire, the operator should ensure that all four radiopaque ends of the FRED are visualized; at this point, it is deployed (▶ Fig. 13.1c).

13.5 Recapturing Wire

After the device has been deployed, the distal support wire is left in place during an initial control angiographic run to evaluate stent apposition. The microcatheter is then advanced

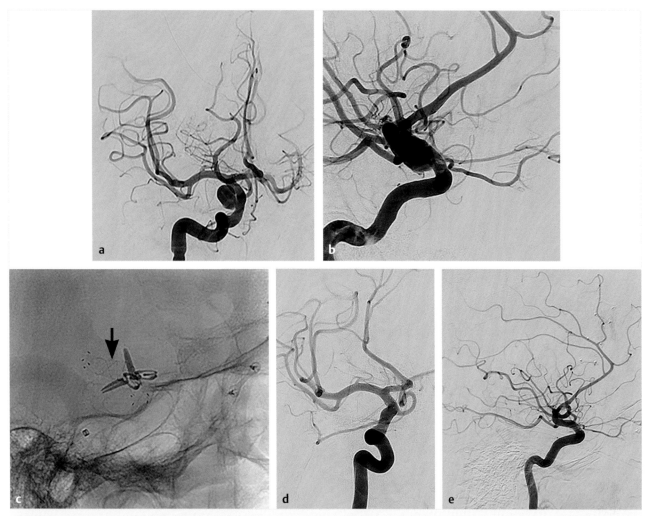

Fig. 13.2 A 55-year-old man presented with a large residual/recurrent 12-mm ophthalmic artery aneurysm after previous treatment with microsurgical clipping (**a,** anteroposterior view; **b,** lateral view). Native image immediately after deployment of the Flow Re-direction Endoluminal Device (FRED) (*arrow*) (**c**); 1 year later, follow-up angiography demonstrated no residual aneurysm (**d,** anteroposterior view; **e,** lateral view). (Used with permission from Barrow Neurological Institute, Phoenix, AZ.)

through the stent to recapture the wire. If incomplete wall apposition is observed, percutaneous angioplasty can then be performed over an exchange length microwire.

13.6 Discussion

To date, four series including 81 patients with 93 aneurysms treated with the FRED have been published (▶ Table 13.1).[8,9,10,11] Across these series, 79 of 93 aneurysms were located on the ICA (85%), predominantly in the ophthalmic segment. Other described locations included the posterior circulation in 11 of 93 (12%) aneurysms and the anterior cerebral artery in 4 of 93 (4%) aneurysms. The aneurysm morphology was most commonly small and saccular with a wide neck (55/93, 59%). Other treated aneurysm types included fusiform, dissecting, or blister in 19 of 93 aneurysms (20%) and large or giant in 19 of 93 (20%). One early series focused on presenting technically successful deployment in 13 of 13 patients without complication;

angiographic follow-up data were not available.[9] Two other series described no deployment issues in 35 patients with 42 aneurysms.[10,11] In one series, the authors described a case in which two stents could not be advanced through the proximal hub of the microcatheter; the stents were exchanged uneventfully for a new one.[8] The authors described another case of an oversized stent that would not deploy; they ultimately undersized the stent, which resulted in foreshortening of the stent postprocedurally.[8] Möhlenbruch et al employed angioplasty after stent deployment in 5 of 29 patients (17%); however, in each case, at least 90% wall apposition of the flow diverter was achieved prior to angioplasty.[10]

Three reported series provided 3-month angiographic follow-up data.[8,10,11] Across these series, complete aneurysm occlusion was reported for 32 of 49 aneurysms (65%); near-complete occlusion was reported for an additional 12 of 49 aneurysms (24%). One of the three series reported aneurysm occlusion in five of five cases with 3-month follow-up and did not provide 6-month angiographic follow-up data.[11] The other

Table 13.1 Published series on the Flow Re-direction Endoluminal Device (FRED)

Series	No. of patients (no. of aneurysms)	Location	Aneurysm type	Occlusion at 3-mo follow-up	Occlusion at 6-mo follow-up	Complications
Diaz et al (2014)[9]	13 (14)	13 ICA 1 PCirc	12 Small 1 F/D/B 1 Lg/G	NR	NR	None
Kocer et al (2014)[8]	33 (37)	34 ICA 1 ACA 2 PCirc	21 Small 11 F/D/B 5 Lg/G	8/10	4/5	1 TIA from dissection 1 ophthalmic TIA
Möhlenbruch et al (2015)[10]	29 (34)	23 ICA 3 ACA 8 PCirc	17 Small 7 F/D/B 10 Lg/G	19/34	22/30	2 strokes, transient symptoms 1 stroke, permanent hemiparesis
Poncyljusz et al (2013)[11]	6 (8)	8 ICA	5 Small 3 Lg/G	5/5	NR	None

Abbreviations: ACA, anterior cerebral artery; F/D/B, fusiform/dissecting/blister; ICA, internal carotid artery; Lg/G, large/giant; NR, not reported; PCirc, posterior circulation; Small, small wide-necked; TIA, transient ischemic attack.

two series, which had 6-month angiographic follow-up data, reported aneurysm occlusion in 26 of 35 cases at this time point (74%); 8 cases were nearly completely occluded (23%), and the one remaining case was occluded at the 12-month follow-up.

No cases of stent stenosis were reported; however, across three series with angiographic follow-up, two cases of asymptomatic stent and parent vessel thrombosis occurred.[8,10,11] One of these two cases was associated with distal stent tine "fishmouthing" (inward crimping of the stent ends).[11] Although one report of 29 patients with 34 aneurysms specifically reported no follow-up evidence of stent fishmouthing or foreshortening,[10] another of 33 patients with 37 aneurysms reported asymptomatic fishmouthing in four cases and foreshortening in one case.[8]

Overall, transiently symptomatic complications were reported in 4 of 81 patients (5%) across the four series. There was one transient ischemic attack (TIA) after an ICA dissection and another ophthalmic TIA without vessel occlusion in a patient with a stent spanning the ophthalmic artery.[8] In another series, one minor stroke occurred in a patient with a superior cerebellar artery aneurysm and another in a patient who was taken off antiplatelet therapy for ventriculoperitoneal shunt revision.[10] One patient had a permanent complication (1%) that was a result of a pontine stroke after treatment of a ruptured basilar trunk aneurysm.[10] The patient was discharged with a Glasgow Coma Scale score of 15 but had permanent hemiparesis. There were no reported cases of posttreatment intracranial hemorrhage or mortality.

Collectively, although the angiographic results and complication rates are quite promising for the FRED, longer follow-up will be necessary to reliably assess the durability and incidence of potentially severe complications. Its improved visibility due to the two helical tantalum markers along the inner mesh is an unquantifiable, though iterative, flow diverter design advantage. The unique dual-layer design with an outer, more porous stent may ultimately facilitate deliverability and reduce technical deployment issues. Furthermore, the incidence of branch occlusions may potentially be mitigated by the presence of the more porous outer stent. In the study by Kocer et al, in 28 patients in whom the ophthalmic artery was covered, only 1 experienced an ophthalmic TIA, but none had occlusion of the vessel or permanent sequelae.[8] Eleven patients had coverage of the anterior choroidal artery (two by the inner flow diverter mesh); in no case was it symptomatic or associated with vessel occlusion.

13.7 Conclusion

The FRED is another promising tool for the neurointerventionalist. Although studies are currently ongoing, the published results to date encourage continued use of the FRED and continued comparison between the various flow diverters available for ease of deployment, angiographic results, complications, and long-term outcomes.

References

[1] Becske T, Kallmes DF, Saatci I, et al. Pipeline for uncoilable or failed aneurysms: results from a multicenter clinical trial. Radiology. 2013; 267(3):858–868

[2] Fiorella D, Lylyk P, Szikora I, et al. Curative cerebrovascular reconstruction with the Pipeline embolization device: the emergence of definitive endovascular therapy for intracranial aneurysms. J Neurointerv Surg. 2009; 1(1):56–65

[3] Gross BA, Frerichs KU. Stent usage in the treatment of intracranial aneurysms: past, present and future. J Neurol Neurosurg Psychiatry. 2013; 84(3):244–253

[4] Kallmes DF, Hanel R, Lopes D, et al. International retrospective study of the pipeline embolization device: a multicenter aneurysm treatment study. AJNR Am J Neuroradiol. 2015; 36(1):108–115

[5] Albuquerque FC, Park MS, Abla AA, Crowley RW, Ducruet AF, McDougall CG. A reappraisal of the Pipeline embolization device for the treatment of posterior circulation aneurysms. J Neurointerv Surg. 2015; 7(9):641–645

[6] Fischer S, Perez MA, Kurre W, Albes G, Bäzner H, Henkes H. Pipeline embolization device for the treatment of intra- and extracranial fusiform and dissecting aneurysms: initial experience and long-term follow-up. Neurosurgery. 2014; 75(4):364–374, discussion 374

[7] Nerva JD, Morton RP, Levitt MR, et al. Pipeline Embolization Device as primary treatment for blister aneurysms and iatrogenic pseudoaneurysms of the internal carotid artery. J Neurointerv Surg. 2015; 7(3):210–216

[8] Kocer N, Islak C, Kizilkilic O, Kocak B, Saglam M, Tureci E. Flow Re-direction Endoluminal Device in treatment of cerebral aneurysms: initial experience with short-term follow-up results. J Neurosurg. 2014; 120(5):1158–1171

[9] Diaz O, Gist TL, Manjarez G, Orozco F, Almeida R. Treatment of 14 intracranial aneurysms with the FRED system. J Neurointerv Surg. 2014; 6(8):614–617

[10] Möhlenbruch MA, Herweh C, Jestaedt L, et al. The FRED flow-diverter stent for intracranial aneurysms: clinical study to assess safety and efficacy. AJNR Am J Neuroradiol. 2015; 36(6):1155–1161

[11] Poncyljusz W, Sagan L, Safranow K, Rać M. Initial experience with implantation of novel dual layer flow-diverter device FRED. Wideochir Inne Tech Maloinwazyjne. 2013; 8(3):258–264

103

14 ADJUVANT TECHNIQUES TO IMPROVE FLOW DIVERSION

WILLIAM R. STETLER JR. and W. CHRISTOPHER FOX

Abstract

Adjuvant techniques to improve flow diversion may be required in certain patients to achieve optimal outcomes. The placement of multiple devices or the use of concurrent adjuvant coil embolization can increase the rate of aneurysm thrombosis and improve reconstruction of the parent artery. These techniques may also lead to a decreased risk of aneurysm rupture and subarachnoid hemorrhage during the latent period and more rapid aneurysm obliteration after flow diversion. With giant aneurysms, the use of adjuvant balloon and/or stent anchor techniques may allow for improved placement of the flow diverter across the anatomic neck of the aneurysm to reconstruct the parent artery.

Keywords: adjuvant treatment, balloon assistance, coiling, flow diversion, intracranial aneurysm, intracranial stent, Pipeline Embolization Device

14.1 Rationale for Multiple Devices

As previously described in earlier chapters, treatment of intracranial aneurysms with flow diversion is accomplished through progressive thrombosis of the aneurysm, as bulk flow is directed through the parent vessel and away from the aneurysm dome.[1] Additionally, this change in hemodynamics between the parent vessel and the aneurysm allows the flow diverter to act as a scaffold for neointimal growth over the stent itself, and as a result, over the neck of the aneurysm.[2,3] Incorporation of the device into the parent artery allows a permanent, durable treatment by reconstructing the parent artery.[4,5,6,7,8,9]

All commercially available flow-diverting stents act as metal sleeves through which native arterial flow preferentially flows. While in vivo studies have shown that there is no immediate change in intra-aneurysmal pressure between pre- and postplacement of a single device,[10] in vitro and computational models have shown that increasing the amount of metal surface area during flow diversion is related to diminished flow into the aneurysm.[11] Because the surface area of metal in the construct is directly related to the number of devices used, placement of additional flow diverters in theory will (1) increase the amount of flow away from the dome of the aneurysm and (2) increase the scaffolding available to promote neointimization. In clinical practice, placement of multiple devices is achieved by placing the initial flow-diverting device, then tracking the microcatheter used to deliver the device back across the stent pusher wire to a position beyond the aneurysm to ready it for deployment of an additional device. Directly overlaying more than one flow diverter increases the coverage across the neck of the aneurysm and diminishes flow into the dome.

The other common reason for using multiple devices is to lengthen the area of vessel reconstructed in large aneurysms, where one device will not adequately span the anatomic neck. In this case, the deploying microcatheter is tracked back over the pusher wire as mentioned earlier, but only a portion of each device is overlapped so as to lengthen the entire construct. This technique of multiple "telescoping" stents for purposes of diversion in a long construct was first described with non–flow-diverting stents,[12,13] and subsequently with flow-diverting devices.[14] In reality, even if the intent is to cover a larger area, the telescoping stent method both lengthens the construct *and* provides increased coverage.

The use of multiple devices initially met with trepidation in the flow diverter era due to concern for perforator occlusion with overlapping stent coverage. However, in vitro models have suggested that placement of multiple flow diverters does not result in small vessel occlusion.[15] Clinically, results have also been favorable and have shown that angiographically visible vessels usually remain open, with complete occlusion being rare,[16] even when multiple stents are used.[17] When internal carotid artery (ICA) branches do become occluded (i.e., ophthalmic artery), this occlusion is usually noted on routine follow-up angiography and is a clinically silent event in most cases (▶ Fig. 14.1).[18]

Nevertheless, placement of multiple devices is not without its own risk. The telescoping stent method increases catheter time and vessel manipulation, both known risk factors for endovascular complications.[19] Furthermore, additional metal surface area achieved with telescoping devices theoretically may lead to increased area for platelet aggregation for thromboembolic events. Multi-institutional series have shown ischemic stroke rates in flow diversion of 4.7%,[20] although a recent meta-analysis of 29 studies showed stroke rate of up to 6% for all cases with the use of the Pipeline Embolization Device (Covidien, Irvine, CA).[21] Similarly, initial reports from the Surpass Study Group also showed ischemic stroke rates of 6%.[7] Despite these relatively high rates of stroke, no series has *directly* linked number of flow diverters placed with increased thromboembolic burden. Rather, the rate of thromboembolism is related to size of the aneurysm treated; patients with larger aneurysms are at increased risk of thromboembolic complications.[20,21] It is reasonable to surmise that the larger the aneurysm, the greater the risk that multiple flow diverters will be required for adequate treatment; however, this cause-and-effect relationship has not been proven, and the mechanism of thromboembolic complications in large aneurysms is not well understood.

We recommend the use of as few flow diverters as is required to properly reconstruct the parent artery. The natural history following flow diverter placement is one of progressive occlusion over time, which has been documented over the evolution of flow diverter development in multiple studies.[4,6,7,8,9,16,22] Therefore, in most cases, we recommend using the minimum number of flow diverters required to adequately achieve aneurysm neck coverage. The placement of additional flow diverters to achieve stasis during the initial implantation is not necessary in most circumstances, given that the expected treatment effect for the majority of aneurysms following flow diversion is progressive aneurysm thrombosis. In our practice, we perform follow-up angiography at 6 months and then at doubling times subsequently until angiographic thrombosis is documented. In

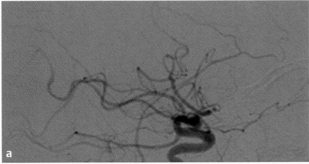
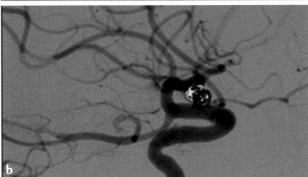
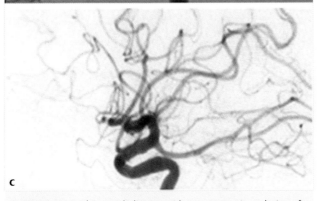

Fig. 14.1 Pre- and Postembolization with asymptomatic occlusion of ophthalmic artery. **(a)** Baseline angiography showing ophthalmic artery aneurysm with normal ophthalmic artery anatomy. **(b)** Post–pipeline-assisted coil embolization image showing patent ophthalmic artery. **(c)** 6-month post-embolization follow-up showing asymptomatic occlusion of ophthalmic artery.

may be encountered when the proximal or distal end of the device ends on an acute turn of the parent vessel. In such a case, the portion of the stent on the inside of the turn may project away from the vessel wall and into the lumen of the parent vessel. Telescoping an additional device to fully appose the stent to the vessel wall around the turn can reconstruct the vessel successfully and prevent an endoleak. If wall apposition is not confirmed adequately with two-dimensional angiography, we use cone beam computed tomography to ensure adequate wall apposition and assess the need for placement of additional devices.

14.2 Rationale for Adjuvant Coil Embolization

A rare, but potentially devastating complication following placement of an intracranial flow diverter is delayed rupture of the treated aneurysm causing subarachnoid hemorrhage (SAH).[7,20,23,24,25,26,27] Rates of rupture causing SAH vary between studies; however, a recent meta-analysis of pooled data suggests that the event occurs in 3% of cases.[21] This complication seems to be directly related to the size of the aneurysm, occurring in 4.5% of giant aneurysm cases, 0.6% of large aneurysm cases (> 10 mm), and 0% of small aneurysm cases (< 10 mm) in one study.[20]

The mechanism for delayed rupture of the treated aneurysm is unknown. Proposed mechanisms include creation of a ball-valve inflow between the stent and the aneurysm that decreases overall blood flow across the stent, but allows some blood into the dome that is unable to exit.[28] This, in theory, creates a slow and steady increase in aneurysmal pressure that could potentiate rupture. Another proposed mechanism is that immediate formation of unstable, erythrocyte-predominant thrombus (red clot) in the dome of the aneurysm after flow diversion leads to an inflammatory reaction that weakens the wall of the aneurysm, potentiating rupture.[23,27] Finally, the change in intra-aneurysmal hemodynamics after flow diversion may lead to increased wall shear stress in areas of the dome that previously had reduced shear stress. This could expose weak portions of the aneurysm to higher hemodynamic stress than prediversion, which could increase the risk of rupture.[23]

Regardless of mechanism by which delayed rupture occurs, many interventionalists feel that placing coils into the aneurysm in addition to placing a flow-diverting device helps promote thrombosis of the aneurysm. In theory, this may lead to reduced risk of delayed rupture and SAH.[29,30] It is hypothesized that coiling in conjunction with flow diversion will lead to formation of a stable platelet-fibrin clot within the aneurysm, instead of the previously described red clot seen after flow diversion alone. This more organized thrombus may, in turn, limit the inflammatory reaction described earlier and thereby decrease delayed rupture.[27]

On a practical level, coiling in conjunction with flow diversion has been shown to lead to a higher rate of occlusion of the aneurysm than when using flow diversion alone. These higher rates of occlusion are seen not only in the immediate periprocedural period but also in the long-term follow-up (6 months).[30] This provides the patient with not only more immediate dome protection (to prevent rupture during the latent period until

some patients, magnetic resonance angiography may substitute for angiography. If progressive thrombosis is not observed over time, placement of additional devices may be necessary. However, by placing the minimum number of devices necessary to reconstruct the parent vessel, regardless of achieving stasis at the time of initial implantation, catheter time is kept to a minimum and metal surface area is reduced, which theoretically reduces the risk of thromboembolic events.

In our experience, should either the neck of the aneurysm extend beyond the length of a single device or the device does not achieve good wall apposition (as may occur when deploying a flow diverter around a tight turn), then additional flow diverters should be placed in a telescoping fashion to achieve full neck coverage and adequate wall apposition. When good wall apposition is not achieved, placing another flow-diverting stent may be necessary to prevent creation of an endoleak. This

thrombosis occurs) but also a more likely chance of treatment success with one intervention. Thus, treatment with coiling and flow diversion may lead to lower retreatment rates and potentially decreased amount of time required for the patient to continue dual-antiplatelet therapy.[29,30]

Another potential benefit of concomitant coiling with flow diversion is that when immediate thrombosis is achieved intraoperatively, the successful angiographic result may prompt the interventionalist to use less flow-diverting stents to achieve stasis from flow diversion alone. As previously discussed, using a single flow-diverting stent reduces the metal surface area placed into the vessel, which may decrease the likelihood of potentiating thromboembolic events.[29] Additionally, when using flow diversion to reconstruct giant aneurysms, concomitant coiling using the jailed technique may also offer the benefit of acting as an intra-aneurysmal scaffold to prevent herniation or prolapse of the flow diverter into the aneurysm itself during deployment.[30]

As a result of the theoretical benefits of coiling concurrently with flow diversion, many interventional surgeons have adopted this practice as first line. For virgin, elective aneurysm treatment with flow diversion at our institution, we routinely place coils loosely for large or giant aneurysms via a jailed microcatheter technique. Care is taken not to densely pack the aneurysm with coils in large aneurysms, given that this has not been shown to be necessary,[29,30] and may even produce mass effect that could lead to in-stent thrombosis.[31]

14.2.1 Technique for Jailed Microcatheter

The most common method for coiling concurrently with placement of a flow diverter is the jailed microcatheter technique. This technique involves placing the flow diverter delivery microcatheter into the distal intracranial vasculature, and subsequently placing a second microcatheter within the aneurysm itself to deliver coils. The flow diverter is then deployed, "jailing" the coiling microcatheter, and the aneurysm subsequently coiled. We describe our jailing technique in detail below.

All patients are treated with aspirin 325 mg and clopidogrel 75 mg daily for 1 week prior to the procedure. VerifyNow (Accriva Diagnostics, San Diego, CA) P2Y12 Reaction Units (PRU) is checked on the morning of the procedure with a goal PRU between 50 and 180. Recently we have been augmenting PRU with the use of platelet mapping thromboelastography (TEG) because our preliminary data indicates this may provide a more accurate picture of platelet inhibition. Femoral access is then achieved in the usual fashion, and systemic heparinization is administered. Point-of-care activated clotting time testing is performed to ensure adequate heparinization. A diagnostic catheter is used to select the vessel to be treated, and then the entire system is exchanged for a 6F Cook Shuttle Sheath (Cook Medical, Bloomington, IN), which is navigated into the distal cervical carotid (▶ Fig. 14.2a).

A 0.72-inch Navien (Covidien, Irvine, CA) guide catheter is then inserted through the shuttle to the cavernous ICA. A Marksman (Covidien) microcatheter is then navigated into the largest distal M2 segment seen. Following this, a smaller microcatheter, such as a SL-10 (Stryker, Kalamazoo, MI) or Prowler-

14 (Codman & Shurtleff, Raynham, MA) is chosen for coiling, and is navigated two-thirds of the way into the dome of the aneurysm. A slightly undersized framing coil is chosen, and the first three to four initial loops are deployed into the dome of the aneurysm. It is important to begin coiling the dome of the aneurysm *before* jailing the microcatheter with the stent so that soft coil loops are present at the end of the microcatheter to prevent rupture, should inadvertent manipulation of the microcatheter occur when deploying the flow diverter itself (▶ Fig. 14.2b).

Following this, the flow diverter is deployed as has been previously described, leaving the coiling microcatheter jailed into the aneurysm itself. When treating giant aneurysms, it is often helpful to partially track the Navien guide catheter over the Marksman (approximately one-fourth to one-third) across the neck of the giant aneurysm before beginning to deploy the flow diverter. Then, after initially deploying the flow diverter in the middle cerebral artery (MCA), the stent may be pulled back into the distal ICA landing zone with the support of the Navien to prevent prolapse into the aneurysm dome. This also allows for a more controlled deployment without contending with the smaller coiling microcatheter, which if left far from the guide catheter can often be hyper-mobile in the pulsatile flow of the giant aneurysm and interfere with the Marksman delivery catheter. After deployment of the flow diverter, the delivery wire is recaptured, and the delivery catheter (Marksman, in this case) is left in the distal M1 or proximal M2 segment to provide distal access if needed. Further coiling of the aneurysm is then performed until the coil mass loosely packs the aneurysm. The coiling microcatheter is then removed either over a coil pusher wire or over a microwire to provide enough support not to disturb the stent (▶ Fig. 14.2c).

It is imperative to maintain distal access until the coiling microcatheter is removed and adequate neck coverage is confirmed on check angiogram. Removing the jailed microcatheter can manipulate and potentially move the flow diverter, and additional stents may be necessary if the neck coverage becomes suboptimal during this process. Once satisfactory results are achieved, the system is removed. The patient is maintained on dual-antiplatelet therapy for 6 months.

14.2.2 Technique for Balloon Coiling followed by Flow Diversion

For practitioners who prefer balloon remodeling for widenecked aneurysms rather than stent-coiling techniques, balloon coiling followed by flow diversion may be a preferred, more comfortable method to achieve concomitant coiling and flow diversion (instead of the jailed microcatheter technique). In these cases, we advocate using a setup appropriate for flow diverter deployment from the start, rather than use the usual balloon-coiling setup and then transitioning to a flow diverter platform.

Balloon coiling followed by flow diversion can also be helpful when treating giant aneurysms, given that one risk of primary flow diverter deployment is prolapse or herniation of the flow diverter into the aneurysm dome. In these cases, use of balloon remodeling to reconstruct the neck of the aneurysm prior to flow diverter placement can be helpful to prevent flow diverter

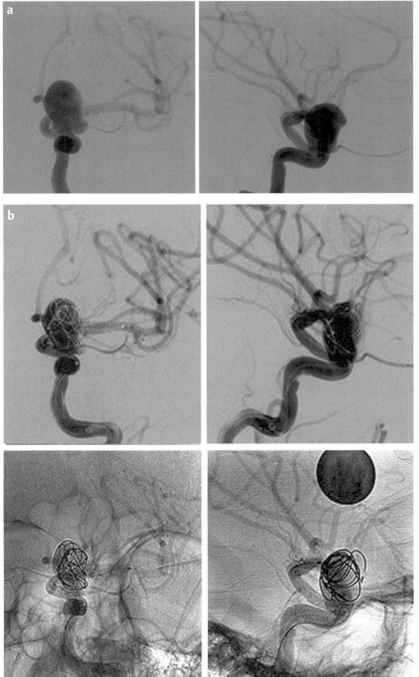

Fig. 14.2 Jailed microcatheter technique example. **(a)** Initial angiography showing large left ophthalmic artery. **(b)** Intraprocedural angiography showing jailed microcatheter technique (*continued*).

prolapse. By placing coils into the dome of the aneurysm with balloon reconstruction of the neck, an intra-aneurysmal scaffold is formed that can provide support for flow diverter deployment to prevent prolapse.

The same preoperative and access is used as described earlier. The Cook Shuttle Sheath is placed into the distal ICA. A 072-inch Navien is placed into the cavernous ICA, and an over-the-wire, compliant intracranial balloon, such as a Scepter XC (MicroVention, Tustin, CA) or Ascent (Codman & Shurtleff) is navigated just beyond the neck of the aneurysm. A conventional coiling catheter as described earlier is then advanced through the guide and placed two-thirds of the way into the dome of the aneurysm. Similar to the jailed microcatheter technique,

three to four coil loops of the initial framing coil (undersized coil is again recommended) are deployed. The balloon is slowly withdrawn to a position across the neck of the aneurysm. Pulling the balloon *back* into position, rather than *pushing* it forward into position, is preferable so that the slack or redundancy in the system is removed immediately before inflation. The balloon is then inflated to reconstruct the neck of the aneurysm, and the remaining portion of the aneurysm is loosely packed with coils. It is not necessary to pack coils close to the neck of the aneurysm because placement of the flow diverter will achieve thrombosis of this typically small residual uncoiled portion of the aneurysm. The balloon is then deflated, but left in place to ensure that the coil mass is stable and will not herniate

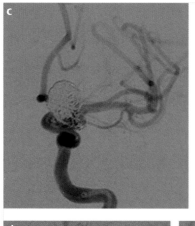
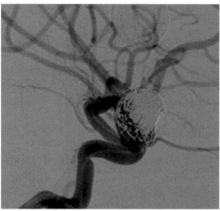

(*continued*) **(c)** Final angiography showing loose coiling of aneurysm with placement of Pipeline flow diverter. **(d)** Six-month follow-up angiography showing complete occlusion of aneurysm.

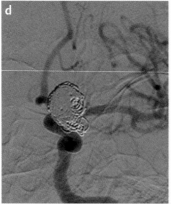
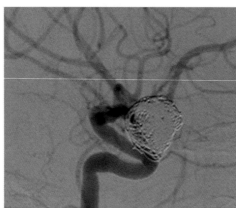

into the parent vessel, and the coiling microcatheter is subsequently removed. The balloon is then removed and replaced with a Marksman microcatheter into the MCA, and the flow diverter is placed as described earlier.

14.3 Other Adjuvant Techniques

14.3.1 Anchor Techniques for Giant Aneurysms

When treating giant ICA aneurysms, gaining sufficient access beyond the aneurysm can prove difficult. It can be hard to navigate a small microcatheter past the large, dysplastic neck of the aneurysm to the MCA when the major vortex of blood flow is into the aneurysm dome and not into the MCA. Often the only way to navigate beyond the aneurysm into the MCA is to loop the microcatheter through the aneurysm itself and then access the MCA. This is a useful technique to guide the microcatheter beyond the aneurysm; however, a complete loop is not amenable to placement of a stent across the neck of the aneurysm. Techniques to anchor the distal catheter and remove the redundant loop within the aneurysm have been described using both a stent[32] and a balloon.[33] We describe our technique for these methods in the following section.

14.3.2 Stent Anchor Technique

The patient is prepared preoperatively as described earlier. Once distal ICA access is achieved with the Cook Shuttle Sheath,

a 044 Distal Access Catheter (DAC) is advanced over a Marksman microcatheter. The Marksman will loop through the aneurysm and then navigate into the distal M1 segment. A size-appropriate Solitaire (Covidien) or Trevo (Stryker) stent retriever is then placed through the Marksman catheter and deployed in the distal M1 segment. At this point, the loop and redundancy of the Marksman is pulled back until it is straight across the anatomic neck of the aneurysm, using the stent as an anchor to maintain distal access. The DAC is then advanced over the Marksman into the M1 segment, and the stent is retrieved back into the Marksman. The DAC helps provide the support necessary to maintain catheter support through the aneurysm without prolapse into the aneurysm dome. Finally, the flow diverter may be deployed through the Marksman catheter as previously described.

14.3.3 Balloon Anchor Technique

As with the stent anchor technique, distal ICA access is achieved with the Cook Shuttle Sheath. Similarly, a 044 DAC is utilized, but instead of primarily using a Marksman microcatheter to gain access to the MCA, an over-the-wire balloon catheter is used. The balloon, like the Marksman in the stent anchor technique, will loop through the aneurysm and navigate into the distal M1 segment. The balloon is then inflated to conform to the size of the M1 and serves as an anchor point. The loop, or redundancy, of the balloon catheter is pulled back until it is straight across the anatomic neck of the aneurysm. The DAC is then advanced over the balloon catheter into the M1 segment.

The balloon is deflated and removed, leaving the DAC across the anatomic neck of the aneurysm with the distal portion of the DAC in the M1 segment. A Marksman microcatheter can then be placed through the DAC into the M2 segment, and a flow diverter deployed through the Marksman as previously described. Should there be significant tortuosity at the carotid siphon, rendering the DAC unstable within the M1 segment without the support of an underlying microcatheter or wire, the balloon catheter can be removed over a 300-cm microwire to offer further support. In such circumstances, we use a wire with additional support, such as a 300-cm Balanced Middle Weight (BMW; Abbott, Santa Clara, CA) wire. This offers additional support to the DAC to maintain distal access when removing the balloon microcatheter.

References

[1] Seong J, Wakhloo AK, Lieber BB. In vitro evaluation of flow diverters in an elastase-induced saccular aneurysm model in rabbit. J Biomech Eng. 2007; 129(6):863–872

[2] Lieber BB, Gounis MJ. The physics of endoluminal stenting in the treatment of cerebrovascular aneurysms. Neurol Res. 2002; 24 Suppl 1:S33–S42

[3] Lieber BB, Sadasivan C. Endoluminal scaffolds for vascular reconstruction and exclusion of aneurysms from the cerebral circulation. Stroke. 2010; 41(10) Suppl:S21–S25

[4] Becske T, Kallmes DF, Saatci I, et al. Pipeline for uncoilable or failed aneurysms: results from a multicenter clinical trial. Radiology. 2013; 267 (3):858–868

[5] Sadasivan C, Cesar L, Seong J, et al. An original flow diversion device for the treatment of intracranial aneurysms: evaluation in the rabbit elastase-induced model. Stroke. 2009; 40(3):952–958

[6] De Vries J, Boogaarts J, Van Norden A, Wakhloo AK. New generation of Flow Diverter (surpass) for unruptured intracranial aneurysms: a prospective single-center study in 37 patients. Stroke. 2013; 44(5):1567–1577

[7] Wakhloo AK, Lylyk P, de Vries J, et al. Surpass Study Group. Surpass flow diverter in the treatment of intracranial aneurysms: a prospective multicenter study. AJNR Am J Neuroradiol. 2015; 36(1):98–107

[8] Nelson PK, Lylyk P, Szikora I, Wetzel SG, Wanke I, Fiorella D. The pipeline embolization device for the intracranial treatment of aneurysms trial. AJNR Am J Neuroradiol. 2011; 32(1):34–40

[9] Fischer S, Vajda Z, Aguilar Perez M, et al. Pipeline embolization device (PED) for neurovascular reconstruction: initial experience in the treatment of 101 intracranial aneurysms and dissections. Neuroradiology. 2012; 54(4):369–382

[10] Tateshima S, Jones JG, Mayor Basto F, Vinuela F, Duckwiler GR. Aneurysm pressure measurement before and after placement of a Pipeline stent: feasibility study using a 0.014 inch pressure wire for coronary intervention. J Neurointerv Surg. 2016; 8(6):603–607

[11] Seshadhri S, Janiga G, Beuing O, Skalej M, Thévenin D. Impact of stents and flow diverters on hemodynamics in idealized aneurysm models. J Biomech Eng. 2011; 133(7):071005

[12] Crowley RW, Evans AJ, Kassell NF, Jensen ME, Dumont AS. Endovascular treatment of a fusiform basilar artery aneurysm using multiple "in-stent stents". Technical note. J Neurosurg Pediatr. 2009; 3(6):496–500

[13] Chalouhi N, Campbell P, Makke Y, et al. Treatment of complex intracranial aneurysms with a telescoping stent technique. J Neurol Surg A Cent Eur Neurosurg. 2012; 73(5):281–288

[14] Cohen JE, Gomori JM, Moscovici S, Itshayek E. Successful endovascular treatment of a growing megadolichoectasic vertebrobasilar artery aneurysm by flow diversion using the "diverter-in-stent" technique. J Clin Neurosci. 2012; 19(1):166–170

[15] Dai D, Ding YH, Kadirvel R, Rad AE, Lewis DA, Kallmes DF. Patency of branches after coverage with multiple telescoping flow-diverter devices: an in vivo study in rabbits. AJNR Am J Neuroradiol. 2012; 33(1):171–174

[16] Szikora I, Berentei Z, Kulcsar Z, et al. Treatment of intracranial aneurysms by functional reconstruction of the parent artery: the Budapest experience with the pipeline embolization device. AJNR Am J Neuroradiol. 2010; 31(6):1139–1147

[17] Vedantam A, Rao VY, Shaltoni HM, Mawad ME. Incidence and clinical implications of carotid branch occlusion following treatment of internal carotid artery aneurysms with the pipeline embolization device. Neurosurgery. 2015; 76(2):173–178, discussion 178

[18] Durst CR, Starke RM, Clopton D, et al. Endovascular treatment of ophthalmic artery aneurysms: ophthalmic artery patency following flow diversion versus coil embolization. J Neurointerv Surg. 2016; 8(9):919–922

[19] Bendszus M, Koltzenburg M, Burger R, Warmuth-Metz M, Hofmann E, Solymosi L. Silent embolism in diagnostic cerebral angiography and neurointerventional procedures: a prospective study. Lancet. 1999; 354 (9190):1594–1597

[20] Kallmes DF, Hanel R, Lopes D, et al. International retrospective study of the pipeline embolization device: a multicenter aneurysm treatment study. AJNR Am J Neuroradiol. 2015; 36(1):108–115

[21] Brinjikji W, Murad MH, Lanzino G, Cloft HJ, Kallmes DF. Endovascular treatment of intracranial aneurysms with flow diverters: a meta-analysis. Stroke. 2013; 44(2):442–447

[22] Briganti F, Napoli M, Leone G, et al. Treatment of intracranial aneurysms by flow diverter devices: long-term results from a single center. Eur J Radiol. 2014; 83(9):1683–1690

[23] Kulcsár Z, Houdart E, Bonafé A, et al. Intra-aneurysmal thrombosis as a possible cause of delayed aneurysm rupture after flow-diversion treatment. AJNR Am J Neuroradiol. 2011; 32(1):20–25

[24] Hampton T, Walsh D, Tolias C, Fiorella D. Mural destabilization after aneurysm treatment with a flow-diverting device: a report of two cases. J Neurointerv Surg. 2011; 3(2):167–171

[25] Fox B, Humphries WE, Doss VT, Hoit D, Elijovich L, Arthur AS. Rupture of giant vertebrobasilar aneurysm following flow diversion: mechanical stretch as a potential mechanism for early aneurysm rupture. J Neurointerv Surg. 2015; 7 (11):e37

[26] Fischer S, Perez MA, Kurre W, Albes G, Bäzner H, Henkes H. Pipeline embolization device for the treatment of intra- and extracranial fusiform and dissecting aneurysms: initial experience and long-term follow-up. Neurosurgery. 2014; 75(4):364–374, discussion 374

[27] Turowski B, Macht S, Kulcsár Z, Hänggi D, Stummer W. Early fatal hemorrhage after endovascular cerebral aneurysm treatment with a flow diverter (SILK-Stent): do we need to rethink our concepts? Neuroradiology. 2011; 53 (1):37–41

[28] Cebral JR, Mut F, Raschi M, et al. Aneurysm rupture following treatment with flow-diverting stents: computational hemodynamics analysis of treatment. AJNR Am J Neuroradiol. 2011; 32(1):27–33

[29] Nossek E, Chalif DJ, Chakraborty S, Lombardo K, Black KS, Setton A. Concurrent use of the Pipeline Embolization Device and coils for intracranial aneurysms: technique, safety, and efficacy. J Neurosurg. 2015; 122(4):904–911

[30] Lin N, Brouillard AM, Krishna C, et al. Use of coils in conjunction with the pipeline embolization device for treatment of intracranial aneurysms. Neurosurgery. 2015; 76(2):142–149

[31] Siddiqui AH, Kan P, Abla AA, Hopkins LN, Levy EI. Complications after treatment with pipeline embolization for giant distal intracranial aneurysms with or without coil embolization. Neurosurgery. 2012; 71(2):E509–E513, discussion E513

[32] Fargen KM, Velat GJ, Lawson MF, Hoh BL, Mocco J. The stent anchor technique for distal access through a large or giant aneurysm. J Neurointerv Surg. 2013; 5(4):e24

[33] Ding D, Starke RM, Evans AJ, Jensen ME, Liu KC. Balloon anchor technique for pipeline embolization device deployment across the neck of a giant intracranial aneurysm. J Cerebrovasc Endovasc Neurosurg. 2014; 16(2):125–130

15 FLOW DIVERTERS FOR BRAIN ANEURYSM TREATMENT: INTRAPROCEDURAL COMPLICATIONS AND MANAGEMENT

BARTLEY MITCHELL, PEDRO AGUILAR-SALINAS, AMIN NIMA AGHAEBRAHIM, ERIC SAUVAGEAU, and RICARDO A. HANEL

Abstract

The recent introduction of flow diverters in the neurointerventional armamentarium is revolutionary. The uniqueness of this technology consists of decreasing the blood flow into the aneurysm sac, which induces changes on the intrasaccular hemodynamics leading to aneurysm thrombosis. This new ability to treat and cure a brain aneurysm with low to no risk of recurrence has been very appealing. Mid- and long-term outcomes in multiple series have demonstrated the safety and effectiveness of flow diverters, especially for wide-necked, large or giant aneurysms that were otherwise challenging to treat by microsurgery or endovascular embolization. However, the neurointerventionalist may face complications at any point during the treatment of aneurysms with the use of this technology. For that reason, the purpose of this chapter is to review the advantages of a triaxial system to provide additional support for flow diverter placement within oftentimes tortuous vascular anatomy; the role of dual-antiplatelet therapy; and potential intraoperative complications, their management, and bail-out techniques.

Keywords: complications, endovascular, flow diverter, intracranial aneurysm, triaxial system

15.1 Introduction

The concept of changing flow to treat brain aneurysms dates back from the technique of Hunterian ligation, when decreasing or stopping flow on the parent vessel would lead to aneurysm thrombosis.[1] There has been an evolution in the treatment of cerebral aneurysms from those early days of microsurgical clipping to endovascular techniques, such as coiling, balloon or stent-assisted coiling, and now flow diversion.

Flow diverters are a group of devices with metal-to-artery coverage of more than 30%, which induce changes on the intrasaccular hemodynamics often leading to thrombosis. Additionally, these devices have small struts and cells that provide a scaffold for endothelial cells to grow over the neck of the aneurysm and ultimately heal the parent vessel defect.[2,3,4]

The purpose of this chapter is to review the intraoperative complications with use of flow diverters, as well as their prevention and management. We will cover events that are common to all flow diverters and also include device-specific issues. There are multiple flow diverter stents on the market today, with some more studied than others. The underlying concept is the same for all of these devices, which is to divert flow away from the aneurysm and to redirect the blood flow to the parent artery. The devices currently on the market for use include Pipeline Embolization Device (PED; Covidien/eV3, Irvine, CA), Silk flow diverter (SILK; Balt Extrusion, Montmorency, France), Flow Redirection Endoluminal Device (FRED; Microvention, Tustin, CA), Surpass (Surpass Medical/Stryker

Medical, Miramar, FL), and p64 (Phenox, Bochum, Germany). To date, the PED is the most studied of these devices and the only one currently available in the United States. There have been more than 20,000 of PEDs implanted worldwide and more than 300 publications related to their use. However, the SILK was actually the first device in this category to become commercially available and has been used over 16,000 times worldwide with 48 publications (▶ Table 15.1).

15.2 Endovascular Access

15.2.1 Catheter Access

In our experience, a triaxial system should be employed when deploying a Pipeline flow diverter. This system consists of a proximal support long sheath, an intermediate catheter to provide additional support, and finally the delivery microcatheter. This progressive triaxial system allows for superior control and device placement when using a flow diverter in often tortuous cerebrovascular anatomy. Device and catheter control are critical in avoiding complications in the deployment of a flow diversion system.

15.2.2 Proximal Long Sheath

The proximal support lays the framework of support for the entire delivery system allowing navigation of oftentimes tortuous vascular anatomy and preventing buildup of forward tension on the system during catheter navigation. Although increased flexibility of the delivery system can offer superior

Table 15.1 Flow diverter usage and publications

FD	PED	Silk	Surpass	FRED	P64
No. of publications (PubMed)[a]	≈ 319	48	5	4	4
No. of cases published	≈ 2,680	694	224	82	140
Devices implanted worldwide[b]	20,000	16,000	1,500	4,341	2,971

Abbreviations: FD, flow diverter; PED, Pipeline Embolization Device; FRED, Flow Redirection Endoluminal Device.
[a]Total number of publications do not reflect the total number of case series but manuscripts obtained with the following search terms: Pipeline Embolization Device, SILK flow diverter, FRED flow diverter, SURPASS flow diverter, p64 flow diverter (PubMed search in June 2016).
[b]Information provided by manufacturer.

trackability, this introduces the possibility of kinking the support catheter around a particularly tight corner. In this situation, a more robust support catheter becomes necessary.

Forward tension can also make delivery of any device treacherous. When pressure is applied for delivery, unsheathing, or recapturing of the device, the operator must apply additional stress on the support system. This can cause the catheters or device to become more difficult to control and move spontaneously or rapidly in an unintended manner due to the high forward tension within the system. Eliminating or reducing the forward tension is an important step in reducing potential complications and allows for superior control in device placement and apposition. This is particularly salient when attempting to avoid coverage over critical vessels while also maintaining an adequate margin of coverage on either side of the aneurysm neck.

The degree of vessel tortuosity often dictates the amount of support necessary for successful navigation of the delivery system. It is incumbent on the operators to have knowledge of the properties and use of a versatile set of delivery catheters. The senior authors (E.S. and R.H.) generally utilize a 6F proximal long sheath, along with an intermediate catheter, such as the 058-inch Navien (Covidien/eV3, Irvine, CA) to offer additional distal support, followed by a 0.027-inch microcatheter (Marksman 027 or Phenom 27). The Arrow-Flex (Teleflex Inc, Wayne, PA) sheath also offers reasonable support for PED placement with moderately more support compared to the Neuron 070 delivery catheter (Penumbra Inc, Irvine, CA). A 6F Shuttle guide sheath (Cook Group; Bloomington, IN) and Fubuki 6F sheath (Asahi Intecc, Aichi, Japan) are even stiffer, more supportive sheaths that allow excellent proximal support. In relatively straightforward access cases for posterior circulation aneurysms, we have found the 6F Neuron 070 or Penumbra Benchmark (Penumbra Inc) to be useful catheters.

15.2.3 Intermediate Catheters

The use of intermediate catheters allows for even more distal support beyond that of the delivery catheter. This additional support is particularly important when the distal arterial anatomy is tortuous, or if the flow diverter device is being placed around a tight turn, such as the carotid siphon. The extra support afforded by an intermediate catheter allows for a more controlled deployment of the device. The intermediate catheter that bridges the gap between the delivery catheter and the distal tip of the microcatheter reduces the amount of forward tension that builds up in the system.

Additionally, if a device becomes distorted or does not deploy in the manner in which an operator intended, it may become necessary to recapture the flow diverter. If the microcatheter has difficulty recapturing the device around serpiginous or nonlinear anatomy, an intermediate catheter can be employed to recapture both the microcatheter and the device. In these instances, the operator will be very thankful for having the foresight to employ an intermediate catheter.

15.2.4 Microcatheters

There are many different options when it comes to selecting a microcatheter to use in the delivery of flow diverter devices.

For instance, the Pipeline Flex flow diverter (Covidien/eV3, Irvine, CA) requires a 0.027-inch inner diameter microcatheter. While the Marksman microcatheter has been a popular choice, different microcatheters may be used depending on one's needs. With particularly tortuous anatomy over long distances, friction on the inside of the microcatheter during device deployment may cause the microcatheter to stretch. This can result in "lock-up" of the device, which can become so pronounced that the device becomes completely lodged in the microcatheter.

Certain rescue strategies are required with this particular complication when the device is partially deployed. It may not be feasible to simply drag the microcatheter and device into the intermediate catheter without risking avulsion or dissection of the parent artery. In this case, the intermediate catheter could be advanced over both the microcatheter and the device, recapturing both at once. Newer microcatheters have certain attributes, which work well with the new Pipeline Flex delivery system's increased pushability and resheathability. More supportive microcatheters, such as the Via 27 (Sequent Medical, Aliso Viejo, CA) and the Phenom 27 (Cathera, Inc.; Mountain View, CA), have been introduced and, in the authors' estimation, seem to perform better when resheathing the Pipeline Flex. Ultimately, user preference and comfort level will influence an operator's choice of microcatheter for delivery of a flow diversion device.

15.3 Platelet Inhibition

Platelet inhibition is a crucial component to the successful use of intravascular stents in the treatment of vascular disease throughout the body. The stakes are often high, particularly with the use of flow diversion in the treatment of aneurysms, where the amount of exposed bare metal is significantly higher compared to other stents. For example, the PED is constructed of a closed-cell woven mesh with 48 strands (75% nitinol, 25% platinum), and typically provides 30 to 35% metal coverage depending on device sizing and vessel curvature.[5] For comparison, the open-cell Neuroform (Stryker Neurovascular, Fremont, CA) and closed-cell Enterprise (Cordis Neurovascular, Miami, FL) stents provide 6.5 to 9.5% metal coverage. This increased metal coverage of flow diverters creates a much larger thrombogenic surface area compared with non–flow diversion stents.

The use of flow diverters comes with the need for dual-antiplatelet use, to prevent acute stent thrombosis, occlusion, and stroke. Patients are typically placed on both aspirin and a P2Y12-receptor antagonist. Patients on standard doses of aspirin and clopidogrel (or any another oral anti-P2Y12 medication) can have a supratherapeutic response, theoretically leading to a higher likelihood of hemorrhage, or a subtherapeutic effect, potentially leading to a higher likelihood of thrombotic events. To this end, platelet function assays have been developed to measure the therapeutic effect of the P2Y12 receptor antagonist. It has been studied in carotid[6] and coronary stenting[7] with positive correlation between high platelet response unit (PRU) values (low level of platelet response to the drug) and thromboembolic events.

Despite this evidence,[8,9,10] the overall usefulness of bedside P2Y12 monitoring has come into question. This was particularly true with the ARCTIC trial,[11] a prospective randomized trial of 2,440 coronary stenting patients with or without P2Y12 response monitoring and medication adjustments. Interestingly, the ARCTIC study showed no improvement in clinical outcomes (primary endpoints: death, MI, in-stent thrombosis, stroke, or urgent revascularization) despite P2Y12 monitoring and medication adjustments compared with standard medication dosing without monitoring or medication adjustments. The monitoring cohort reached the primary endpoint in 34.6% of patients, while the nonmonitoring cohort reached 31.1%. Furthermore, there were no differences in major hemorrhagic events between the two groups. Although the cardiac and carotid stenting literature can offer useful direction with respect to P2Y12 response testing, the overall generalizability of this literature to flow diversion must be approached with caution.

The use of platelet-inhibition testing in flow diversion remains controversial. In the initial Pipeline for Uncoilable or Failed Aneurysms (PUFS)[12] trial, 6 of the 107 patients (5.6%) in the study experienced a major ipsilateral stroke or neurologic death. However, in the study, all patients received a standard dose of aspirin and clopidogrel without routine use of platelet inhibition monitoring. A retrospective analysis of complication rates in patients who underwent platelet testing versus those who did not undergo platelet testing from the International Retrospective Study of Pipeline Embolization Device registry (IntrePED)[13,14] found that platelet testing was associated with higher morbidity. Patients who underwent platelet testing had higher rates of intracranial hemorrhage (2.3 vs. 0% in those with no platelet testing). Neurologic morbidity was 8.2% in those who had platelet testing versus 2.1% in those who did not. Interestingly, the use of multiple devices was also higher in the platelet testing group (38 vs. 27.8%), which potentially increased the density of metal coverage in this group.

In the neurosurgical literature, one retrospective study that examined hemorrhagic and thromboembolic complications during flow diversion demonstrated a combined major complication rate of 9.6% (4% hemorrhagic, 5.6% thromboembolic) in 248 aneurysms treated in 231 patients. Based on their data, the authors concluded that the ideal range for the PRU assay was 70 to 150. A PRU less than 60 was a significant predictor of hemorrhagic complications, whereas a PRU higher than 240 was a predictor of thromboembolic events.[15] These findings are echoed in other smaller retrospective studies, which also demonstrate a higher risk of symptomatic thromboembolic events in patients with elevated PRU test results (indicating lower platelet inhibition) and a higher risk of intracranial hemorrhages in patients with PRU less than 60.[15,16,17]

Hemorrhagic complications following flow diversion while on dual-antiplatelet medication can be potentially devastating, particularly when trying to negotiate a delicate balancing act between hemorrhage prevention and device thrombosis. This particular conundrum is true with the use of any bare-metal stent placed, which requires pretreatment with dual-antiplatelet therapy prior to treatment. Our protocol involves at least 3 months of continuous aspirin and clopidogrel or ticagrelor following flow diversion.[18,19] Following that, patients generally remains on aspirin for the rest of their life.

In our practice, we routinely check a P2Y12 level preoperatively in all patients. Those patients with an elevated P2Y12 (>200), despite at least 5 days of an aspirin and clopidogrel

regimen, are typically switched to ticagrelor. In those patients who have had less time to take the aspirin/clopidogrel regimen and have a borderline P2Y12 level (200–240), we typically redose an additional oral bolus of clopidogrel (150–450 mg) followed by recheck of the P2Y12 levels. With supratherapeutic levels (30–60), the authors suggest dose adjustment, occasionally with doses as low as 5 mg of clopidogrel daily, to decrease hemorrhagic complications. Despite this, the use of platelet-inhibition testing remains controversial, likely due to our inadequate understanding of the mechanisms behind both stent-induced thrombosis and posttreatment hemorrhagic complications. Prospective analyses of these certainly seem warranted.

15.4 Periprocedural Technical Events and Complications

15.4.1 Intraoperative In-Stent Thrombosis and Side-Branch Occlusion

Although a rare occurrence if patients have been adequately pretreated with antiplatelet medication prior to flow diverter placement, in-stent thrombosis occurs. It is critical to recognize this complication to act quickly to prevent thrombus migration and stroke. Additional intravenous antiplatelet medications, glycoprotein IIb/IIIa inhibitors, should be administered such as Integrilin (eptifibatide, Millenium Pharmaceuticals) or ReoPro (Abciximab, Janssen Pharmaceuticals) with close monitoring with additional angiographic runs. If this is ineffective, then direct thrombus aspiration may be necessary.

Additionally, the device can occlude side branches, which may pose significant complications. When this is detected perioperatively, the authors suggest initially checking for collateral flow that may create competition for flow through that side branch mimicking occlusion. If occlusion is detected, the use of a glycoprotein IIb/IIIa-inhibitor agent is indicated. We routinely check angiograms after partial deployment of the device across critical side branches. If side-branch occlusion is detected, the device can be resheathed. Mild induced hypertension may also be employed in this situation.

15.4.2 Intraoperative Aneurysm Rupture

Intraoperative aneurysm rupture is particularly daunting during flow diversion due to the routine use of dual-antiplatelet medications. Dealing with these hemorrhagic complications is likely more challenging in this situation. Having a treatment strategy ahead of time, however, can make the difference between stopping the bleeding from the ruptured aneurysm quickly and sustaining a catastrophic bleed requiring surgical evacuation.

When an aneurysm rupture is detected, the first maneuver should be to lower the patient's blood pressure. If the device has been deployed and extravasation from the aneurysm continues, then placing multiple devices across the aneurysm may stop the bleeding by diverting all flow away from the aneurysm dome. This can also be accomplished temporarily by using a balloon catheter inflated over the neck of the aneurysm. There are obviously risks with both strategies, from increasing the likelihood of side branch occlusion from multiple devices to developing strokes from prolonged balloon occlusion.

If the flow diverter has not yet been deployed following an intraoperative rupture, then coil embolization along with placement of the flow diverter is an excellent option. The operator may choose to employ balloon remodeling during coil embolization followed by flow diversion or jail a second coiling microcatheter into the aneurysm during flow diversion.

Finally, parent vessel occlusion can be used as a final endovascular solution to intra-aneurysmal ruptures during flow diversion. It is beneficial to know the preoperative collateral circulation pattern within the circle of Willis prior to parent artery sacrifice. The blood pressure should be raised following sacrifice, especially if one initially lowered it to control the initial hemorrhage. Vessel occlusion can be accomplished via any number of options, including coil embolization, the use of liquid embolics (NBCA, Onyx), or the use of a device specifically designed for vessel occlusion (Amplatzer, St Jude Medical; EV3 MVP microvascular plug system).

When all other endovascular methods have been exhausted, microsurgical clipping can be considered. However, there is a very real danger of excessive and potentially life-threatening bleeding both during and after surgery in the face of significant platelet inhibition. Furthermore, the transfusion of platelets in the setting of a recent device deployment increases the risk of in-stent thrombosis with subsequent stroke. However, this calculated risk may be necessary in a patient who does not have sufficient collateral circulation to an area of the brain supplied by the parent vessel.

15.4.3 Delayed Aneurysm Rupture

Delayed rupture of the aneurysm can be devastating in patients on dual-antiplatelet therapy. Eighty-one cases of delayed aneurysm rupture were identified in a recent review article with 76% of those occurring within the first month following flow diversion (▶ Table 15.2).[20] The outcomes in these cases were generally poor with 81% of patients experiencing death or severe neurologic disability. Additionally, giant aneurysms accounted for a large proportion (46.3%) of delayed rupture.

Larger aneurysms have been noted to have higher rates of rupture with giant aneurysms having the highest probability of rupture. Fortunately, the overall rate of delayed aneurysm rupture following flow diversion has been relatively low (0.6–1.6%, ▶ Table 15.3).[12,14] In the ASPIRe (Aneurysm Study of Pipeline in

Table 15.2 Timing of delayed aneurysmal rupture following treatment with flow diverter devices

Time from treatment	Number of cases
<1 d	6 (10.3%)
1–7 d	19 (32.8%)
7–30 d	20 (34.5%)
>30 d	13 (22.4%)

Source: Permission obtained from Rouchaud et al.[20]

Table 15.3 Summary of delayed aneurysm rupture following flow diverter deployment in prospective trials

ASPIRe	IntrePED	PUFS
3/191 (1.6%)	5/793 (0.6%)	1/107 (0.9%)

Abbreviations: ASPIRe, Aneurysm Study of Pipeline in an Observational Registry; IntrePED, International Retrospective Study of the Pipeline Embolization Device; PUFS, Pipeline for Uncoilable or Failed Aneurysms.

an Observational Registry) study, a larger proportion of giant aneurysms (>25 mm) experienced delayed rupture (9.5%) compared with aneurysms less than 25 mm (0.6%). Similarly, the IntrePED study identified five delayed aneurysm ruptures of which three were giant and the remaining two were large.

Several possible mechanisms have been posited for delayed aneurysm rupture following flow diversion as listed below.
1. Abrupt flow change: possibly from uneven neck coverage with different pore densities generating a different flow pattern.
2. Intraluminal wall manipulation during flow diverter placement.
3. Poor device apposition.
4. Device migration.
5. Intra-aneurysmal thrombus formation/expansion ("fat man pants syndrome"; ▶ Fig. 15.1, ▶ Fig. 15.2).
6. Thrombolytic cascade leading to mural destabilization.

A more complete discussion of this topic can be found in Chapter 16.

15.4.4 In-Stent Stenosis

The high percentage of metal coverage attained by flow diverters allows for flow stasis and the subsequent thrombosis of target aneurysms. With the PED (35% metal coverage), aneurysm thrombosis/obliteration was seen in upward of 93% of the cases by 6-month posttreatment.[21] However, the occurrence of in-stent stenosis is also seen in a significant proportion of cases. Lylyk et al[21] also reported in-stent stenosis in 7 out of 38 cases (18%). Fortunately, none of these cases required additional treatment and three of the seven cases improved spontaneously. In-stent stenosis has been reported in up to 7% of cases overall.[22] In-stent stenosis was identified in 39% of PEDs and 57% of SILK flow diverters, although the vast majority of patients remained asymptomatic with high rates of spontaneous resolution.[23,24]

In some cases, in-stent stenosis can be severe enough to limit flow warranting treatment with angioplasty.[25] However, caution must be taken regarding the use of angioplasty to treat in-stent stenosis. When the stenotic region is proximal to the aneurysm, augmenting distal flow with balloon angioplasty can potentially change the flow dynamics within the aneurysm. Indeed, Cebral et al[26] reported two paraclinoidal giant aneurysms that ruptured within 1 week of angioplasty treatment to treat a proximal stenotic portion of the parent vessel/device.

A more complete discussion of this topic can be found in Chapter 16.

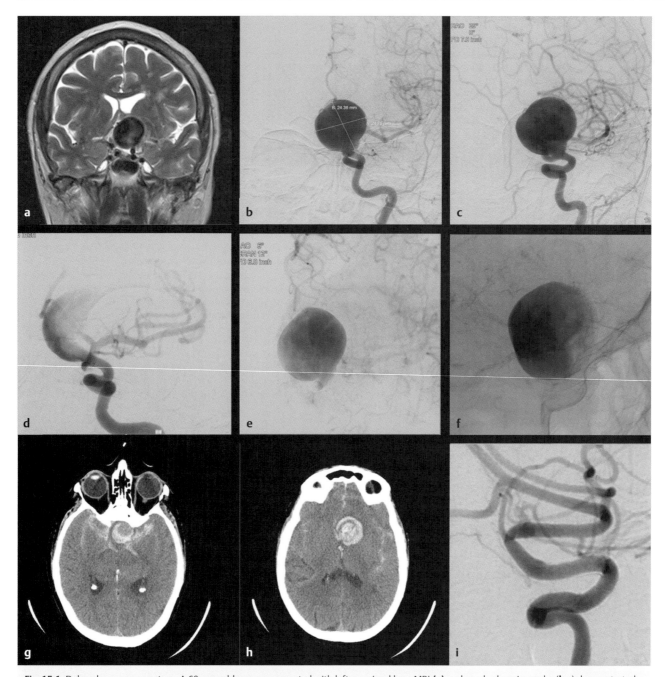

Fig. 15.1 Delayed aneurysm rupture: A 68-year-old woman presented with left eye visual loss. MRI **(a)** and cerebral angiography **(b,c)** demonstrated a giant left internal carotid artery ophthalmic segment aneurysm. The patient was treated with a single Pipeline Embolization Device (PED) placement. Note the contrast stasis induced by device placement **(d–f)**. Five-days posttreatment, the patient presented with delayed aneurysm ruptured demonstrated by CT head **(g,h)**. The patient survived the event and underwent retreatment with an additional PED. A 10-month follow-up angiography demonstrated complete aneurysm occlusion **(i)**.

15.4.5 Device Apposition

Complete device apposition to the vessel wall during initial PED deployment is a central component in achieving successful flow diversion and allows for the eventual neointimalization over the exposed area of the flow diverter. Likewise, incomplete device apposition can create a false lumen, allow for endoleak with persistent aneurysm filling, or potentially facilitate in-stent stenosis or thrombosis leading to delayed ischemic events.[27]

Fortunately, intraprocedural C-Arm CT can now be utilized to successfully visualize device apposition in cases where there is ambiguity with standard digital subtraction angiography techniques.[28,29,30] Balloon angioplasty can be used adjunctively during initial PED deployment to maximize device apposition. This concept is, by no means, new and the importance of good stent

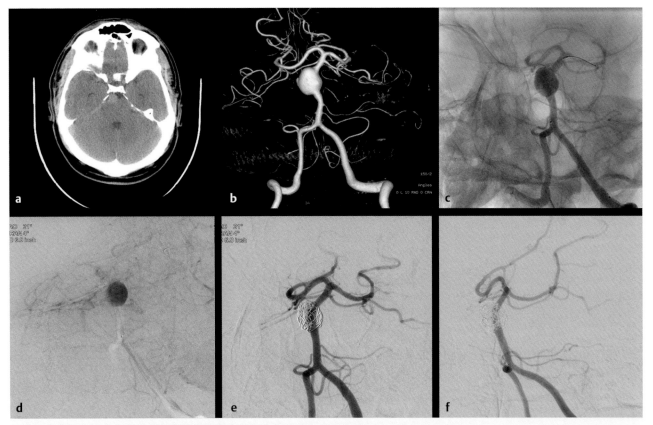

Fig. 15.2 Coiling to reduce delayed aneurysm rupture: A 44-year-old man presented with acute onset of headache. CT head **(a)** showed no evidence of hemorrhage. Cerebral angiography demonstrated a mid-basilar aneurysm with daughter sac **(b)**. Decision was made for Pipeline Embolization Device (PED)-assisted coiling. Microcatheter is jailed in the aneurysm **(c)**. PED is placed with good stasis of contrast within the aneurysm **(d)**. Adjuvant coiling is performed to reduce risk of delayed aneurysm rupture with immediate posttreatment result **(e)** shown. Twelve-month follow-up angiography with complete aneurysm occlusion **(f)**.

apposition with flow diversion has been widely recognized since the publication of the PUFS trial.

15.4.6 Choosing the Right Size

The PED can be expected to expand an extra 0.25-mm beyond its primary size under most circumstances. This can be useful in the setting of vessel diameter variability or irregularity allowing for additional expansion in these areas. Additionally, accurate measurement of the vessel diameter from angiographic runs or three-dimensional reconstructions can have inherent errors based on the calibration and image thresholding. When in doubt, our recommendation would be to oversize the device to mitigate the risk of device mal-apposition as described earlier.

Oversizing, however, can lead to overall lengthening of the constrained portion of the device, as well as decreasing the metal coverage with the PED from geometric "stretching" of the closed-cell design. With the PED, there is a predictable parabolic variability in device porosity based on the device-to-vessel diameter mismatch, as well as with high degrees of vessel curvature.[5] Vessel curvature is especially relevant around the tight turn of the carotid artery near the ophthalmic artery and can lead to the need to place more than one device in this region to adequately treat an ophthalmic segment aneurysm. This

inherent characteristic is reportedly minimized with the Surpass flow diverter.

The best strategy, however, is always choosing the appropriately sized device, as opposed to grossly oversizing for the sake of ensured apposition. The AngioSuite Calculator (Angiosuite.com) was developed to assist with the selection of an appropriately sized device. This smartphone application calculates the device size based on the proximal, mid-, and distal parent artery diameters and calculates the expanded length of the device once deployed in the parent vessel to ensure the best fit.

Despite our best efforts, there may be circumstances that ultimately prevent full apposition. A device deployed in the setting of vasospasm may initially appear to be well fit. However, once the vessel normalizes in caliber, the initial device sizing and apposition may be inappropriate. This could easily precipitate device migration and subsequent thrombosis of the vessel. Treatment options at this point are limited, as device retrieval is difficult or impossible. Furthermore, angioplasty or placement of additional devices may be futile in the setting of a grossly undersized device. The remaining definitive option, in this case, would be parent artery sacrifice to prevent propagation of any thrombus and subsequent stroke. This final option relies on the collateral circulation with augmented blood pressure to prevent misery perfusion. If artery occlusion is not feasible, a bypass surgery may be necessary to regain blood flow to the distal perfusion territory. To mitigate the risk of vasospasm, some authors advocate the routine use of pre–device deployment, intra-arterial verapamil in the planned area of treatment. After an intra-arterial dose (5–20 mg) is given, measurements of the parent vessel are taken from a new angiogram, reducing the likelihood of undersizing.

Accurate sizing of the device can be difficult in certain situations, especially if there is a significantly smaller distal vessel diameter compared with a more proximal diameter. This can lead to oversizing in the distal outflow region. Poor apposition of the device can occur during deployment due to the mismatch between the distal vessel diameter and the size of the device. In these situations, we use balloon angioplasty to ensure the best apposition. The balloon is initially inflated along the unapposed region to further expand the device. This is followed by inflation at the proximal end of the device with subsequent forward pressure to allow for better expansion to the vessel walls. However, excessive forward pressure can potentially lead to herniation of the device into the aneurysm or cause the device to buckle or "accordion" along the vessel wall.[31] However, when properly performed, this method can greatly improve the fit of the device along the vessel wall.

15.4.7 Foreign Body Retrieval

Flow diversion presents an often unique set of complications during deployment compared with traditional endovascular aneurysm treatment strategies. Technical difficulties during deployment of a flow diverter can precipitate serious complications, including vessel thrombus, vessel rupture, endothelial damage during retrieval, or dislodging of embolic material with subsequent stroke.

Foreign body retrieval may be necessary during any endovascular case and developing a contingency plan is critical to minimizing complications. Snare-loops, balloon catheters, curved catheters, and stone baskets have all been employed successfully for this purpose. In a recent comprehensive review of all reported cases of retrieval of malposition endovascular devices, it was found that endovascular methods of retrieval predominated (94% of cases) with high rates of success.[32] Combined open/endovascular methods of retrieval have also been used if endovascular retrieval is not possible or successful.

Additionally, severe twisting resulting in significant in-stent deformity after deployment of a flow diverter has been reported[33] and may present a more significant physical barrier to blood flow compared with other intracranial stents (i.e., Neuroform, Enterprise). In this instance, the device was retrieved using a 4-mm Amplatz Goose-Neck microsnare-loop (Covidien/EV3, Plymouth, MN) followed by the successful deployment of a second device. This early report, however, involved the use of a Pipeline Classic, which could not be resheathed unlike the newer Pipeline Flex.

15.5 Conclusion

Flow diverters not only have problems common to other stents but also possess their own unique set of problems. While the safety and efficacy of flow diverters have been demonstrated in recent trials and multiple case series, it is important to have an understanding of the difficulties that may arise during deployment. One should possess the basic strategies for complication avoidance and management during endovascular procedures, generally, and flow diversion, specifically. The authors stress the importance of the use of a triaxial delivery system, the careful use of dual-antiplatelet therapy, the need for correct device size selection, and the confirmation of good wall apposition in any case of flow diversion.

References

[1] Cooper B. Lectures on the Principles and Practice of Surgery. 2nd ed. Philadelphia, PA: Blanchard & Lee; 1852

[2] Sadasivan C, Cesar L, Seong J, et al. An original flow diversion device for the treatment of intracranial aneurysms: evaluation in the rabbit elastase-induced model. Stroke. 2009; 40(3):952–958

[3] Sadasivan C, Cesar L, Seong J, Wakhloo AK, Lieber BB. Treatment of rabbit elastase-induced aneurysm models by flow diverters: development of quantifiable indexes of device performance using digital subtraction angiography. IEEE Trans Med Imaging. 2009; 28(7):1117–1125

[4] Kadirvel R, Ding YH, Dai D, Rezek I, Lewis DA, Kallmes DF. Cellular mechanisms of aneurysm occlusion after treatment with a flow diverter. Radiology. 2014; 270(2):394–399

[5] Shapiro M, Raz E, Becske T, Nelson PK. Variable porosity of the pipeline embolization device in straight and curved vessels: a guide for optimal deployment strategy. AJNR Am J Neuroradiol. 2014; 35(4):727–733

[6] Sorkin GC, Dumont TM, Wach MM, et al. Carotid artery stenting outcomes: do they correlate with antiplatelet response assays? J Neurointerv Surg. 2014; 6(5):373–378

[7] Stone GW, Witzenbichler B, Weisz G, et al. ADAPT-DES Investigators. Platelet reactivity and clinical outcomes after coronary artery implantation of drug-eluting stents (ADAPT-DES): a prospective multicentre registry study. Lancet. 2013; 382(9892):614–623

[8] Breet NJ, van Werkum JW, Bouman HJ, et al. Comparison of platelet function tests in predicting clinical outcome in patients undergoing coronary stent implantation. JAMA. 2010; 303(8):754–762

[9] Price MJ, Endemann S, Gollapudi RR, et al. Prognostic significance of post-clopidogrel platelet reactivity assessed by a point-of-care assay on thrombotic events after drug-eluting stent implantation. Eur Heart J. 2008; 29(8):992–1000

[10] Delgado Almandoz JE, Crandall BM, Scholz JM, et al. Last-recorded P2Y12 reaction units value is strongly associated with thromboembolic and hemorrhagic complications occurring up to 6 months after treatment in patients with cerebral aneurysms treated with the pipeline embolization device. AJNR Am J Neuroradiol. 2014; 35(1):128–135

[11] Collet JP, Cuisset T, Rangé G, et al. ARCTIC Investigators. Bedside monitoring to adjust antiplatelet therapy for coronary stenting. N Engl J Med. 2012; 367 (22):2100–2109

[12] Becske T, Kallmes DF, Saatci I, et al. Pipeline for uncoilable or failed aneurysms: results from a multicenter clinical trial. Radiology. 2013; 267 (3):858–868

[13] Brinjikji W, Lanzino G, Cloft HJ, et al. Risk factors for ischemic complications following Pipeline Embolization Device treatment of intracranial aneurysms: results from the IntrePED study. AJNR Am J Neuroradiol. 2016; 37(9):1673–1678

[14] Kallmes DF, Hanel R, Lopes D, et al. International retrospective study of the pipeline embolization device: a multicenter aneurysm treatment study. AJNR Am J Neuroradiol. 2015; 36(1):108–115

[15] Daou B, Starke RM, Chalouhi N, et al. P2Y12 reaction units: effect on hemorrhagic and thromboembolic complications in patients with cerebral aneurysms treated with the Pipeline Embolization Device. Neurosurgery. 2016; 78 (1):27–33

[16] Tan LA, Keigher KM, Munich SA, Moftakhar R, Lopes DK. Thromboembolic complications with Pipeline Embolization Device placement: impact of procedure time, number of stents and pre-procedure P2Y12 reaction unit (PRU) value. J Neurointerv Surg. 2015; 7(3):217–221

[17] Delgado Almandoz JE, Crandall BM, Scholz JM, et al. Pre-procedure P2Y12 reaction units value predicts perioperative thromboembolic and hemorrhagic

complications in patients with cerebral aneurysms treated with the Pipeline Embolization Device. J Neurointerv Surg. 2013; 5 Suppl 3:iii3–iii10

[18] Hanel RA, Taussky P, Dixon T, et al. Safety and efficacy of ticagrelor for neuro-endovascular procedures. A single center initial experience. J Neurointerv Surg. 2014; 6(4):320–322

[19] Nordeen JD, Patel AV, Darracott RM, et al. Clopidogrel resistance by P2Y12 platelet function testing in patients undergoing neuroendovascular proce-dures: incidence of ischemic and hemorrhagic complications. J Vasc Interv Neurol. 2013; 6(1):26–34

[20] Rouchaud A, Brinjikji W, Lanzino G, Cloft HJ, Kadirvel R, Kallmes DF. Delayed hemorrhagic complications after flow diversion for intracranial aneurysms: a literature overview. Neuroradiology. 2016; 58(2):171–177

[21] Lylyk P, Miranda C, Ceratto R, et al. Curative endovascular reconstruction of cerebral aneurysms with the pipeline embolization device: the Buenos Aires experience. Neurosurgery. 2009; 64(4):632–642, discussion 642–643, quiz N6

[22] Gross BA, Frerichs KU. Stent usage in the treatment of intracranial aneu-rysms: past, present and future. J Neurol Neurosurg Psychiatry. 2013; 84 (3):244–253

[23] Cohen JE, Gomori JM, Moscovici S, Leker RR, Itshayek E. Delayed complica-tions after flow-diverter stenting: reactive in-stent stenosis and creeping stents. J Clin Neurosci. 2014; 21(7):1116–1122

[24] Lubicz B, Van der Elst O, Collignon L, Mine B, Alghamdi F. Silk flow-diverter stent for the treatment of intracranial aneurysms: a series of 58 patients with emphasis on long-term results. AJNR Am J Neuroradiol. 2015; 36(3):542–546

[25] Kan P, Siddiqui AH, Veznedaroglu E, et al. Early postmarket results after treat-ment of intracranial aneurysms with the pipeline embolization device: a U.S.

multicenter experience. Neurosurgery. 2012; 71(6):1080–1087, discussion 1087–1088

[26] Cebral JR, Mut F, Raschi M, et al. Aneurysm rupture following treatment with flow-diverting stents: computational hemodynamics analysis of treatment. AJNR Am J Neuroradiol. 2011; 32(1):27–33

[27] Heller R, Calnan DR, Lanfranchi M, Madan N, Malek AM. Incomplete stent apposition in Enterprise stent-mediated coiling of aneurysms: persistence over time and risk of delayed ischemic events. J Neurosurg. 2013; 118 (5):1014–1022

[28] Ding D, Starke RM, Durst CR, et al. DynaCT imaging for intraprocedural evalu-ation of flow-diverting stent apposition during endovascular treatment of intracranial aneurysms. J Clin Neurosci. 2014; 21(11):1981–1983

[29] Heran NS, Song JK, Namba K, Smith W, Niimi Y, Berenstein A. The utility of DynaCT in neuroendovascular procedures. AJNR Am J Neuroradiol. 2006; 27 (2):330–332

[30] Moskowitz SI, Kelly ME, Haynes J, Fiorella D. DynaCT evaluation of in-stent restenosis following Wingspan stenting of intracranial stenosis. J Neurointerv Surg. 2010; 2(1):2–5

[31] Martínez-Galdámez M, Ortega-Quintanilla J, Hermosín A, Crespo-Vallejo E, Ailagas JJ, Pérez S. Novel balloon application for rescue and realignment of a proximal end migrated pipeline flex embolization device into the aneurysmal sac: complication management. BMJ Case Rep. 2016; 2016

[32] Schechter MA, O'Brien PJ, Cox MW. Retrieval of iatrogenic intravascular for-eign bodies. J Vasc Surg. 2013; 57(1):276–281

[33] Mitchell B, Jou LD, Mawad M. Retrieval of distorted pipeline embolic device using snare-loop. J Vasc Interv Neurol. 2014; 7(5):1–4

16 POSTPROCEDURAL COMPLICATIONS

M. YASHAR S. KALANI, MIN S. PARK, PHILIPP TAUSSKY, and CAMERON G. McDOUGALL

Abstract

Flow-diverting stents have allowed for anatomical reconstruction of diseased vasculature using a minimally invasive approach, but their use is associated with unique complications. The introduction of foreign material, its interaction with the endothelium and clotting cascade, and even restoration of normal flow patterns can result in injury and complication. This chapter includes a review of postprocedural complications associated with the use of flow-diverting technology, focusing on thrombotic and hemorrhagic complications.

Keywords: aneurysm, complications, flow diversion, flow-diverting stents, occlusion, rupture

16.1 Introduction

Flow-diverting stents have revolutionized the care of cerebral aneurysms. Although the transition from Hunterian ligation to aneurysm clipping heralded an era of improved outcome for patients,[1] it was the introduction of endovascular techniques in the form of the Guglielmi detachable coil,[2,3] the improvements on the basic design of this technology and the advent of stents and flow-altering technology allowed for anatomical reconstruction of diseased vasculature using a minimally invasive approach.[4,5,6,7] The bare metal nature of flow-diverting stents provides a scaffold on which endothelial cells can grow, thereby excluding the aneurysm sac from the parent artery flow, but this very nature predisposes flow-diverting stents to a set of unique complications. Although flow-diverting stents allow for restoration of more physiological flows within diseased vasculature, the introduction of foreign material, its interaction with the endothelium and clotting cascade, and perhaps even restoration of normal flow patterns, can result in injury and complication. Soon after the first use of flow-diverting stents, it became clear that this technology is by no means benign and is associated with a nonnegligible complication rate, both intra- and postprocedural.[8] In this chapter, we review the data on the postprocedural complications associated with the use of flow-diverting technology, focusing on thrombotic and hemorrhagic complications.

16.2 Complication Rates after Flow Diversion

Flow diversion, like most disruptive technologies, has revolutionized the treatment of cerebral aneurysms. With the introduction and widespread use of flow diversion, however, a new battery of complications that are seldom noted with simple coiling or stent-assisted coiling of cerebral aneurysms has been reported.[9] These include, broadly, thrombotic[10,11,12,13] and hemorrhagic[14,15,16,17,18] complications. The overall perioperative morbidity and mortality rates associated with flow diversion range from 8 to 10%.[19,20] A recent pooled analysis of the International Retrospective study of the Pipeline Embolization Device (IntrePED),[21] Pipeline for Uncoilable or Failed Aneurysms (PUFS),[4] and Aneurysm Study of Pipeline in an Observational Registry (ASPIRe)[22] studies reported a major ipsilateral intracranial hemorrhage rate of 2%, major ipsilateral ischemic stroke rate of 3.7%, major morbidity rate of 5.7%, and mortality rate of 3.3% in a cohort of 1,092 patients with 1,221 aneurysms.[23] Despite small reports on factors predisposing to these complications, the cause of the majority of these complications remains unknown.[17,18] Common to these complications is the temporal window in which most of these events occur—limited, generally, to the first month after deployment of the device—and the often-poor outcome associated with these complications, which is frequently due to the accompanying dual-antiplatelet regimens.

16.3 Thrombotic Complications of Flow Diversion

16.3.1 Occlusion of Device and Stroke

Although uncommon, ischemic stroke is the leading cause of complications after treatment of aneurysms using flow diverters and is identified in 3 to 6% of patients.[4,20,21] In the PUFS trial, the rate of acute ischemic stroke within 6 months of treatment was 6.5%. In this cohort, 2.8% of patients had stroke secondary to in-stent thrombosis or occlusion.[24] The rate of stroke after 6 months was 0% in this cohort. Review of the IntrePED registry noted an incidence of 4.5% of ischemic stroke (36/793 patients with 906 aneurysms).[25] In this series, 72.2% of all strokes occurred within 30 days of treatment (median, 3.5 days; range, 0–397 days), resulting in 10 deaths and 26 major neurological deficits. On multivariate analysis, fusiform aneurysm was the only predictor of postprocedural ischemic stroke. Larger fusiform aneurysms had a higher rate of complications than smaller fusiform aneurysms.

Park et al[26] reported four permanent complications resulting in death or permanent morbidity in a cohort of 126 patients treated at the Barrow Neurological Institute (mortality rate of 3.2%). There were four cerebrovascular accidents in the absence of device occlusion (► Fig. 16.1), one of which resulted in death. A second patient had clot in the device and underwent uneventful clot removal. Six patients had complete occlusion of their flow diverters on follow-up imaging. Two had devastating neurological deficits as a result of occlusion and died. The remaining four had no deficits or neurological sequelae.

One noted cause of thrombotic complication is the resistance of a subset of the population to aspirin and clopidogrel.[27,28] This resistance is further complicated by lack of consistency and agreement with regard to the appropriate antiplatelet regimen after flow diverter placement.[29] Tan et al[30] reported thromboembolic complications in 6.8% of patients treated with a Pipeline Embolization Device (PED). In this cohort, patients with P2Y12 reaction unit values of more than 208 were more likely to have thromboembolic complications. In a meta-analysis of 19 studies, Skukalek et al[31] identified that the use of high-dose aspirin less than 6 months post–PED deployment was

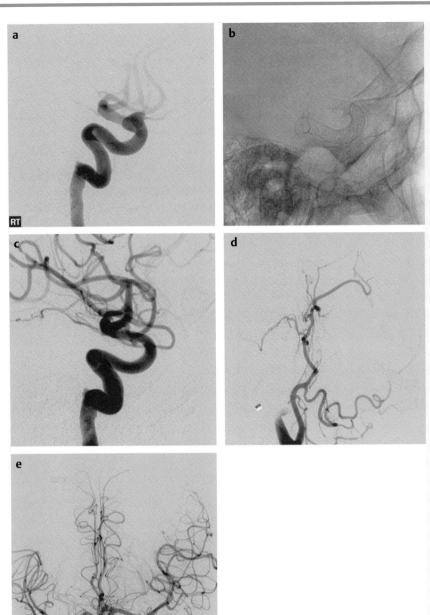

Fig. 16.1 Delayed occlusion of Pipeline Embolization Device (PED). **(a)** Working angle projection of a right ophthalmic segment aneurysm. **(b)** Native projection following deployment of two PEDs. **(c)** Final angiography after treatment of aneurysm. **(d)** Follow-up angiography 2 weeks after deployment of PED demonstrates occlusion of left internal carotid artery. **(e)** Left internal carotid artery injection demonstrates filling across the anterior communicating artery. (Reproduced with permission from Park et al.[26])

associated with fewer thrombotic events than when low-dose aspirin was used. A higher rate of thrombotic events was observed with the use of clopidogrel less than 6 months post–PED deployment.

Other mechanisms of ischemia in a delayed fashion include acute and subacute in-stent thrombosis during the procedure resulting in postoperative occlusion of the stent with or without distal emboli, exacerbated by inappropriate dual-antiplatelet regimens and the bare metal nature of the stent.

16.3.2 Occlusion of Side Branches and Perforators

Occlusion of side branches or perforating vessels can cause devastating strokes when these vessels represent end vessels without redundant or anastomotic circulations. Posterior circulation aneurysms or those aneurysms with perforating vessels emanating from the diseased portion of the vessel (e.g., lenticulostriate arteries from the M1 segment of the middle cerebral artery) are at a higher risk of complication with perforator strokes.[32,33] A recent meta-analysis noted a perforator infarction rate of 3.0% across all aneurysms studied and a higher rate in aneurysms in the posterior circulation.[20] The higher complication rate of thrombosis in the treatment of dolichoectatic and fusiform basilar artery aneurysms with the use of flow diverters provides a cause for pause in the use of these devices for this subset of aneurysms.[34] The higher complication rate in this group is likely caused by poor wall apposition of flow diverters in the setting of fusiform aneurysms. Poor wall apposition results in delayed endothelialization of stents and increased likelihood of in-stent thrombosis and embolization. Other factors include the larger size of these aneurysms, use of multiple flow diverters, and nonuniform use of dual-antiplatelet medications.[12,21,34,35]

Occlusion of the anterior choroidal artery can have potentially devastating complications, but fortunately it appears that anterior choroidal artery loss after flow diversion is a rare event. Brinjikji et al[36] reported their experience with flow diversion for ICA aneurysms in which the anterior choroidal artery was covered by the stent. In the immediate postprocedure setting, all 15 patients in this study had patency of the anterior choroidal artery. At 6-month follow-up, only a single anterior choroidal artery was occluded, and this patient did not suffer any complications from the loss of this artery. In a cohort of 49 patients treated with flow diversion in whom branch vessels of the internal carotid artery were covered by the flow-diverting stents, the overall rate of branch vessel occlusion was 4% for the ophthalmic artery, 7.1% for the posterior communicating artery, and 0% for the anterior choroidal artery. None of these patients had neurological deficits secondary to the occlusion of the covered vessel. Branch occlusion was not associated with the number of flow diverters used.[37] A second larger cohort of 82 patients was recently described by the Buffalo group.[38] In this cohort, 127 arterial branches were covered by flow diverters. At a mean angiographic follow-up of 10 months, arterial branch occlusion occurred in 15.8% and included occlusion of the anterior cerebral arteries ($n = 2$), ophthalmic arteries ($n = 8$), and posterior communicating arteries ($n = 3$). There were no anterior choroidal artery occlusions in this series, and none of the patients experienced neurological deficits.

Occlusion of the ophthalmic artery in a delayed fashion has been reported,[39,40] although in most cases this occlusion is of no consequence because of the redundant collateral circulation provided to the territory by branches of the external carotid artery. In rare cases, occlusion of the ophthalmic artery can cause visual disturbances.[41]

16.4 Hemorrhagic Complications of Flow Diversion

16.4.1 Delayed Aneurysm Rupture

Delayed rupture of cerebral aneurysm is a poorly understood complication of flow diversion. Rouchaud et al[42] recently presented a systematic review on delayed hemorrhagic complications after flow diversion. They identified 81 cases of delayed aneurysm rupture and 101 cases of delayed intraparenchymal hemorrhage. In this cohort, the majority of delayed aneurysm ruptures (76.6%) occurred within 1 month of treatment, and most (81.3%) were associated with a poor outcome (death or severe neurological deficits). Giant aneurysm size is one of the strongest predictors of delayed aneurysm rupture after flow diversion.[16,17,21] In the same cohort, aneurysms of all rupture status accounted for 46.3% of all cases of delayed ruptured aneurysms.[42] Interestingly, giant aneurysms represent a small subset of all aneurysms treated with flow diversion; in the IntrePED cohort, giant

aneurysms comprised 16% of all treated aneurysm but accounted for a disproportionate number of cases of delayed aneurysm rupture.[21] A minority of giant aneurysms treated with flow diversion and concomitant coiling (17.8%) accounted for delayed cases of ruptured, reaffirming the notion that addition of coils decreases the likelihood of delayed ruptures,[18,43,44] but documenting that a minority of cases of giant aneurysms go on to rupture even in the presence of adjunctive coiling. The decision to use coiling in an aneurysm in which flow diversion has already been completed should include an assessment of the added risk associated with coiling relative to coil/flow diversion and the increased time of the procedure associated with concomitant coiling, which could increase the risk of complications.[45] What is not clear is the relative packing density of the aneurysms that ruptured with flow diversion despite coiling. It is possible that denser packing of the aneurysm sac, which is associated with its own challenges, may decrease the risk of rupture in this subset.

The cause of delayed aneurysm rupture remains enigmatic. Computational flow dynamic studies suggest that alterations of flow within the aneurysm could result in intra-aneurysmal pressure elevation, predisposing to aneurysm rupture.[14] Others propose that sudden thrombosis of the aneurysm sac can result in the release of proteases that result in rapid breakdown of weakened aneurysmal wall and hemorrhage.[46,47,48,49,50,51,52,53]

16.4.2 Distal Lobar Hemorrhages

Delayed intraparenchymal hemorrhages are a devastating complication of flow diversion that has occurred in 2 to 3% of cases.[20,21] In a cohort of 793 patients with 906 cerebral aneurysms in the IntrePED registry, 20 (2.5%) had intraparenchymal hemorrhages.[25] In a recent meta-analysis of all reported cases in the literature of cases of delayed intraparenchymal hemorrhage, 82.2% were ipsilateral to the site of treatment. The majority occurred within 1 month of treatment (86%),[42] and a quarter of these hemorrhages occurred within 24 hours of flow diversion. In one study, all cases of delayed hemorrhages occurred within 6 months of treatment, and higher risk of hemorrhage correlated with the use of three or more flow-diverting devices.[25] Interestingly, one in five cases of delayed intraparenchymal hemorrhage was in the contralateral hemisphere to the side treated. Given that this hemisphere is unlikely to be hemodynamically affected[14,54,55] by the placement of the flow diverter and is likely free of thrombotic events, the dual-antiplatelet regimen has been proposed to have a role as a causative driver of this complication. It is interesting to note that dual-antiplatelet regimens appear safer in the setting of stroke prevention (annual risk of hemorrhage: 1.5%) and in the setting of stent-assisted coiling (annual risk of hemorrhage: 2.2%).[56] The coincident timing of hemorrhage, with most cases occurring during the first month after treatment, and the fact that patients are maintained on dual-antiplatelet regimens for at least 3 months cannot be overlooked. Studies suggest that a P2Y12 reaction unit value of less than 60 portends a higher risk of hemorrhage, and care must be taken to maintain the patient in a therapeutic and non-supratherapeutic window.[57,58] Despite this, no study to date has documented a lower risk of hemorrhage secondary to titration of dual-antiplatelet medication after P2Y12 testing.

The increased metal surface area of flow diverters has been suggested as a contributor to activation of the clotting cascade despite antiplatelet use. This theory is supported by the higher incidence of hemorrhages with use of multiple flow-diverting stents for treatment of a single lesion.

The contribution to delayed hemorrhage of intraprocedural exposure to the foreign material coating (polyvinylpyrrolidone) of the shuttle guide sheath has been reported (▶ Fig. 16.2), but this effect has been questioned by other studies.[25,59] The possibility that these hemorrhages are the result of hemorrhagic conversion of microthrombi has also been proposed but is not well validated.[60,61] The increased association of these types of hemorrhage with treatment of giant aneurysms has been noted (23%) and has been attributed to hemodynamic factors (Windkessel effect),[54,55] prolonged procedure times, and increased complexity of the treatment paradigms used to treat giant lesions.[20,42]

Of these factors, the theory of hyperperfusion (Windkessel effect)[54,55] after flow diversion requires some discussion. This theory postulates that increased flow into distal arterial territory, secondary to exclusion of flow into the aneurysm sac, overwhelms the system and results in hemorrhage. Interestingly, similar changes are noted after aneurysmal clipping of giant aneurysms.[62]

Regardless of the cause, delayed intraparenchymal hemorrhage was associated with a significant rate of morbidity and mortality (68.5%), although a minority of hemorrhages were documented in patients with giant aneurysms (23%). Tomas et al[61] suggested that evacuation of hematomas in patients with delayed hemorrhages may result in improved outcomes and is safe despite the presence of dual-antiplatelet medications.

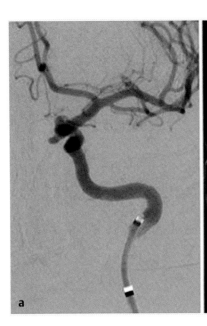
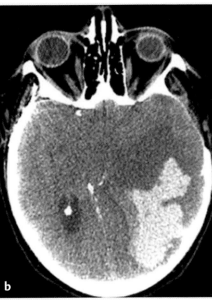

Fig. 16.2 Delayed intraparenchymal hemorrhage after deployment of Pipeline Embolization Device (PED). **(a)** Pretreatment angiography demonstrates a left paraophthalmic aneurysm. **(b)** Axial computed tomography obtained after intracranial hemorrhage in this patient (*continued*).

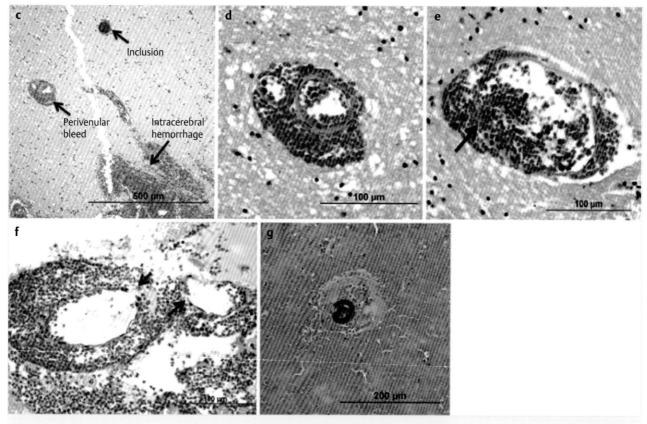

Fig. 16.2 (*continued*) **(c–g)** Photomicrographs showing a foreign body inclusion (*arrows*) near the region of intracerebral hemorrhage. (Reproduced with permission from Hu et al.[59])

16.5 Conclusion

Flow diversion has changed the treatment paradigm for cerebral aneurysms. Many aneurysms that were previously not amenable to standard microsurgical or endovascular treatment are now readily treated using flow diversion. Despite these advances, the 5 to 10% rate of complications associated with the use of flow diverters raises a flag of caution that this technology should be used judiciously and its overzealous application can result in preventable complications in patients.

References

[1] Polevaya NV, Kalani MY, Steinberg GK, Tse VC. The transition from hunterian ligation to intracranial aneurysm clips: a historical perspective. Neurosurg Focus. 2006; 20(6):E3

[2] Guglielmi G, Viñuela F, Dion J, Duckwiler G. Electrothrombosis of saccular aneurysms via endovascular approach. Part 2: Preliminary clinical experience. J Neurosurg. 1991; 75(1):8–14

[3] Guglielmi G, Viñuela F, Sepetka I, Macellari V. Electrothrombosis of saccular aneurysms via endovascular approach. Part 1: Electrochemical basis, technique, and experimental results. J Neurosurg. 1991; 75(1):1–7

[4] Becske T, Kallmes DF, Saatci I, et al. Pipeline for uncoilable or failed aneurysms: results from a multicenter clinical trial. Radiology. 2013; 267 (3):858–868

[5] Grotenhuis JA, de Vries J, Tacl S. Angioscopy-guided placement of balloon-expandable stents in the treatment of experimental carotid aneurysms. Minim Invasive Neurosurg. 1994; 37(2):56–60

[6] Nelson PK, Lylyk P, Szikora I, Wetzel SG, Wanke I, Fiorella D. The pipeline embolization device for the intracranial treatment of aneurysms trial. AJNR Am J Neuroradiol. 2011; 32(1):34–40

[7] Saatci I, Yavuz K, Ozer C, Geyik S, Cekirge HS. Treatment of intracranial aneurysms using the pipeline flow-diverter embolization device: a single-center experience with long-term follow-up results. AJNR Am J Neuroradiol. 2012; 33(8):1436–1446

[8] van Rooij WJ, Sluzewski M. Perforator infarction after placement of a pipeline flow-diverting stent for an unruptured A1 aneurysm. AJNR Am J Neuroradiol. 2010; 31(4):E43–E44

[9] Ravindra VM, Mazur MD, Park MS, et al. Complications in endovascular neurosurgery: critical analysis and classification. World Neurosurg. 2016; 95:1–8

[10] Cirillo L, Leonardi M, Dall'olio M, et al. Complications in the treatment of intracranial aneurysms with silk stents: an analysis of 30 consecutive patients. Interv Neuroradiol. 2012; 18(4):413–425

[11] Fiorella D, Hsu D, Woo HH, Tarr RW, Nelson PK. Very late thrombosis of a pipeline embolization device construct: case report. Neurosurgery. 2010; 67 3 Suppl Operative:E313–E314, discussion E314

[12] Klisch J, Turk A, Turner R, Woo HH, Fiorella D. Very late thrombosis of flow-diverting constructs after the treatment of large fusiform posterior circulation aneurysms. AJNR Am J Neuroradiol. 2011; 32(4):627–632

[13] Phillips TJ, Wenderoth JD, Phatouros CC, et al. Safety of the pipeline embolization device in treatment of posterior circulation aneurysms. AJNR Am J Neuroradiol. 2012; 33(7):1225–1231

[14] Cebral JR, Mut F, Raschi M, et al. Aneurysm rupture following treatment with flow-diverting stents: computational hemodynamics analysis of treatment. AJNR Am J Neuroradiol. 2011; 32(1):27–33

[15] Cruz JP, Chow M, O'Kelly C, et al. Delayed ipsilateral parenchymal hemorrhage following flow diversion for the treatment of anterior circulation aneurysms. AJNR Am J Neuroradiol. 2012; 33(4):603–608

[16] Kulcsár Z, Houdart E, Bonafé A, et al. Intra-aneurysmal thrombosis as a possible cause of delayed aneurysm rupture after flow-diversion treatment. AJNR Am J Neuroradiol. 2011; 32(1):20–25

[17] Kulcsár Z, Szikora I.. The ESMINT Retrospective Analysis of Delayed Aneurysm Ruptures after flow diversion (RADAR) study. EJMINT. 2012; 2012:1244000088

[18] Turowski B, Macht S, Kulcsár Z, Hänggi D, Stummer W. Early fatal hemorrhage after endovascular cerebral aneurysm treatment with a flow diverter (SILK-Stent): do we need to rethink our concepts? Neuroradiology. 2011; 53 (1):37–41

[19] Arrese I, Sarabia R, Pintado R, Delgado-Rodriguez M. Flow-diverter devices for intracranial aneurysms: systematic review and meta-analysis. Neurosurgery. 2013; 73(2):193–199, discussion 199–200

[20] Brinjikji W, Murad MH, Lanzino G, Cloft HJ, Kallmes DF. Endovascular treatment of intracranial aneurysms with flow diverters: a meta-analysis. Stroke. 2013; 44(2):442–447

[21] Kallmes DF, Hanel R, Lopes D, et al. International retrospective study of the pipeline embolization device: a multicenter aneurysm treatment study. AJNR Am J Neuroradiol. 2015; 36(1):108–115

[22] Aneurysm Study of Pipeline in an Observational Registry (ASPIRE). Available at: https://clinicaltrials.gov/ct2/show/NCT01557036. Accessed December 28, 2016

[23] Kallmes DF, Brinjikji W, Cekirge S, et al. Safety and efficacy of the Pipeline embolization device for treatment of intracranial aneurysms: a pooled analysis of 3 large studies. J Neurosurg. 2016 Oct 28:1–6 [Epub ahead of print]

[24] Kallmes DF, Ding YH, Dai D, Kadirvel R, Lewis DA, Cloft HJ. A new endoluminal, flow-disrupting device for treatment of saccular aneurysms. Stroke. 2007; 38(8):2346–2352

[25] Brinjikji W, Lanzino G, Cloft HJ, et al. Risk factors for ischemic complications following Pipeline Embolization Device treatment of intracranial aneurysms: results from the IntrePED study. AJNR Am J Neuroradiol. 2016; 37(9):1673–1678

[26] Park MS, Albuquerque FC, Nanaszko M, et al. Critical assessment of complications associated with use of the Pipeline Embolization Device. J Neurointerv Surg. 2015; 7(9):652–659

[27] Delgado Almandoz JE, Kadkhodayan Y, Crandall BM, Scholz JM, Fease JL, Tubman DE. Variability in initial response to standard clopidogrel therapy, delayed conversion to clopidogrel hyper-response, and associated thromboembolic and hemorrhagic complications in patients undergoing endovascular treatment of unruptured cerebral aneurysms. J Neurointerv Surg. 2014; 6(10):767–773

[28] Jones GM, Twilla JD, Hoit DA, Arthur AS. Prevention of stent thrombosis with reduced dose of prasugrel in two patients undergoing treatment of cerebral aneurysms with pipeline embolisation devices. J Neurointerv Surg. 2013; 5 (5):e38

[29] Faught RW, Satti SR, Hurst RW, Pukenas BA, Smith MJ. Heterogeneous practice patterns regarding antiplatelet medications for neuroendovascular stenting in the USA: a multicenter survey. J Neurointerv Surg. 2014; 6(10):774–779

[30] Tan LA, Keigher KM, Munich SA, Moftakhar R, Lopes DK. Thromboembolic complications with Pipeline Embolization Device placement: impact of procedure time, number of stents and pre-procedure P2Y12 reaction unit (PRU) value. J Neurointerv Surg. 2015; 7(3):217–221

[31] Skukalek SL, Winkler AM, Kang J, et al. Effect of antiplatelet therapy and platelet function testing on hemorrhagic and thrombotic complications in patients with cerebral aneurysms treated with the pipeline embolization device: a review and meta-analysis. J Neurointerv Surg. 2016; 8(1):58–65

[32] Gawlitza M, Januel AC, Tall P, Bonneville F, Cognard C. Flow diversion treatment of complex bifurcation aneurysms beyond the circle of Willis: a single-center series with special emphasis on covered cortical branches and perforating arteries. J Neurointerv Surg. 2016; 8(5):481–487

[33] Peschillo S, Caporlingua A, Cannizzaro D, et al. Flow diverter stent treatment for ruptured basilar trunk perforator aneurysms. J Neurointerv Surg. 2016; 8 (2):190–196

[34] Siddiqui AH, Abla AA, Kan P, et al. Panacea or problem: flow diverters in the treatment of symptomatic large or giant fusiform vertebrobasilar aneurysms. J Neurosurg. 2012; 116(6):1258–1266

[35] Szikora I, Turányi E, Marosfoi M. Evolution of flow-diverter endothelialization and thrombus organization in giant fusiform aneurysms after flow diversion: a histopathologic study. AJNR Am J Neuroradiol. 2015; 36(9):1716–1720

[36] Brinjikji W, Kallmes DF, Cloft HJ, Lanzino G. Patency of the anterior choroidal artery after flow-diversion treatment of internal carotid artery aneurysms. AJNR Am J Neuroradiol. 2015; 36(3):537–541

[37] Vedantam A, Rao VY, Shaltoni HM, Mawad ME. Incidence and clinical implications of carotid branch occlusion following treatment of internal carotid

[38] Rangel-Castilla L, Munich SA, Jaleel N, et al. Patency of anterior circulation branch vessels after Pipeline embolization: longer-term results from 82 aneurysm cases. J Neurosurg. 2017 Apr; 126(4):1064–1069 Epub 2016 Jun 10

[39] Moon K, Albuquerque FC, Ducruet AF, Webster Crowley R, McDougall CG. Treatment of ophthalmic segment carotid aneurysms using the pipeline embolization device: clinical and angiographic follow-up. Neurol Res. 2014; 36(4):344–350

[40] Puffer RC, Kallmes DF, Cloft HJ, Lanzino G. Patency of the ophthalmic artery after flow diversion treatment of paraclinoid aneurysms. J Neurosurg. 2012; 116(4):892–896

[41] Szikora I, Berentei Z, Kulcsar Z, et al. Treatment of intracranial aneurysms by functional reconstruction of the parent artery: the Budapest experience with the pipeline embolization device. AJNR Am J Neuroradiol. 2010; 31(6):1139–1147

[42] Rouchaud A, Brinjikji W, Lanzino G, Cloft HJ, Kadirvel R, Kallmes DF. Delayed hemorrhagic complications after flow diversion for intracranial aneurysms: a literature overview. Neuroradiology. 2016; 58(2):171–177

[43] Berge J, Biondi A, Machi P, et al. Flow-diverter silk stent for the treatment of intracranial aneurysms: 1-year follow-up in a multicenter study. AJNR Am J Neuroradiol. 2012; 33(6):1150–1155

[44] Velioglu M, Kizilkilic O, Selcuk H, et al. Early and midterm results of complex cerebral aneurysms treated with Silk stent. Neuroradiology. 2012; 54 (12):1355–1365

[45] Park MS, Kilburg C, Taussky P, et al. Pipeline Embolization Device with or without adjunctive coil embolization: analysis of complications from the IntrePED Registry. AJNR Am J Neuroradiol. 2016; 37(6):1127–1131

[46] Adolph R, Vorp DA, Steed DL, Webster MW, Kameneva MV, Watkins SC. Cellular content and permeability of intraluminal thrombus in abdominal aortic aneurysm. J Vasc Surg. 1997; 25(5):916–926

[47] Carrell TW, Burnand KG, Booth NA, Humphries J, Smith A. Intraluminal thrombus enhances proteolysis in abdominal aortic aneurysms. Vascular. 2006; 14(1):9–16

[48] Fontaine V, Jacob MP, Houard X, et al. Involvement of the mural thrombus as a site of protease release and activation in human aortic aneurysms. Am J Pathol. 2002; 161(5):1701–1710

[49] Frösen J, Piippo A, Paetau A, et al. Remodeling of saccular cerebral artery aneurysm wall is associated with rupture: histological analysis of 24 unruptured and 42 ruptured cases. Stroke. 2004; 35(10):2287–2293

[50] Houard X, Rouzet F, Touat Z, et al. Topology of the fibrinolytic system within the mural thrombus of human abdominal aortic aneurysms. J Pathol. 2007; 212(1):20–28

[51] Michel JB, Rouer M, Alsac JM. Regarding "A multilayer stent in the aorta may not seal the aneurysm, thereby leading to rupture". J Vasc Surg. 2013; 57 (2):605

[52] Rossignol P, Fontaine V, Meilhac O, Anglés-Cano E, Jacob MP, Michel JB. Physiopathology of aortic aneurysm [in French]. Rev Prat. 2002; 52(10):1061–1065

[53] Tulamo R, Frösen J, Hernesniemi J, Niemelä M. Inflammatory changes in the aneurysm wall: a review. J Neurointerv Surg. 2010; 2(2):120–130

[54] Mitha AP, Mynard JP, Storwick JA, Shivji ZI, Wong JH, Morrish W. Can the Windkessel hypothesis explain delayed intraparenchymal haemorrhage after flow diversion? A case report and model-based analysis of possible mechanisms. Heart Lung Circ. 2015; 24(8):824–830

[55] Velat GJ, Fargen KM, Lawson MF, Hoh BL, Fiorella D, Mocco J. Delayed intraparenchymal hemorrhage following pipeline embolization device treatment for a giant recanalized ophthalmic aneurysm. J Neurointerv Surg. 2012; 4(5):e24

[56] Diener HC, Bogousslavsky J, Brass LM, et al. MATCH investigators. Aspirin and clopidogrel compared with clopidogrel alone after recent ischaemic stroke or transient ischaemic attack in high-risk patients (MATCH): randomised, double-blind, placebo-controlled trial. Lancet. 2004; 364(9431):331–337

[57] Chalouhi N, Zanaty M, Jabbour PM, et al. Intracerebral hemorrhage after pipeline embolization: management of antiplatelet agents and the case for point-of-care testing–case reports and review of literature. Clin Neurol Neurosurg. 2014; 124:21–24

[58] Delgado Almandoz JE, Crandall BM, Scholz JM, et al. Pre-procedure P2Y12 reaction units value predicts perioperative thromboembolic and hemorrhagic complications in patients with cerebral aneurysms treated with the Pipeline Embolization Device. J Neurointerv Surg. 2013; 5 Suppl 3:iii3–iii10

[59] Hu YC, Deshmukh VR, Albuquerque FC, et al. Histopathological assessment of fatal ipsilateral intraparenchymal hemorrhages after the treatment of

supraclinoid aneurysms with the Pipeline Embolization Device. J Neurosurg. 2014; 120(2):365–374

[60] Iosif C, Camilleri Y, Saleme S, et al. Diffusion-weighted imaging-detected ischemic lesions associated with flow-diverting stents in intracranial aneurysms: safety, potential mechanisms, clinical outcome, and concerns. J Neurosurg. 2015; 122(3):627–636

[61] Tomas C, Benaissa A, Herbreteau D, Kadziolka K, Pierot L. Delayed ipsilateral parenchymal hemorrhage following treatment of intracranial aneurysms with flow diverter. Neuroradiology. 2014; 56(2):155–161

[62] Murakami H, Inaba M, Nakamura A, Ushioda T. Ipsilateral hyperperfusion after neck clipping of a giant internal carotid artery aneurysm. Case report. J Neurosurg. 2002; 97(5):1233–1236

17 FLOW DIVERSION GRADING SCALES

MIN S. PARK, MARCUS MAZUR, M. YASHAR S. KALANI, and PHILIPP TAUSSKY

Abstract

While flow diversion has become a standard part of the neuro-interventionalist's armamentarium, there is no commonly agreed upon system to grade results. Recently, four different grading systems (OKM scale, Kamran-Byrne scale, SMART scale, and the flow-diverting stent scale) have been published to help address this shortcoming. We review these four different systems in detail and compare and contrast the features among one another. While all of the scales have some merits, currently, no one system has been widely accepted by the neurointervention world.

Keywords: cerebral aneurysm, flow diversion, flow diverting stents, grading systems

17.1 Introduction

As the popularity of flow-diverting stents (FDSs) as an accepted endovascular treatment for large and giant cerebral aneurysms has grown, more and more practitioners are using FDSs for "off-label" indications, including smaller aneurysms and posterior and distal anterior circulation aneurysms.[1,2,3] This increased usage necessitates a common language to describe the results of treatment and to provide a uniform reporting structure for short-, mid-, and long-term radiographic results.

Because flow diversion represents a vastly different strategy than coil embolization for treatment of cerebral aneurysms, there are concerns that the Roy and Raymond scale, which is used to grade outcomes after endovascular treatment of saccular aneurysms,[4] will be inadequate for classifying these aneurysms. While the initial results after coil embolization are often dramatic with, ideally, complete or near-complete occlusion of the aneurysm, the same cannot be said for aneurysms treated with flow diversion. Often, there is still significant filling of the aneurysm sac that resolves as occlusion occurs over a period of time.[5] Using the Roy and Raymond scale, almost all aneurysms treated with flow diversion would be classified as having residual aneurysm filling.

While the three-point scale of Roy and Raymond has gained wide acceptance as an angiographic classification scheme for assessment after coil embolization, the same cannot be said for the several competing grading scales proposed for flow diversion.[6,7,8,9] These scales, thus far, have not yet reached a critical mass with neurointerventional surgeons and are not widely employed in the literature at the time of this writing.

17.2 Grading Scales

17.2.1 O'Kelly-Marotta Scale

In 2010, O'Kelly et al attempted to address a deficit in outcome assessment by proposing the first grading scale for the angiographic assessment of aneurysms following flow diversion (▶ Fig. 17.1).[6] The O'Kelly-Marotta (OKM) scale was designed to

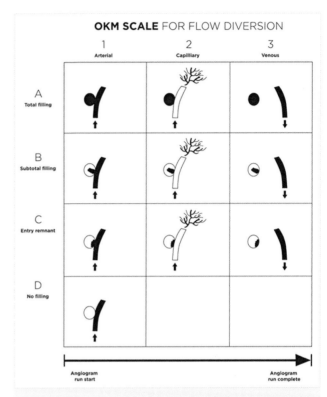

Fig. 17.1 OKM scale for flow diversion of cerebral aneurysms. (Reproduced with permission from O'Kelly et al.[6])

account for both the degree of aneurysm filling and the amount of contrast stasis after FDS deployment. This scale requires an angiographic run that continues into the venous phase. O'Kelly et al described two main components for their classification scheme: the amount of aneurysm filling and the phase in which the aneurysm clears (▶ Table 17.1).

The degree of aneurysm filling is classified from A to D after the deployment of the FDS. Aneurysms receive a grade of A if greater than 95% of the aneurysm fills, grade B for 5 to 95%, grade C for neck remnant (< 5%), and grade D for no filling of the aneurysm. The time to contrast clearance from the aneurysm is represented in the stasis grade and is measured on a three-point scale: grade 1, clearing in the arterial phase; grade 2, clearing in the capillary phase; and grade 3, clearing in the venous phase. Thus, aneurysms in the OKM scale are described with both a letter and a number grade (▶ Fig. 17.1, ▶ Fig. 17.2, ▶ Fig. 17.3). Grades may be given to both pre- and posttreatment angiograms of aneurysms.

17.2.2 Kamran-Byrne Scale

One year later, Kamran et al published their proposed grading scheme for outcomes after deployment of an FDS after analyzing the data from the SILK registry (Balt Extrusion,

Table 17.1 Comparison of four grading scales

Scale	Filling grade	Stasis grade	Vessel patency	Inter- and intraobserver variability
OKM	Four grades from A to D	Three grades from 1 to 3	None	κ = 0.74 κ = 0.99
Kamran-Byrne	Five grades from 0 to 4, with separate measurements for saccular and fusiform aneurysms	None	Three grades from A to C	Aneurysm occlusion κ = 0.89 Parent artery patency κ = 0.90
SMART	Five grades from 0 to 4, with separate measurements for saccular and fusiform aneurysms	Only for grade 0 aneurysms from A to C	5 grades from 0 to 4	
Flow-diverting stent scale (FDSS)	3 grades from 1 to 3 based on the Raymond score	None	None	Kendall's W 0.61

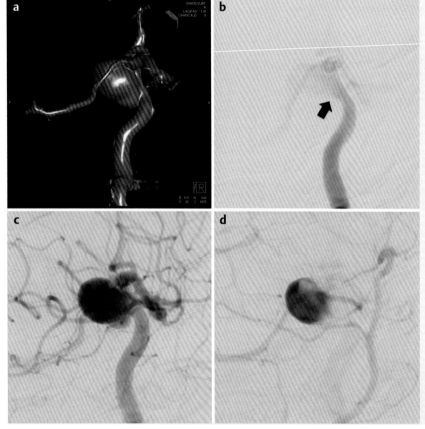

Fig. 17.2 (a) Right cavernous internal carotid artery aneurysm measuring 16 × 13 × 9 mm in size. **(b)** Early arterial-phase angiography demonstrating a coherent, inflow jet (*black arrow*) after deployment of a Pipeline Embolization Device. **(c)** Late arterial-phase angiography demonstrating complete filling of the aneurysm after treatment. There is no evidence of parent artery stenosis. **(d)** Late venous-phase angiography demonstrating contrast stasis. By the OKM scale, this would be graded as an A3 aneurysm. By the Kamran-Byrne scale, this would be graded as an Axis I grade 0 and Axis II grade A aneurysms. By the SMART scale, this would be graded as a grade 0c and ISS grade 0 aneurysms.

Montmorency, France)[7] (▶ Fig. 17.4, ▶ Table 17.1). Their scale is a two-part classification system that grades the extent of aneurysm occlusion (Axis I) and the parent vessel patency (Axis II). The classification system includes criteria for both saccular and fusiform aneurysms.

Axis I measurements of degree of occlusion in saccular aneurysms are graded on a five-point scale from 0 to 4: grade 0, no occlusion of the aneurysm; grade 1, more than 50% of pretreatment aneurysm filling; grade 2, less than 50% filling of pretreatment aneurysm filling; grade 3, neck remnant only;

and grade 4, complete occlusion of the aneurysm (▶ Fig. 17.2 and ▶ Fig. 17.4a).

While the Axis I grading scheme for the degree of aneurysm occlusion in saccular aneurysms is straightforward, the measurement of degree of filling in fusiform aneurysms is somewhat more complex, requiring both a length and width determination of the filling portion of the fusiform aneurysm. Grades 0 and 4 again indicate no occlusion and complete occlusion, respectively, but for fusiform aneurysms, grade 1 indicates more than 50% filling in both length and width of the

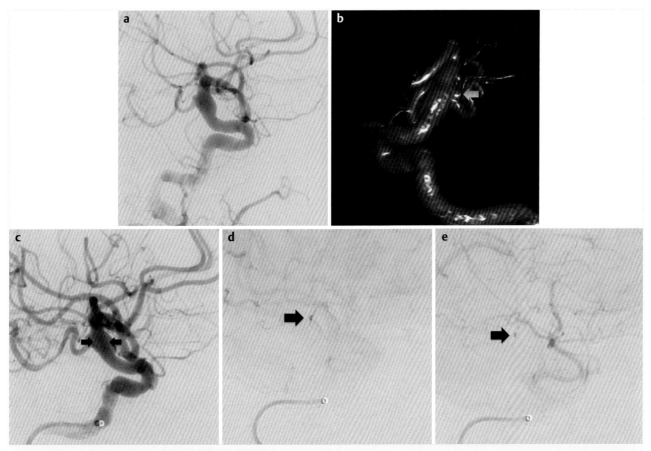

Fig. 17.3 **(a)** Fusiform right internal carotid artery aneurysm with a small dorsal daughter sac. **(b)** Three-dimensional rotational angiogram of the fusiform right internal carotid artery aneurysm with a daughter sac (*arrow*) adjacent to the posterior communicating artery origin. **(c)** Late arterial-phase angiography demonstrating complete filling of the aneurysm after deployment of a Pipeline Embolization Device (outlined by the *black arrows*). **(d)** Capillary-phase angiography demonstrating contrast stasis within the daughter sac of the aneurysm (*black arrow*). **(e)** Late venous-phase angiography demonstrating contrast stasis within the daughter sac of the fusiform aneurysm (*black arrow*). By the OKM scale, this would be graded as an A3 aneurysm. By the Kamran-Byrne scale, this would be graded as an Axis I grade 0 and Axis II grade A aneurysms. By the SMART scale, this would be graded as a grade 1 and ISS grade 0 aneurysms.

aneurysm, grade 2 indicates less than 50% filling of either the length or width, and grade 3 indicates less than 50% filling of both length and width (▶ Fig. 17.3 and ▶ Fig. 17.4b).

In their development of the grading scale, Kamran et al also stressed the importance of the state of the parent vessel after FDS deployment. Axis II patency is measured on a three-point scale from A to C: A, no change in the parent artery diameter; B, narrowing of the parent artery; and C, occlusion of the parent artery.

17.2.3 SMART Scale

In 2011, a third grading scale for the evaluation of cerebral aneurysms treated with FDS was published (▶ Fig. 17.5, ▶ Table 17.1).[8] The SMART scale prioritizes the degree and location of the contrast stasis in the aneurysm after treatment and the inflow characteristics. Additionally, the developers also considered the final patency of the parent vessel in the scale. This scale shares certain similarities with the Kamran-Byrne scale previously described, which is not surprising considering that

two of the creators of the Kamran-Byrne scale are also authors on the SMART scale.[7,8]

The degree of residual flow of the aneurysm is measured on a five-point scale from 0 to 4. Grade 0 represents an aneurysm with a coherent inflow jet in the arterial phase, regardless of residual filling. If no inflow jet is identified, assessments are performed during the venous phase of the angiogram: grade 1 aneurysms are completely patent with a diffuse inflow of contrast; grade 2 aneurysms exhibit residual filling that reaches the wall or dome of the aneurysm; grade 3 aneurysms exhibit filling limited to the neck of the aneurysm (saccular aneurysms) or residual filling not reaching the former aneurysm boundaries (fusiform aneurysms); and grade 4 is reserved for aneurysms that are completely occluded. While grade 0 aneurysms are graded in the early arterial phase, all other grades are determined during venous phase angiograms (▶ Fig. 17.2, ▶ Fig. 17.3, ▶ Fig. 17.5).

One of the critiques of the Kamran-Byrne scale was that it failed to consider contrast stasis.[10] The SMART scale addresses this shortcoming with a three-point grading scale to assess flow dynamics for grade 0 aneurysms. A letter modifier is added to

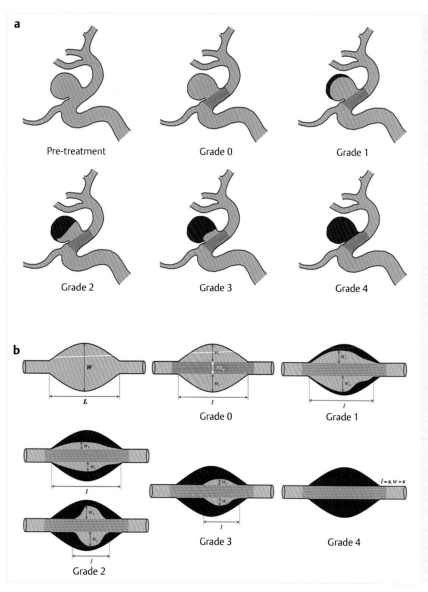

Fig. 17.4 (a) Kamran–Byrne scale for residual filling of saccular aneurysms. **(b)** Kamran–Byrne scale for residual filling of fusiform aneurysms. (Reproduced with permission from Kamran et al. [7])

the assigned grade of the aneurysm: A, no contrast stasis; B, stasis in the capillary phase; and C, stasis in the venous phase (▶ Fig. 17.2d).

The degree of parent artery patency after treatment is graded on an expanded five-point scale of in-stent stenosis (ISS): ISS grade 0, no stenosis; ISS grade 1, mild, not hemodynamically significant stenosis; ISS grade 2, moderate, 50 to 70% stenosis; ISS grade 3, severe, hemodynamically significant stenosis greater than 70%; and ISS grade 4, occluded parent vessels.

17.2.4 Flow-Diverting Stent Scale (FDSS)

More recently, we published a grading scale based on the long-term outcomes following flow diversion (▶ Table 17.1 and ▶ Table 17.2).[9] In a retrospective review of 171 patients treated with flow diversion at two institutions, we identified statistically significant factors related to failure of aneurysm occlusion. An initial post-treatment Raymond score of 2 or 3, age ≥ 60

years, size > 15 mm, and presence of a side branch associated with the aneurysm were found to be statistically significant factors in aneurysm patency after one year.

The FDSS uses the Raymond score as the basis of the grading system with an initial occlusion score of 1 (complete occlusion), 2 (residual neck filling), or 3 (residual dome filling). An additional point is added for any patient ≥ 60 years of age, for any aneurysm > 15 mm, and for any aneurysm with an associated side branch at the neck, sidewall, or dome. This results in a scoring system from 1 (young patient with an aneurysm < 15 mm without a side branch that completely occludes following flow diversion) to a 6 (older patient with an aneurysm > 15 mm with an associated side branch and residual filling to the dome after flow diversion).

17.3 Validation

Any grading scale must have a high degree of reproducibility to provide a meaningful language for common use. This is largely

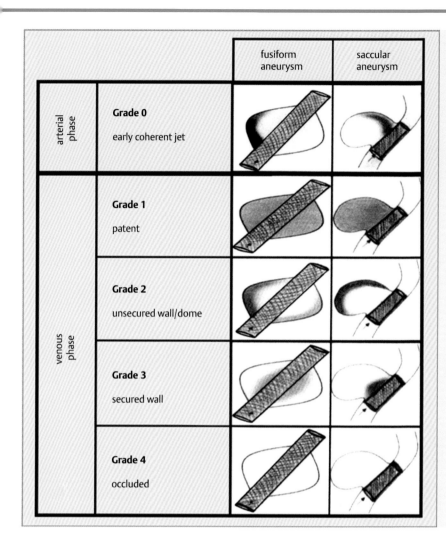

		fusiform aneurysm	saccular aneurysm
arterial phase	**Grade 0** early coherent jet		
venous phase	**Grade 1** patent		
	Grade 2 unsecured wall/dome		
	Grade 3 secured wall		
	Grade 4 occluded		

Fig. 17.5 Residual filling grading for saccular and fusiform aneurysms on the SMART scale. (Reproduced with permission from Grunwald et al.[8])

Table 17.2 The flow-diverting stent scale (FDSS)

Raymond score	Age	Aneurysm size	Side branch
1 – complete occlusion	0 – Age < 60 years	0 – Size < 15 mm	0 – No side branch
2 – residual neck filling	1 – Age ≥ 60 years	1 – Size > 15 mm	1 – Side branch
3 – residual dome filling			

incumbent on having a discrete and well-defined classification system that is also easy to use.

In a follow-up publication to the original OKM scale, Joshi et al[10] rated the inter- and intraobserver reliability with multiple raters. Thirty-one neurointerventional practitioners from neuroradiology and neurosurgery rated 14 aneurysms treated with FDS. They found substantial (κ= 0.74) and almost perfect agreement (κ= 0.99) for inter- and intraobserver reliability, respectively, using the OKM scale. Additionally, there was no statistically significant difference between different specialties (neuroradiology vs. neurosurgery) or levels of training (fellow

vs. attending physician). The one area that presented the raters with the most difficulty was with filling grade C, where there was only a 45% correct response rate compared with at least 80% for all other categories.

Kamran et al[7] also measured the reliability of the Kamran-Byrne grading scale using two experienced interventional neuroradiologists as raters. They reviewed 55 angiographies (39 saccular and 16 fusiform aneurysms). Kamran et al noted a high degree of interobserver reliability with their two-axis grading scale (Axis I, κ= 0.89; Axis II, κ= 0.90) between the two raters.

The FDSS reliability was assessed by three raters: one endovascular neurosurgeon and two neuroradiologists.[9] The interrater reliability of the grading scale (Kendall's W) was 0.61 (p = 0.005). Additionally, the two cohorts identified in the study (patients with complete occlusion and patients with aneurysm residuals) had statistically significant differences in the immediate post-treatment scores. Patients with occluded aneurysms had an average score of 3.6±1.0, whereas patients with an aneurysm residual had an average score of 4.4±0.7 (p < 0.01). Using a cutoff of FDSS 4 resulted in a specificity of 50.9% and a positive predictive value of 40.5% for having a residual aneurysm after flow diversion. The internal validity was tested using a bootstrapping technique from samples from the residual aneurysm cohort. The mean calculated FDSS for this cohort was 4.44±0.10 (95% CI, 4.24 to 4.64).

17.4 Discussion of Grading Scales

The goal of any grading scale is to create a common language, ensuring uniformity in the medical literature and to create a standardized outcome report to allow for comparisons between different published reports. There are several factors that would likely influence a scale's adoption into standard use. Like the Roy and Raymond scale for coiled aneurysms, first and foremost, the scale must be easy to use. Greater complexity will likely result in less use. Additionally, the scale must be sensitive enough to distinguish between appropriate subgroups and reproducible to ensure a high level of observer agreement (▶ Table 17.1). Ultimately, the scales should be able to provide a meaningful prediction of defined outcomes to validate the creation of the subgroups within the grading system.

There are several obvious differences between the four grading systems. Because the low-porosity metal braids of the FDS are designed to disrupt inflow into the aneurysm, the OKM and SMART scales consider contrast stasis to be a key factor in their grading systems. The OKM scale is more descriptive of the degree of contrast stasis (arterial, capillary, and venous phase), while the SMART scale measures the degree of residual filling strictly in the venous phase. The SMART scale, as described, sets up an interesting situation where an aneurysm without an early, coherent inflow jet, but with complete aneurysm filling in the arterial phase and early clearance before the venous phase, would be graded as a 4 (occluded aneurysm). This would seem counterintuitive and in marked contrast to the OKM scale (Grade A3). The Kamran-Byrne scale and FDSS do not consider contrast stasis; however, when we developed the FDSS, contrast stasis was not identified as a statistically significant variable in predicting aneurysm occlusion (p = 0.33).

The authors of the Kamran-Byrne and SMART scales also stress the importance of ISS in their respective grading scales.

While ISS serves as a measure of the patency of the stent and a marker of potential complications, it is not well delineated how this relates to eventual aneurysm occlusion.

As it stands now, there has not been one widely accepted grading scale that has captured the attention of neurointerventional practitioners to become the standard language for flow diversion.

References

[1] Becske T, Kallmes DF, Saatci I, et al. Pipeline for uncoilable or failed aneurysms: results from a multicenter clinical trial. Radiology. 2013; 267(3):858–868

[2] Nelson PK, Lylyk P, Szikora I, Wetzel SG, Wanke I, Fiorella D. The pipeline embolization device for the intracranial treatment of aneurysms trial. AJNR Am J Neuroradiol. 2011; 32(1):34–40

[3] Park MS, Albuquerque FC, Nanaszko M, et al. Critical assessment of complications associated with use of the Pipeline Embolization Device. J Neurointerv Surg. 2015; 7(9):652–659

[4] Roy D, Milot G, Raymond J. Endovascular treatment of unruptured aneurysms. Stroke. 2001; 32(9):1998–2004

[5] Fiorella D, Lylyk P, Szikora I, et al. Curative cerebrovascular reconstruction with the Pipeline embolization device: the emergence of definitive endovascular therapy for intracranial aneurysms. J Neurointerv Surg. 2009; 1(1):56–65

[6] O'Kelly CJ, Krings T, Fiorella D, Marotta TR. A novel grading scale for the angiographic assessment of intracranial aneurysms treated using flow diverting stents. Interv Neuroradiol. 2010; 16(2):133–137

[7] Kamran M, Yarnold J, Grunwald IQ, Byrne JV. Assessment of angiographic outcomes after flow diversion treatment of intracranial aneurysms: a new grading schema. Neuroradiology. 2011; 53(7):501–508

[8] Grunwald IQ, Kamran M, Corkill RA, et al. Simple measurement of aneurysm residual after treatment: the SMART scale for evaluation of intracranial aneurysms treated with flow diverters. Acta Neurochir (Wien). 2012; 154(1):21–26, discussion 26

[9] Park MS, Mazur MD, Moon K, et al. An outcomes-based grading scale for the evaluation of cerebral aneurysms treated with flow diversion. J Neurointerv Surg. 2016 Oct 19. DOI: doi:10.1136/neurintsurg-2016–012688

[10] Joshi MD, O'Kelly CJ, Krings T, Fiorella D, Marotta TR. Observer variability of an angiographic grading scale used for the assessment of intracranial aneurysms treated with flow-diverting stents. AJNR Am J Neuroradiol. 2013; 34 (8):1589–1592

18 RADIOGRAPHIC IMAGING AFTER FLOW DIVERSION

SCOTT McNALLY

Abstract

Prior to treatment, aneurysms can be diagnosed and selected for endovascular treatment or surgery using a variety of radiology techniques. Imaging can detect markers of aneurysm rupture risk, including size, location, irregularity, and wall enhancement. In addition to detecting and guiding treatment of unruptured and ruptured intracranial aneurysms, imaging can be used after treatment to determine success and failure. The primary goals of imaging include (1) diagnosis of acute subarachnoid hemorrhage; (2) detection of an intracranial aneurysm or other source of bleeding; (3) determination of aneurysm type (e.g., saccular, blister), location, and geometry for rupture risk calculation or treatment planning; and (4) follow-up to ensure appropriate treatment. By using lumen methods such as digital subtraction angiography, computed tomography angiography, and magnetic resonance angiography, one can identify residual aneurysm filling and monitor treatment response after flow diversion. Novel methods characterizing hemodynamics may detect important changes that occur with flow diversion. In addition, vessel wall imaging techniques may be helpful to monitor aneurysm wall inflammation in response to treatment.

Keywords: CTA, DSA, flow-diverting stent, intracranial aneurysm, MRA, MRI, vessel wall imaging

18.1 Digital subtraction angiography

Digital subtraction angiography (DSA) is usually performed via femoral access with a biplane unit with rotational/three-dimensional (3D) capabilities. Intra-arterial injection is performed using iodinated contrast after guiding the catheter to each of the four main vessels of the neck. Using X-rays, 2D views are taken, with rotational radiography used to create 3D models useful for treatment planning. DSA has the highest spatial resolution of all imaging modalities and is considered the gold standard for evaluating intracranial aneurysms. The high spatial resolution allows for aneurysm neck characterization to guide

endovascular versus open surgical treatment and better visualization of associated branch vessels. Furthermore, DSA has temporal resolution for evaluation of arterial, capillary, and venous phases. In addition to conventional DSA, 3D rotational angiography (3DRA) further increases the sensitivity of small aneurysms less than 3 mm in size and can identify aneurysms missed by computed tomography angiography (CTA)/magnetic resonance angiography (MRA) or DSA alone.[1,2] These factors make DSA the gold standard in evaluating treatment response after flow diversion. While initial results showed a small but significant mortality of 0.06% and a more worrisome stroke rate of 4%,[3] more recent reports show DSA complication rates below 0.3%.[4] Because DSA is an invasive procedure, the information acquired from this study must be weighed against the small procedural risk associated with it. Certainly, DSA and 3DRA are essential for treatment planning (▶ Fig. 18.1) and immediate evaluation of successful flow diversion (▶ Fig. 18.2).

18.2 Computed Tomography Angiography)

On CTA, contrast fills the aneurysm lumen and allows easy detection of pre- and posttreatment status. For treatment planning, CTA can accurately determine aneurysm lumen location and geometry, with measurements of size, shape, neck size, presence of daughter sacs, and other concerning features including wall irregularities or, rarely, active contrast extravasation diagnostic of aneurysm rupture (▶ Fig. 18.3). CTA is performed on multi-row detector helical scanners in the axial plane from which multiplanar reformats, maximum intensity projections, and 3D reconstructions are produced (see ▶ Table 18.1 for our institutional protocol). Early CT technology lacked sensitivity for detecting aneurysms 3 mm and smaller, with sensitivity as low as 84% using four-channel multi-row detector CT scanners.[5] Several investigators and a recent meta-analysis have demonstrated that current CTA protocols with multidetector scanners have a spatial resolution that can reliably diagnose aneurysms compared to DSA, with sensitivity approaching 100%.[6,7,8,9,10]

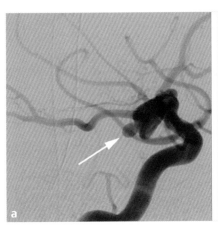
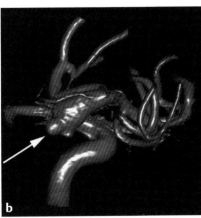

Fig. 18.1 Digital subtraction angiography (DSA) pretreatment planning in patient 1, a 75-year-old asymptomatic woman. DSA (**a**) and 3DRA (**b**) demonstrate a wide-necked, irregular 7 × 8 mm posterior communicating artery aneurysm with an associated daughter sac (*arrows*).

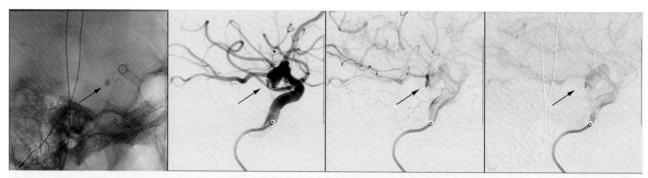

Fig. 18.2 Immediate posttreatment digital subtraction angiography in patient 1. Status post deployment of a Pipeline Flex device, there is successful flow diversion through the stent lumen with more stagnant flow in the aneurysm sac. Contrast from a prior injection pools within the dependent aneurysm sac and is subtracted on the current injection (*arrows*).

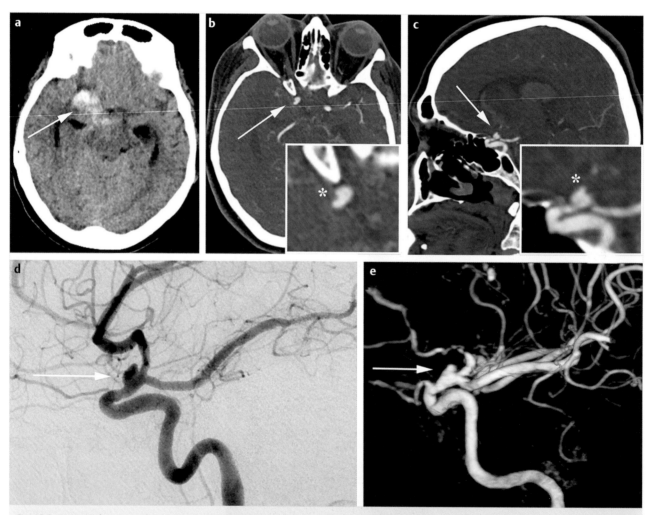

Fig. 18.3 Computed tomography angiography (CTA) aneurysm detection in patient 2, a 45-year-old woman presenting with worst headache of life. Noncontrast CT (**a**) shows subarachnoid hemorrhage and intraparenchymal hemorrhage localized to the right Sylvian fissure and right frontal lobe (*arrow*). Axial CTA (**b**) and sagittal CTA reformat (**c**) shows an irregular outpouching along the right internal carotid artery (ICA) consistent with a dorsal variant blister aneurysm (*arrow, asterisk*). Digital subtraction angiography (**d**) and 3DRA (**e**) via right ICA injection confirm the dorsal variant blister aneurysm.

CTA can also be used to monitor aneurysms following treatment, though one must be aware of potential artifacts related to metallic hardware, including some stents, coils, and clips. These can result in extensive beam hardening from the metal.

This is due to the use of multiple X-ray energies and the "hardening" of the beam after it passes through any high attenuation material leaving only the high energy X-rays. While this can limit the evaluation of aneurysms adjacent to metallic

Table 18.1 CTA imaging protocol

CTA protocol[a]	Isovue 370	Injection rate	Injection delay	Slice thickness
CTA brain	100 mL	4 mL/s	10 s	0.625 mm

[a]All CTA images were performed with a 64-section Siemens scanner (Definition or Definition AS), with dose modulation and 100–120 kVp. Intravenous access was through an antecubital vein by using an 18- or 20-gauge angiocatheter. Bolus monitoring used an ROI in the ascending aorta and trigger at 100 Hounsfield units (HU). Multiplanar reformats were created and images obtained from a PACS workstation. Images were initially reviewed on CTA settings (window 96, level 150 HU), and modified as required to depict lumen separate from stent.

hardware, current flow-diverting stents produce little, if any, beam-hardening artifact (▶ Fig. 18.4). Following flow diversion, the lumen internal to the stent can be evaluated with appropriate windowing and leveling to maximize differences between the contrast within the lumen and the stent. In addition, posttreatment CTA can also show progressive thrombosis of the aneurysm which can occasionally be detected as a high attenuation crescent on noncontrast CT. However, in the subacute setting, from 6 hours to 1 week after clot formation, the ability to detect blood products drops dramatically.

One drawback to CTA imaging is the radiation dose imparted to the patient. This results in a small, but significant, risk of carcinogenesis as extrapolated from certain studies. Over the past 30 years, medical radiation sources have increased the average radiation dose per person in the United States from an average of 3.6 mSv in the 1980s to 6.2 mSv in 2006.[11] Extrapolating data from radiation exposure at Hiroshima, Three Mile Island, and Chernobyl and radiation workers to current CT use, it has been estimated that about 1.5 to 2.0% of all cancers in the United Stated may be attributable to CT radiation.[12] A noncontrast CT and CTA of the head results in a mean effective dose of approximately 3.6 versus 4.3 mSv between two studies (1.7 vs. 2.7 mSv for noncontrast head CT and 1.9 vs. 1.6 mSv for head CTA) using estimations from CT phantoms, dosimeters during CT scans on patients, and dose-length products (DLPs) to estimate the effective dose.[13,14] This imparts an overall low cancer risk to patients undergoing noncontrast CT and CTA of the brain. As a comparison, the radiation dosages for flow diversion follow-up are significantly less than that during workup of acute ischemic stroke with additional CTA neck and CT perfusion studies (which is estimated at 1 in 1,200 patients).[14]

The effective dose is calculated from the DLP (mGy–cm) and takes into account the radiosensitivity of imaged organs, 80% of which is attributed to the thyroid.[15] One reason for this low risk is that most patients undergoing scanning for aneurysms are often within the sixth to ninth decades, and exposure in this age group carries a lower risk of excess cancer mortality due to decreased DLP conversion factors. Although the individual risk of cancer with CT/CTA aneurysm workup is likely small, databases have been developed for future large-scale epidemiologic studies addressing CT radiation risk.[16]

18.3 Magnetic Resonance Imaging and Magnetic Resonance Angiography

For sequential follow-up imaging, magnetic resonance imaging/magnetic resonance angiography (MRI/MRA) has certain advantages over DSA and CTA. First, MRI/MRA does not use ionizing radiation, and MRA sequences can image aneurysms without the need for contrast. This avoids the repeat ionizing radiation from DSA or CTA. In addition, noncontrast MRA sequences avoid any potential risk of contrast dye.

18.3.1 MRI/MRA Aneurysm Imaging

The 3D time-of-flight (TOF) sequence on MRA eliminates the need for contrast, which is prohibitive in patients with renal failure or contrast allergy. This technique can be used without or with contrast, and can identify and characterize aneurysms prior to (▶ Fig. 18.5) and after treatment (▶ Fig. 18.6). A meta-analysis of MRA studies for evaluating aneurysms demonstrated that contrast-enhanced MRA (CEMRA) and TOF had similar abilities at detection of aneurysms.[17] CEMRA, however, was found to be superior to TOF due to its ability to eliminate flow-related artifacts and spin saturation.[18] Although CEMRA had a lower spatial resolution compared to DSA, qualitative grading of images is similar.[19] Despite lower spatial resolution, small branch vessels are better visualized on 3 T MRA compared to CTA due to the lack of venous contrast contamination.[20]

As MRA technology continues to improve, spatial resolution and sensitivity to smaller aneurysms are also expected to improve. With current sequences, the spatial resolution at 1.5 T is often as low as 1 mm,[21] whereas at 3 T the spatial resolution can be as low as 0.6 mm while preserving signal to noise,[22] with radiologists unanimously reporting significantly better visualization of aneurysms at 3 T. A meta-analysis studying the sensitivity of MRA for detection of cerebral aneurysms performed by Sailer et al found a trend toward significance in better detection of smaller aneurysms on 3 T versus 1.5 T scanners ($p = 0.054$)[17] with a pooled sensitivity of 1.5 T and 3 T scanners of approximately 95% for all aneurysms. These results suggest that MRA, especially 3 T, can be used to follow up flow-diverted aneurysms.

18.3.2 Magnetic Resonance Imaging Safety

Because of the potential advantages of noncontrast 3D TOF in patients with renal failure and the lack of ionizing radiation, MRI/MRA can be useful for follow-up after flow diversion. And as MRI sequences continue to advance, its use will likely increase in the future. It is therefore important to consider the potential risks related to contrast agents and the magnetic field with MRI use. All MRI studies should be performed following American College of Radiology (ACR) guidelines to minimize any inherent risks and with the following considerations for patient safety.[23]

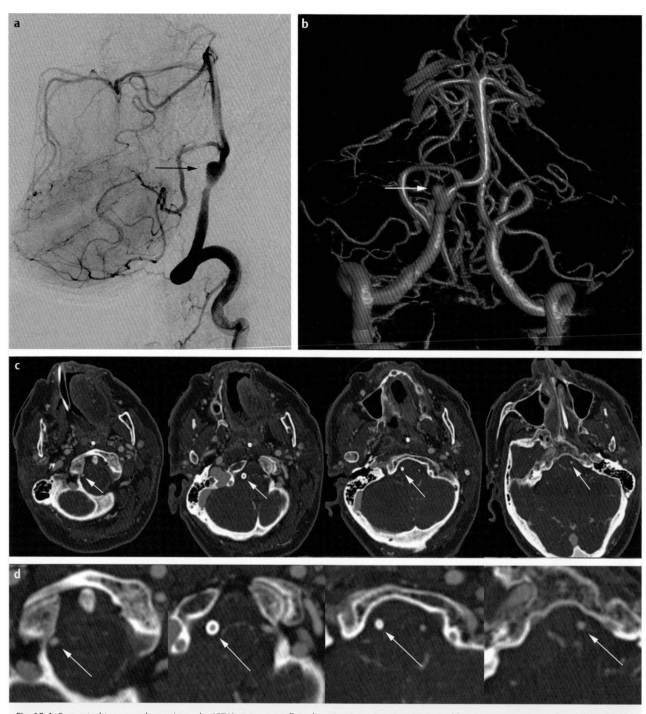

Fig. 18.4 Computed tomography angiography (CTA) status post–flow diversion in patient 3, a 57-year-old woman presenting with acute SAH and a dissecting pseudoaneurysm. Digital subtraction angiography (**a**) and 3DRA (**b**) via a right vertebral artery injection demonstrate a right V4 segment pseudoaneurysm (*arrow*) just proximal to the right PICA origin. CTA (**c**) shows posttreatment appearance of the right vertebral artery (*arrow*) with preserved lumen from inferior (**c**, left) to superior (**c**, right) as well as magnified CTA images demonstrating the treated right vertebral artery (*arrow*) (**d**). CTA window ~2,500, level ~600.

Recent studies have suggested that injection of intravenous MRI contrast, specifically gadolinium-based contrast agents (GBCA), in patients with impaired kidney function may rarely be associated with nephrogenic systemic fibrosis (NSF), a potentially fatal disease characterized by progressive skin and soft-tissue thickening. Patients should be screened for acute kidney disease and chronic kidney disease and should not receive gadolinium if estimated glomerular filtration rate is less than 30 mL/min/1.73 m². Of the available contrast agents, gadopentetate dimeglumine (MultiHance, 0.1 mmol/kg) is associated with a significantly lower incidence of NSF relative to other GBCA (4 in 100,000 vs. 36.5 in 100,000).[24,25] In addition, newer agents such as gadofosveset trisodium (Ablavar, 0.03 mmol/kg) have had no NSF cases reported in more than 90,000 studies.

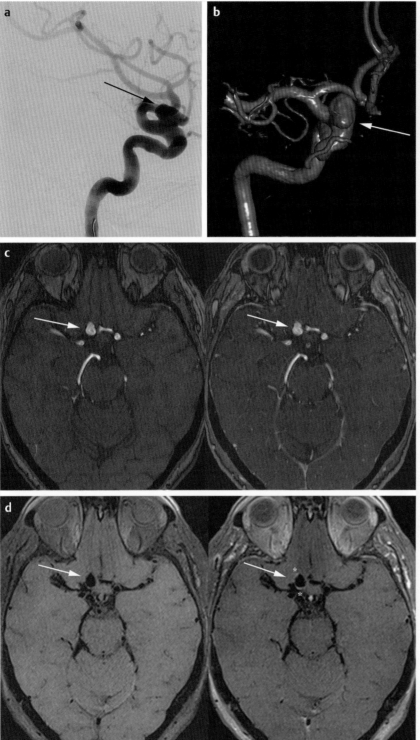

Fig. 18.5 MRI/MRA pretreatment planning in patient 4, a 70-year-old woman with a right ophthalmic artery aneurysm. Pretreatment DSA (**a**), 3DRA (**b**), and MRA pre- and postcontrast 3D time of flight (**c**, left and right, respectively) demonstrate a wide-necked, irregular 10 × 7 mm right ophthalmic artery aneurysm (*arrow*). Pretreatment HRMRI pre- and postcontrast black blood images (**d**, left and right, respectively) demonstrate the aneurysm (*arrow*) and areas of wall enhancement (*asterisks*) consistent with wall inflammation and sites of rupture risk.

An additional risk of GBCA is contrast allergy. It is estimated that 1 to 2% of patients have a minor transient reaction, including nausea, local warmth, headache, and dizziness. Severe anaphylactic reactions are exceedingly rare (< 0.005%). Because of these potential reactions, gadolinium should always be administered under the supervision of a radiologist.

Another major risk is the presence of MRI-incompatible hardware. Patients should be screened for potential MRI-

incompatible hardware, including pacemakers, orbital shrapnel, or vascular stents placed within the past 8 weeks. If after alternate imaging (e.g., CTA, DSA) has been exhausted, MRI may be the only way to answer the clinical question. The presence of a pacemaker is not necessarily an absolute contraindication to MRI scanning. If the patient is not pacemaker dependent and the patient agrees after informed consent, MRI can be performed in select circumstances after appropriate radiology

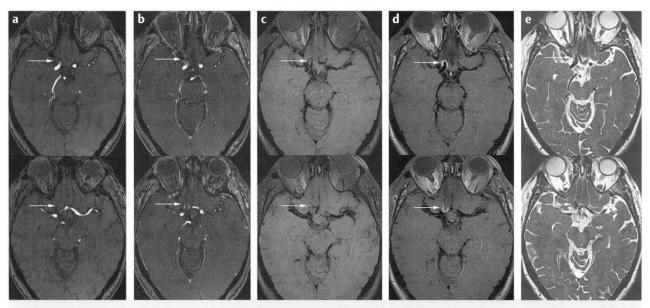

Fig. 18.6 Posttreatment aneurysm evaluation with MRI/MRA in patient 4. Status post–flow diversion, MRA pre- (**a**, top = inferior at aneurysm neck, bottom = superior at aneurysm dome) and postcontrast 3D time of flight (**b**) demonstrate absent filling of the aneurysm sac with contrast (*arrows*). Posttreatment HRMRI pre- (**c**) and postcontrast (**d**) T1-weighted black-blood images demonstrate new wall thickening and enhancement (*arrow*) within the aneurysm neck (top) and sac (bottom) consistent with organizing thrombus. Thrombus is also seen on T2-weighted images (**e**) as hyperintense signal along the neck (top) and within the sac (bottom).

screening and under close monitoring by a cardiologist. Additionally, patients should also be screened for pregnancy. While MRI is considered safe in pregnant patients, many questions remain with GBCA.

18.4 Beyond Lumen Imaging

While pre- and posttreatment aneurysms can be assessed with lumen-imaging methods, aneurysm rupture risk does not solely depend on lumen-imaging findings. Structural changes occurring within aneurysm walls are oftentimes not captured by lumen imaging. Advanced imaging studies have suggested that the identification of hemodynamic or inflammatory factors may allow for a better prediction model of aneurysm rupture. Blood flow also impacts endothelial function and can be beneficial or harmful to aneurysm stability. In addition, wall inflammation plays an essential role in aneurysm instability. It is thought that a delicate balance exists between aneurysm geometry, blood flow, and wall pathophysiology in the pathophysiology of aneurysm formation.[26] Recent advances in the literature highlight the ability to measure (1) hemodynamic predictors and (2) inflammatory markers of aneurysm vulnerability. As imaging technology evolves and allows us to gather more detailed information, it may allow us to better predict the efficacy of aneurysm treatment after flow diversion. However, further study is needed before any definitive predictions can be made.

18.4.1 Hemodynamic Predictors

Fluid dynamics are known to play an important role in aneurysm formation, growth, and rupture, and may aid in identifying the inflow zone to guide endovascular treatment.[27,28]

Computational flow dynamics (CFD) has been applied to lumen images (DSA, CTA, MRA) to simulate true flow conditions. Multiple hemodynamic forces can be calculated (tensional stress, compressional stress, shear stress/oscillatory shear index [OSI]) using these models. Wall shear stress, OSI, inflow jet, and the impingement zone have all been shown to be important in predicting aneurysm rupture risk.[29] OSI, a measure of directional change in wall shear stress during diastole and systole, can be a surrogate marker for rupture risk.[30,31] Inflow jets have also been shown to be important.[32] CFD may be important in identifying changes between pre– and post–flow diversion shear stress and OSI with the potential for modulation of the aneurysm rupture risk.[26,30,33] Additionally, specific features now discernable on 4D-CTA, such as aneurysm pulsations, may indicate higher risk of aneurysm growth and rupture and could be modeled pre- and posttreatment.[34] New MRI protocols can also define aneurysmal wall motion abnormalities associated with higher risk of rupture.[35]

18.4.2 MRI Vessel Wall Imaging

The pathophysiology of aneurysm growth, wall thinning, and rupture involves multiple changes on histology, including endothelial disruption, collagen loss, and inflammatory cell migration. While previous lumen imaging could not detect these pathologic changes, newly developed black-blood T1-weighted MRI sequences are able to detect contrast leakage at 3 T and identify unstable aneurysms or rupture sites in patients with aneurysmal subarachnoid hemorrhage (▶ Fig. 18.5, ▶ Table 18.2). These techniques can identify an aneurysm rupture site in patients with multiple intracranial aneurysms (present in 15–20% of cases), allowing for more accurate and timely treatment.[36] Aneurysmal wall enhancement also

Table 18.2 MRI sequence parameters

MRI sequence[a]	TR/TE (ms)	FOV (mm²)	Matrix	Slice thickness (mm)	Time (min:s)
3D TOF	22/3.6	200 × 181	384 × 331	0.5	6:50
3D DANTE T1w BB SPACE	800/21	162 × 162	196 × 192	0.8	5:47
3D T2w BB SPACE	1,000/118	200 × 200	384 × 380	0.5	4:18

Abbreviations: FOV, field of view; TOF, time of flight; TR/TE, repetition time/echo time.

[a]All MRI images were obtained at 3 T on Siemens Verio, Trio, or Prisma platforms with standard head coils and standard contrast dose of MultiHance, 0.1 mmol/kg. Images were obtained in the following order: TOF pre, T1w BB pre, contrast injection, TOF post, T2w BB post, T1w BB post. TOF uses a saturation slab to image only inflowing blood.

correlates with a history of rupture. Aneurysm wall enhancement was identified in 98.4% of ruptured aneurysms, while there was no wall enhancement in 81.9% of unruptured aneurysms.[37] Aneurysm wall permeability can also be quantified using dynamic contrast-enhanced (DCE) MRI and the perfusion parameter K^{trans}, a size-independent predictor of rupture risk.[38]

While wall enhancement and inflammation predicts pre-treatment aneurysm instability, this enhancement can also be seen within excluded aneurysms after endovascular treatment. In this case, enhancement of the neck and within the sac after treatment may additionally predict treatment response. This finding can be detected using HR-MRI after flow diversion (▶ Fig. 18.6).

18.5 Conclusion

Multiple imaging tools are available not only to diagnose intracranial aneurysms but also to guide treatment and assess treatment success after flow diversion. These techniques can be used to assess residual aneurysm lumen and monitor growth. Future advances in imaging, including vessel wall imaging, may allow better characterization of vessel wall vulnerability in aneurysms prior to treatment and may assess healing and decreased rupture risk after flow diversion.

References

[1] van Rooij WJ, Sprengers ME, de Gast AN, Peluso JP, Sluzewski M. 3D rotational angiography: the new gold standard in the detection of additional intracranial aneurysms. AJNR Am J Neuroradiol. 2008; 29(5):976–979

[2] Bechan RS, van Rooij SB, Sprengers ME, et al. CT angiography versus 3D rotational angiography in patients with subarachnoid hemorrhage. Neuroradiology. 2015; 57(12):1239–1246

[3] Hankey GJ, Warlow CP, Molyneux AJ. Complications of cerebral angiography for patients with mild carotid territory ischaemia being considered for carotid endarterectomy. J Neurol Neurosurg Psychiatry. 1990; 53(7):542–548

[4] Fifi JT, Meyers PM, Lavine SD, et al. Complications of modern diagnostic cerebral angiography in an academic medical center. J Vasc Interv Radiol. 2009; 20(4):442–447

[5] Teksam M, McKinney A, Casey S, Asis M, Kieffer S, Truwit CL. Multi-section CT angiography for detection of cerebral aneurysms. AJNR Am J Neuroradiol. 2004; 25(9):1485–1492

[6] Uysal E, Yanbuloğlu B, Ertürk M, Kilinç BM, Başak M. Spiral CT angiography in diagnosis of cerebral aneurysms of cases with acute subarachnoid hemorrhage. Diagn Interv Radiol. 2005; 11(2):77–82

[7] McKinney AM, Palmer CS, Truwit CL, Karagulle A, Teksam M. Detection of aneurysms by 64-section multidetector CT angiography in patients acutely suspected of having an intracranial aneurysm and comparison with digital subtraction and 3D rotational angiography. AJNR Am J Neuroradiol. 2008; 29 (3):594–602

[8] Prestigiacomo CJ, Sabit A, He W, Jethwa P, Gandhi C, Russin J. Three dimensional CT angiography versus digital subtraction angiography in the detection of intracranial aneurysms in subarachnoid hemorrhage. J Neurointerv Surg. 2010; 2(4):385–389

[9] Xing W, Chen W, Sheng J, et al. Sixty-four-row multislice computed tomographic angiography in the diagnosis and characterization of intracranial aneurysms: comparison with 3D rotational angiography. World Neurosurg. 2011; 76(1–2):105–113

[10] Guo W, He XY, Li XF, et al. Meta-analysis of diagnostic significance of sixty-four-row multi-section computed tomography angiography and three-dimensional digital subtraction angiography in patients with cerebral artery aneurysm. J Neurol Sci. 2014; 346(1–2):197–203

[11] Smith-Bindman R, Lipson J, Marcus R, et al. Radiation dose associated with common computed tomography examinations and the associated lifetime attributable risk of cancer. Arch Intern Med. 2009; 169(22):2078–2086

[12] Brenner DJ, Hall EJ. Computed tomography–an increasing source of radiation exposure. N Engl J Med. 2007; 357(22):2277–2284

[13] Cohnen M, Wittsack HJ, Assadi S, et al. Radiation exposure of patients in comprehensive computed tomography of the head in acute stroke. AJNR Am J Neuroradiol. 2006; 27(8):1741–1745

[14] Mnyusiwalla A, Aviv RI, Symons SP. Radiation dose from multidetector row CT imaging for acute stroke. Neuroradiology. 2009; 51(10):635–640

[15] Jessen KA, Shrimpton PC, Geleijns J, Panzer W, Tosi G. Dosimetry for optimisation of patient protection in computed tomography. Appl Radiat Isot. 1999; 50(1):165–172

[16] Kim KP, Berrington de González A, Pearce MS, et al. Development of a database of organ doses for paediatric and young adult CT scans in the United Kingdom. Radiat Prot Dosimetry. 2012; 150(4):415–426

[17] Sailer AM, Wagemans BA, Nelemans PJ, de Graaf R, van Zwam WH. Diagnosing intracranial aneurysms with MR angiography: systematic review and meta-analysis. Stroke. 2014; 45(1):119–126

[18] Nael K, Michaely HJ, Villablanca P, Salamon N, Laub G, Finn JP. Time-resolved contrast enhanced magnetic resonance angiography of the head and neck at 3.0 tesla: initial results. Invest Radiol. 2006; 41(2):116–124

[19] Nael K, Krishnam M, Nael A, Ton A, Ruehm SG, Finn JP. Peripheral contrast-enhanced MR angiography at 3.0 T, improved spatial resolution and low dose contrast: initial clinical experience. Eur Radiol. 2008; 18(12):2893–2900

[20] Goto M, Kunimatsu A, Shojima M, et al. Depiction of branch vessels arising from intracranial aneurysm sacs: time-of-flight MR angiography versus CT angiography. Clin Neurol Neurosurg. 2014; 126:177–184

[21] Schellinger PD, Richter G, Kohrmann M, Dorfler A. Noninvasive angiography (magnetic resonance and computed tomography) in the diagnosis of ischemic cerebrovascular disease. Techniques and clinical applications. Cerebrovasc Dis. 2007; 24 Suppl 1:16–23

[22] Bernstein MA, Huston J, III, Lin C, Gibbs GF, Felmlee JP. High-resolution intracranial and cervical MRA at 3.0T: technical considerations and initial experience. Magn Reson Med. 2001; 46(5):955–962

[23] Kanal E, Barkovich AJ, Bell C, et al. ACR Blue Ribbon Panel on MR Safety. ACR guidance document for safe MR practices: 2007. AJR Am J Roentgenol. 2007; 188(6):1447–1474

[24] Kaewlai R, Abujudeh H. Nephrogenic systemic fibrosis. AJR Am J Roentgenol. 2012; 199(1):W17–23

[25] Prince MR, Zhang H, Morris M, et al. Incidence of nephrogenic systemic fibrosis at two large medical centers. Radiology. 2008; 248(3):807–816

[26] Meng H, Tutino VM, Xiang J, Siddiqui A. High WSS or low WSS? Complex interactions of hemodynamics with intracranial aneurysm initiation, growth, and rupture: toward a unifying hypothesis. AJNR Am J Neuroradiol. 2014; 35 (7):1254–1262

[27] Futami K, Sano H, Misaki K, Nakada M, Ueda F, Hamada J. Identification of the inflow zone of unruptured cerebral aneurysms: comparison of 4D flow MRI and 3D TOF MRA data. AJNR Am J Neuroradiol. 2014; 35(7):1363–1370

[28] Schneiders JJ, Marquering HA, van Ooij P, et al. Additional value of intra-aneurysmal hemodynamics in discriminating ruptured versus unruptured intracranial aneurysms. AJNR Am J Neuroradiol. 2015; 36(10):1920–1926

[29] Wong GK, Lau JC, Poon WS. Flow diverting stents for cerebral aneurysm treatment: time to replace coiling? J Clin Neurosci. 2011; 18(8):1143

[30] Can A, Du R. Association of hemodynamic factors with intracranial aneurysm formation and rupture: systematic review and meta-analysis. Neurosurgery. 2016; 78(4):510–520

[31] Xiang J, Natarajan SK, Tremmel M, et al. Hemodynamic-morphologic discriminants for intracranial aneurysm rupture. Stroke. 2011; 42(1):144–152

[32] Cebral JR, Castro MA, Burgess JE, Pergolizzi RS, Sheridan MJ, Putman CM. Characterization of cerebral aneurysms for assessing risk of rupture by using patient-specific computational hemodynamics models. AJNR Am J Neuroradiol. 2005; 26(10):2550–2559

[33] Munarriz PM, Gómez PA, Paredes I, Castaño-Leon AM, Cepeda S, Lagares A. Basic principles of hemodynamics and cerebral aneurysms. World Neurosurg. 2016; 88:311–319

[34] Hayakawa M, Tanaka T, Sadato A, et al. Detection of pulsation in unruptured cerebral aneurysms by ECG-gated 3D-CT angiography (4D-CTA) with 320-row area detector CT (ADCT) and follow-up evaluation results: assessment based on heart rate at the time of scanning. Clin Neuroradiol. 2014; 24 (2):145–150

[35] Vanrossomme AE, Eker OF, Thiran JP, Courbebaisse GP, Zouaoui Boudjeltia K. Intracranial aneurysms: wall motion analysis for prediction of rupture. AJNR Am J Neuroradiol. 2015; 36(10):1796–1802

[36] Matouk CC, Mandell DM, Günel M, et al. Vessel wall magnetic resonance imaging identifies the site of rupture in patients with multiple intracranial aneurysms: proof of principle. Neurosurgery. 2013; 72(3):492–496, discussion 496

[37] Nagahata S, Nagahata M, Obara M, et al. Wall enhancement of the intracranial aneurysms revealed by magnetic resonance vessel wall imaging using three-dimensional turbo spin-echo sequence with motion-sensitized driven-equilibrium: a sign of ruptured aneurysm? Clin Neuroradiol. 2016; 26(3):277–283

[38] Vakil P, Ansari SA, Cantrell CG, et al. Quantifying intracranial aneurysm wall permeability for risk assessment using dynamic contrast-enhanced MRI: a pilot study. AJNR Am J Neuroradiol. 2015; 36(5):953–959

19 MANAGEMENT OF ANEURYSM RESIDUALS FOLLOWING TREATMENT WITH FLOW DIVERTERS

R. WEBSTER CROWLEY and ROBERT M. STARKE

Abstract

When compared to aneurysms previously treated with other endovascular techniques, or even most surgical techniques, those already treated with flow diversion have substantially limited options when aneurysms persist. This chapter begins by discussing many of the reasons why flow diversion may fail to completely occlude an aneurysm. Treatment failures can largely be attributed to suboptimal or inappropriate device positioning, device failure, or the involvement of a branch vessel demanding flow. The second half of the chapter discusses the available treatment options for residual aneurysms following prior treatment with flow diverters. Endovascular options include first and foremost the placement of additional flow diverters. Other options that may be feasible for some aneurysms include parent vessel sacrifice, or even occasionally coil embolization of the aneurysm. It is also important to recognize the utility of microsurgery for some aneurysms. Microsurgical options may include clip reconstruction, or trapping/parent vessel sacrifice with or without bypass.

Keywords: cerebral aneurysm, endovascular techniques, flow diversion, Pipeline Embolization Device, treatment failure

19.1 Introduction

The management of residual aneurysms following prior treatment is a difficult task regardless of the initial treatment modality. Whether an aneurysm was previously managed surgically or endovascularly, aneurysms that go on to fail or recur following prior treatment often carry an increased degree of complexity when compared to its initial treatment. This increased degree of complexity is, perhaps, never more true then when the prior treatment involved a flow diverter. Unlike standard coil embolization, stent-assisted coil embolization, or even surgical clipping, placement of a flow diverter generally precludes one from accessing the aneurysm should this be needed in future cases. Therefore, many of the tools in the neurointerventionalist's armamentarium are rendered useless once a flow diverter has been placed across an aneurysm. Unfortunately, for patients with residual aneurysm filling despite previous flow-diverting stents, therapeutic options are not only more limited, they may also be associated with increased morbidity and mortality.

Clearly, there is a substantial difference between aneurysm recurrence and aneurysm residual. Residuals are typically present at the completion of the aneurysm treatment, and may be monitored with observation or retreated depending on a number of variables, including the size of the residual, growth or progressive occlusion of the residual, aneurysm location, rupture status, and physician preference. Conversely, recurrent aneurysms are those that were previously determined to be occluded, yet later developed aneurysmal filling. Flow diverters, by their very nature, result in substantial aneurysm residual upon completion of the procedure when used as a standalone treatment. Yet once an aneurysm treated with flow diversion is angiographically occluded, the chance that it later recurs is extremely low.[1] In other words, with very few exceptions,[2] treatment failures for flow diverters are not aneurysm recurrences, but residuals that never went away.

19.2 Reasons for Treatment Failure

When assessing an aneurysm residual following flow diversion, the most important factor in determining the next step is to identify the reasons the initial treatment did not lead to complete occlusion. This information not only shapes the modality of any future treatment but also helps in deciding whether subsequent treatment is even needed in the first place. There are many reasons treatment with flow diverters may result in residual aneurysm. Included among these reasons is the presence of associated side branches, inadequate wall apposition, stent migration or contraction, overall aneurysm size and morphology, and previous aneurysm treatment. In general, these reasons for persistent aneurysm filling can be broken down into three categories: aneurysm residual due to inappropriate device position; aneurysm residual due to device failure; or aneurysm residual that is necessary for maintenance of blood flow elsewhere. While the categories are meant to define the underlying cause for the persistence of aneurysm residual, they also carry different implications regarding the potential, or need for, future treatment. It is therefore paramount that the treating physician accurately determines the cause for treatment failure.

19.2.1 Aneurysm Residual Due to Inappropriate Device Position

Inappropriate device position is a rather broad term that can include a number of actual problems with the device construct. However, it is very important to recognize that of all the different etiologies behind failed flow diverter treatment, residual aneurysms that are felt to be secondary to inappropriate device position should theoretically be the easiest to retreat. The main reason for this is simply that the flow diverter construct that had been previously created is not expected to be successful if it is not placed in a manner that maximizes its flow-diverting properties.

If the flow diverter from the original treatment was undersized with regard to its diameter, particularly at the proximal aspect of the construct, inadequate wall apposition of the flow diverter can result in an endoleak, with subsequent continued filling of the aneurysm. Other reasons for inadequate wall apposition include placement of the proximal end of the stent within a sharp curve, as can be seen with the anterior genu of the cavernous internal carotid artery, and placement of the stent within an irregular, atherosclerotic segment of artery. Finally, incomplete opening of an appropriately sized stent can result in an endoleak. Unfortunately, incomplete stent opening can also result in acute thrombus formation within the lumen of the parent artery. Largely due to this concerning risk, great efforts are made to recognize and manage incomplete stent opening at the time of initial treatment with balloon angioplasty or other manipulations. Therefore, it is unlikely to be the cause of a residual aneurysm as seen on later follow-up angiography. Occasionally, however, it is not immediately clear if a stent is not opened uniformly because of an issue with the stent itself, or if it is as a result of irregularity in the parent artery. Therefore, if there is any question regarding the adequacy of stent apposition, we generally perform a computed tomography angiography, such as Dyna CT (Siemens, Malvern, PA), in the angiography suite. This may help differentiate areas of the stent construct that may benefit from angioplasty, and those that are simply not fully expanded due to areas of stenotic artery.

While, in theory, inadequate wall apposition is something that can be detected during the initial treatment procedure, occasionally the stent configuration or location can change at some point of time after completion of the procedure. Complete migration of a flow diverter, in which the entire stent moves distally, is a rare complication that can be seen with undersizing of the device. Fortunately, this has become more of a theoretical concern, given that our understanding of flow diverters has improved. Nevertheless, it can occur, and certainly if the stent migrates past the aneurysm neck, it would result in an incompletely treated aneurysm, and possibly occlusion of the vessel that it migrates to.

Another more common cause for flow diverter malposition is contraction, or partial migration of the device.[3,4] Unlike complete migration in which the whole stent moves, contraction involves a portion of the stent contracting or foreshortening while the remainder of the stent stays in a relatively stable position. This may more likely occur in particularly tortuous arteries when a vector of force is directing the stent into the aneurysm, and in general is a result of deploying the flow diverter with an insufficient length and apposition on either side of the aneurysm. Unfortunately, it may be difficult to determine the exact amount of stent that should be deployed in the normal artery proximal and distal to the aneurysm to ensure that it does not eventually contract, as it likely varies on an individual basis. However, it may more likely occur with particularly tortuous arteries or those that require significant tension buildup to pass the stent into the desired location. For this reason, it may be reasonable to select longer stents for those aneurysms in which one anticipates potential issues with contraction.

Contraction may also be seen with telescoping flow-diverting stents. This is generally avoided by ensuring that a significant portion of the stent (30–50%) is overlapping, and by choosing a diameter for the inner stent that is at least as large as the outer one. In other words, deploying a smaller stent within a larger stent may greatly increase the chances of contraction and disconnection of a stent construct.

19.2.2 Aneurysm Residual Due to Device Failure

Unlike residual aneurysms that are secondary to inappropriate device positioning, a number of aneurysms may have device constructs that are perfectly positioned and sized, but yet still result in incomplete occlusion of the target aneurysm. These are aneurysms that fail not because of technical issues with the treatment but rather because of something inherent to the aneurysm, which for some reason may make them less likely to respond to treatment with flow diversion.

Aneurysm size and morphology certainly play a large role in the likelihood that the aneurysm goes on to complete occlusion. Decreased rates of complete occlusion are seen with fusiform or dissecting aneurysms.[5,6,7] Aneurysms that are associated with particularly sharp curves of the parent artery may have a jet stream of flow into the aneurysm that may not correct with flow diversion. Another group of aneurysms that are less likely to have successful treatment with a flow-diverting stent are those aneurysms that have already been previously treated, particularly those with a history of prior stent placement.[6,8,9,10,11] There may be a number of reasons for this. Passage of the microcatheter through a preexisting stent can be problematic because if the microcatheter unknowingly passes through a cell of the existing stent, a subsequent point of restriction is created upon deployment of a flow diverter. Assuming the true lumen of the stent is maintained by the microcatheter, in the process of deployment the distal end of the flow diverter may catch on the prior stent leading to stretching of the device and less ideal results.[12] In addition, placement of a flow-diverting stent within another stent may be associated with an increased risk of in-stent or stent-adjacent stenosis.[13]

There is reasonable literature regarding the effect that prior treatments have on flow diverters. Heiferman et al reported their series of 25 aneurysms that had failed stent-assisted embolization.[11] Following subsequent treatment with flow-diverting stents, complete occlusion was seen in only 38% of cases. Nelson et al reported in their series of 31 aneurysms that of the two aneurysms not initially occluded with a flow-diverting stent, one was treated with another stent. In this small series, the authors noted that prior stent placement makes apposition of a flow-diverting stent more challenging and may decrease neointimal formation and endothelialization required for aneurysm obliteration.[14] In a review of 63 aneurysms treated with flow diversion, Lylyk et al found that the only aneurysm remaining patent at 12-month follow-up had been previously treated with stent-assisted coiling.[15] The authors concluded that the prior stent likely decreased the apposition of the flow-diverting stent to the parent vessel, which created an endoleak and likely decreased endothelialization.

In a matched cohort analysis, 21 patients with previously stented recurrent aneurysms who later underwent Pipeline Embolization Device placement (group 1) were compared with 63 patients who had treatment with the Pipeline Embolization Device with no prior stent placement (group 2).[16] Pipeline Embolization Device treatment resulted in complete aneurysm occlusion in significantly fewer patients in groups 1 (55.6%) versus group 2 (80.4%). The rate of good clinical outcome at the latest follow-up in group 1 was 81.0 versus 93.2% in group 2 ($p = 0.1$), and complications were observed in 14.3% of patients in group 1 and 9.5% of patients in group 2 ($p = 0.684$). Intrinsically, it appears that the use of the Pipeline Embolization Device in the management of previously stented aneurysms is less effective than the use of this device in nonstented aneurysms. Prior stent placement may also worsen the safety and efficacy profile of this device. It is also reasonable to suggest that aneurysms that require further stent placement may be more complex aneurysms that may already have a higher risk of morbidity and lower occlusion rate. Nevertheless, recurrent stent placement following previously stented aneurysms is challenging and must be performed cautiously.

19.2.3 Necessary Aneurysm Residual

While the primary goal of most aneurysm treatments is complete occlusion of the target aneurysm, there are certain aneurysms in which it may actually be beneficial to leave a portion of the aneurysm. This is centered on the premise that for some aneurysms, complete obliteration may actually be more harmful than incomplete occlusion. This has been well described for the flow diversion of ophthalmic artery segment aneurysms; however, it can be seen with any aneurysm that incorporates an important arterial branch (▶ Fig. 19.1). For these aneurysms,

true angiographic obliteration would include sacrifice of the associated branch, with the high possibility of downstream ischemic injury. When these aneurysms are treated surgically, clip reconstruction may allow for preservation of the vessel of concern, while excluding as much of the aneurysm as possible. However, even for surgically clipped aneurysms, when a branch arises from the aneurysm itself, maintenance of blood flow through an associated branch by definition requires the presence of residual aneurysm.

When treating these aneurysms endovascularly, there are generally two potential outcomes. Either the aneurysm goes on to occlude completely along with the associated branch or the branch remains patent through a subtotally occluded aneurysm. Fortunately, experience with flow diversion suggests that those aneurysms that develop complete occlusion of both the aneurysm and branch vessel do so silently, presumably due to sufficient collateral supply to the affected territory that prevents any clinical sequelae.[17,18] For those aneurysms that maintain preserved flow to the associated branch, there is typically near-complete occlusion of the aneurysm, with development of a channel through the aneurysm that supplies the branch (▶ Fig. 19.2). It is often difficult to accurately predict which aneurysms will occlude completely and which ones will form

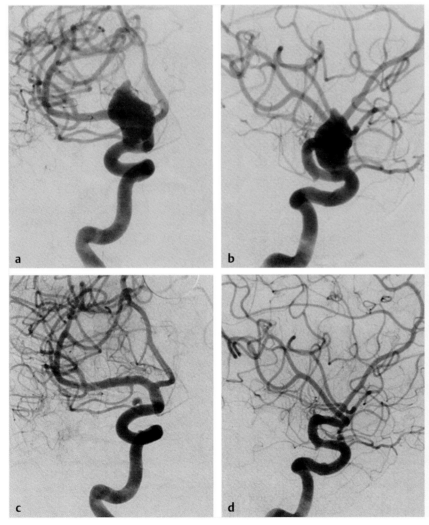

Fig. 19.1 Angiographic images of a large unruptured right ophthalmic artery aneurysm. Pretreatment posteroanterior **(a)** and lateral **(b)** images are seen demonstrating possible origin of the ophthalmic artery arising from the aneurysm neck. The patient was treated with a single Surpass flow-diverting stent (Stryker Neurovascular, Fremont, CA). A posttreatment angiography **(c,d)** performed 1 year posttreatment demonstrated near-complete obliteration (> 99%) of the aneurysm, with a small amount of residual aneurysm associated with a patent ophthalmic artery.

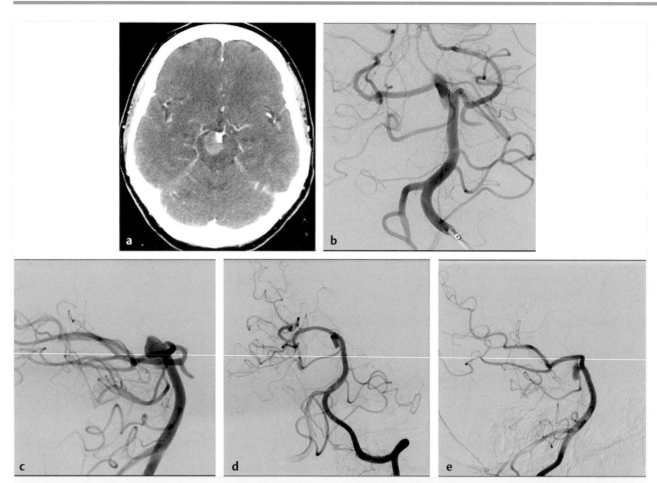

Fig. 19.2 Large partially thrombosed aneurysm involving the right posterior cerebral and superior cerebellar arteries. CT scan **(a)** shows extent of aneurysmal size that is partially thrombosed. Pretreatment angiographic images **(b,c)** demonstrate the portion of the aneurysm that actively fills. Also seen is the origin of the superior cerebellar artery arising from the aneurysm. The patient underwent treatment using a single Pipeline Embolization Device. Posttreatment follow-up angiographic images **(d,e)** show complete occlusion of the superior portion of the majority of the aneurysm, with a small amount of residual associated with a patent superior cerebellar artery. Of note, the left posterior cerebellar artery no longer fills from the vertebral artery; instead blood flow is supplied from the left posterior communicating artery, with no resultant neurological symptoms.

this channel. However, lack of negative sequelae related to these branch artery occlusions suggests that those aneurysms that go on to occlude completely have sufficient collateral to the territory in question, while those aneurysms with continued flow do not. In other words, the aneurysm residuals seen in many of these cases are necessary residuals that are preventing ischemic events. This is a very important distinction, given that additional treatment for small, stable residuals associated with preserved branch vessels may be of little use, and could in fact be harmful. Therefore, retreatment of small aneurysm residuals that exist because of continued flow through an important branch vessel should not be performed, unless, for some reason, the re-rupture risk of the aneurysm remnant remains a substantial concern.

19.3 Retreatment of Previously Treated Aneurysms

When a physician decides to treat an aneurysm endovascularly, it is helpful to give thought to future treatments should they be necessary. Paramount in this decision process is an understanding of the reasons for any residual aneurysm as outlined earlier, and an appreciation of the fact that not all residuals require treatment. With the exception of parent vessel sacrifice, perhaps no endovascular aneurysm treatment modality limits future treatment options as substantially as flow diversion does. Once a flow diverter is in place, the general convention is that future treatment options are limited to either placement of additional stents or surgical management. While this is not quite accurate for every residual aneurysm, it remains true that most of the tools available to cerebrovascular surgeons are rendered useless once a flow-diverting stent has been incorporated into a patient's treatment.

19.3.1 Additional Devices

For those residual aneurysms that are deemed to require additional treatment, the most obvious option following flow diversion is simply placement of additional flow-diverting stents. This is almost without questioning the treatment of choice for aneurysms whose initial treatment failed due to inappropriate device positioning. However, it is frequently also the first-line retreatment option for any residual aneurysm that has already been treated with a flow diverter.

Additional devices are placed depending on the reason of the initial treatment failure. Endoleaks are treated by placing additional stents in a telescoping fashion. These failures are usually due to poor wall apposition at the proximal end of the device construct, and the stents placed during retreatment are sized accordingly to ensure adequate wall apposition at the end of the revised construct where the endoleak exists. As noted earlier, the additional stents should never be of smaller diameter than the stents they are being placed within.

When treatment has failed due to device migration or contraction, additional stents are placed ideally to reconstitute the device construct that was originally planned. It is necessary to take into account the reason for change in the initial stent configuration, a concern that is often obviated by building a longer device construct with more substantial purchase on both sides of the aneurysm neck.

For those aneurysms that persist despite well-devised flow diversion constructs, additional stents are usually placed completely within the existing stents to increase the stent coverage across the neck of the aneurysm. This decreases the porosity of the device construct, and subsequently increases flow diversion away from the aneurysm (▶ Fig. 19.3).

19.3.2 Coil Embolization

Coil embolization following flow diversion may be carried out in very limited settings, but is often not considered as a viable therapeutic option. If there is a large endoleak that supplies blood flow to the residual aneurysm, a microcatheter might be advanced outside of the stent into the aneurysm. Additional flow-diverting stents would ultimately be necessary to eliminate the endoleak, after successful catheterization and coil embolization of the aneurysm. Additionally, a suitable side branch for aneurysm access, such as posterior communicating artery aneurysm, may allow for catheterization of the aneurysm through a cross-circulation approach after initial flow diversion.

19.3.3 Parent Artery Sacrifice

In patients with continued filling of an aneurysm despite prior flow diversion, parent vessel sacrifice may be a reasonable option. In fact, historically, before the development of flow diverters, many of these aneurysms would have been treated with parent artery occlusion. Parent vessel sacrifice can be associated with thromboembolic complications in up to 20% of patients, although rates of morbidity and mortality are significantly lower in patients passing a balloon occlusion test.[19,20,21,22,23,24] Long-term risks of parent vessel sacrifice must be weighed against both the potential risks and failure of aneurysm obliteration of further treatments with alternative strategies.

While we prefer to perform parent vessel sacrifice endovascularly, it can be performed either surgically or endovascularly.

19.3.4 Microsurgical Treatment

Microsurgical alternatives for persistent residual aneurysms following flow diversion are limited. Flow-diverting stents have been such a substantial technological advance largely because they allow for the treatment of many large or giant aneurysms that previously had only high-risk options, including highly morbid open surgical procedures. Failed treatment using flow diverters does not, all of a sudden, make these complex cases any easier should open surgery become the best remaining option, and it could potentially make those surgeries more dangerous, especially when factoring in the need for antiplatelet therapy. Clip reconstruction may be possible, but the residual aneurysm is often fragile and may not provide a significant aneurysm neck to allow for placement of clips. As the use of flow diverters, particularly Pipeline (ev3), has expanded past the on-label indications to include aneurysms that may also be reasonable surgical candidates, microsurgery would likely still remain an option should flow diversion fail—of course, again with an increased potential risk due to the need for performing open cerebrovascular surgery while on antiplatelet therapy.

Another interesting consideration is that aneurysms may continue to enlarge despite no residual filling of the aneurysm from the parent vessel or even complete occlusion of the parent vessel following treatment with a flow-diverting stent.[2,25,26,27] The most common etiologies of this include progressive inflammation and growing thrombus from blood supply from the parent vessel or parasitized blood flow to the aneurysm dome from small perforators that lead to the growing thrombus. A continuous cycle of mural hemorrhage and thrombosis by the vasa vasorum may result in progressive enlargement of occluded giant aneurysms. At this stage, these aneurysms begin to resemble neoplastic rather than vascular lesions, and there are usually no or limited endovascular options. In select cases, microsurgical resection or decompression of the aneurysm may be necessary if there is significant mass effect, persistent edema, or parent vessel obstruction.[2,16,26] For these cases, microsurgical trapping and possibly removal of the aneurysm with or without bypass is one of the few remaining treatment options. When absolutely necessary, flow diverters have been removed and the aneurysm treated microsurgically both with and without direct cerebral bypass.[26,28] However, these surgeries are associated with significant risk and probably should carried out only in the event that all other therapeutic options, including observation, are not viable.

19.4 Future Directions

Many new endovascular technologies are being invented and tested for the treatment of cerebral aneurysms. Further options are necessary to allow for safe and effective therapies of aneurysms previously treated with flow diversion. These should be less invasive or associated with lower risk of morbidity and mortality than the aforementioned options. Owing to the small number of patients with residual aneurysms following flow diversion, prospective multicenter collaborations will be necessary to determine the optimal treatments for these patients.

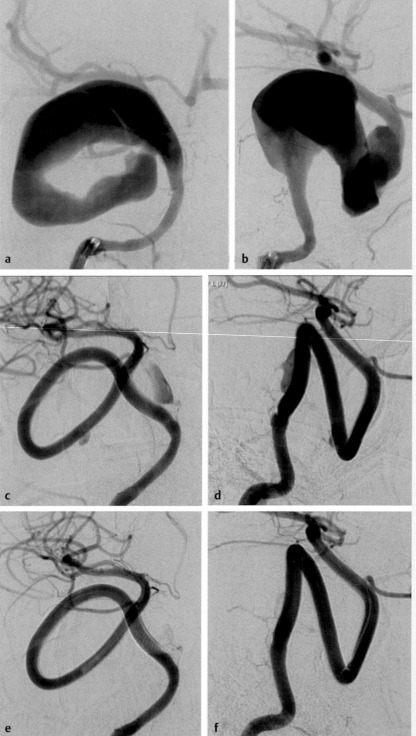

Fig. 19.3 Angiographic images of a giant, partially thrombosed aneurysm of the right cavernous internal carotid artery. Pretreatment images **(a,b)** demonstrate the filling component of the aneurysm as it created a channel within the aneurysm. The aneurysm was treated with telescoping Pipeline flow-diverting stents. Follow-up imaging **(c,d)** showed that the aneurysm was largely thrombosed, with the exception of continued filling in two distinct locations. One additional Pipeline was placed across each of the two areas of continued aneurysmal filling, after which follow-up imaging **(e,f)** demonstrated complete occlusion of the aneurysm. (Credit: Cameron G. McDougall, MD.)

References

[1] Becske T, Potts MB, Shapiro M, et al. Pipeline for uncoilable or failed aneurysms: 3-year follow-up results. J Neurosurg. 2016 Oct 14:1–8 –[Epub ahead of print]

[2] Abla AA, Zaidi HA, Crowley RW, et al. Optic chiasm compression from mass effect and thrombus formation following unsuccessful treatment of a giant supraclinoid ICA aneurysm with the Pipeline device: open surgical bailout with STA-MCA bypass and parent vessel occlusion. J Neurosurg Pediatr. 2014; 14(1):31–37

[3] Chalouhi N, Satti SR, Tjoumakaris S, et al. Delayed migration of a pipeline embolization device. Neurosurgery. 2013; 72(2) Suppl Operative:ons229–ons234, discussion ons234

[4] Chalouhi N, Tjoumakaris SI, Gonzalez LF, et al. Spontaneous delayed migration/shortening of the pipeline embolization device: report of 5 cases. AJNR Am J Neuroradiol. 2013; 34(12):2326–2330

[5] Fischer S, Perez MA, Kurre W, Albes G, Bäzner H, Henkes H. Pipeline embolization device for the treatment of intra- and extracranial fusiform and dissecting aneurysms: initial experience and long-term follow-up. Neurosurgery. 2014; 75(4):364–374, discussion 374

[6] Jabbour P, Chalouhi N, Tjoumakaris S, et al. The Pipeline Embolization Device: learning curve and predictors of complications and aneurysm obliteration. Neurosurgery. 2013; 73(1):113–120, discussion 120

[7] Kerolus M, Kasliwal MK, Lopes DK. Persistent aneurysm growth following pipeline embolization device assisted coiling of a fusiform vertebral artery aneurysm: a word of caution! Neurointervention. 2015; 10(1):28–33

[8] Chalouhi N, Starke RM, Yang S, et al. Extending the indications of flow diversion to small, unruptured, saccular aneurysms of the anterior circulation. Stroke. 2014; 45(1):54–58

[9] Chalouhi N, Tjoumakaris S, Phillips JL, et al. A single pipeline embolization device is sufficient for treatment of intracranial aneurysms. AJNR Am J Neuroradiol. 2014; 35(8):1562–1566

[10] Chalouhi N, Tjoumakaris S, Starke RM, et al. Comparison of flow diversion and coiling in large unruptured intracranial saccular aneurysms. Stroke. 2013; 44(8):2150–2154

[11] Heiferman DM, Billingsley JT, Kasliwal MK, et al. Use of flow-diverting stents as salvage treatment following failed stent-assisted embolization of intracranial aneurysms. J Neurointerv Surg. 2016; 8(7):692–695

[12] Chalouhi N, Chitale R, Starke RM, et al. Treatment of recurrent intracranial aneurysms with the Pipeline Embolization Device. J Neurointerv Surg. 2014; 6(1):19–23

[13] Chalouhi N, Polifka A, Daou B, et al. In-Pipeline stenosis: incidence, predictors, and clinical outcomes. Neurosurgery. 2015; 77(6):875–879, discussion 879

[14] Nelson PK, Lylyk P, Szikora I, Wetzel SG, Wanke I, Fiorella D. The pipeline embolization device for the intracranial treatment of aneurysms trial. AJNR Am J Neuroradiol. 2011; 32(1):34–40

[15] Lylyk P, Miranda C, Ceratto R, et al. Curative endovascular reconstruction of cerebral aneurysms with the pipeline embolization device: the Buenos Aires experience. Neurosurgery. 2009; 64(4):632–642, discussion 642–643, quiz N6

[16] Daou B, Starke RM, Chalouhi N, et al. The use of the Pipeline Embolization Device in the management of recurrent previously coiled cerebral aneurysms. Neurosurgery. 2015; 77(5):692–697, discussion 697

[17] Burrows AM, Brinjikji W, Puffer RC, Cloft H, Kallmes DF, Lanzino G. Flow diversion for ophthalmic artery aneurysms. AJNR Am J Neuroradiol. 2016 [Epub ahead of print]

[18] Moon K, Albuquerque FC, Ducruet AF, Webster Crowley R, McDougall CG. Treatment of ophthalmic segment carotid aneurysms using the pipeline embolization device: clinical and angiographic follow-up. Neurol Res. 2014; 36(4):344–350

[19] Barr JD, Lemley TJ. Endovascular arterial occlusion accomplished using microcoils deployed with and without proximal flow arrest: results in 19 patients. AJNR Am J Neuroradiol. 1999; 20(8):1452–1456

[20] Chalouhi N, Starke RM, Tjoumakaris SI, et al. Carotid and vertebral artery sacrifice with a combination of Onyx and coils: technical note and case series. Neuroradiology. 2013; 55(8):993–998

[21] Graves VB, Perl J, II, Strother CM, Wallace RC, Kesava PP, Masaryk TJ. Endovascular occlusion of the carotid or vertebral artery with temporary proximal flow arrest and microcoils: clinical results. AJNR Am J Neuroradiol. 1997; 18 (7):1201–1206

[22] Sorteberg A, Bakke SJ, Boysen M, Sorteberg W. Angiographic balloon test occlusion and therapeutic sacrifice of major arteries to the brain. Neurosurgery. 2008; 63(4):651–660, discussion 660–661

[23] Tjoumakaris SI, Dumont AS, Gonzalez LF, Rosenwasser RH, Jabbour PM. A novel endovascular technique for temporary balloon occlusion and permanent vessel deconstruction with a single microcatheter. World Neurosurg. 2013; 79(5–6):798.E13:798.E1–6

[24] Zussman B, Gonzalez LF, Dumont A, et al. Endovascular management of carotid blowout. World Neurosurg. 2012; 78(1–2):109–114

[25] Dehdashti AR, Thines L, Willinsky RA, Tymianski M. Symptomatic enlargement of an occluded giant carotido-ophthalmic aneurysm after endovascular treatment: the vasa vasorum theory. Acta Neurochir (Wien). 2009; 151 (9):1153–1158

[26] Ding D, Starke RM, Liu KC. Microsurgical strategies following failed endovascular treatment with the pipeline embolization device: case of a giant posterior cerebral artery aneurysm. J Cerebrovasc Endovasc Neurosurg. 2014; 16 (1):26–31

[27] Wajnberg E, Silva TS, Johnson AK, Lopes DK. Progressive deconstruction: a novel aneurysm treatment using the pipeline embolization device for competitive flow diversion: case report. Neurosurgery. 2014; 10 Suppl 1:E161–E166, discussion E166

[28] Ding D, Liu KC. Microsurgical extraction of a malfunctioned pipeline embolization device following complete deployment. J Cerebrovasc Endovasc Neurosurg. 2013; 15(3):241–245

20 HEMODYNAMIC MODIFICATIONS OF FLOW-DIVERTING STENTS

SHERVIN RAHIMPOUR, PRIYA NAIR, DAVID FRAKES, and L. FERNANDO GONZALEZ

Abstract

Recently, the endovascular treatment paradigm of cerebral aneurysms has shifted from intrasaccular therapies, where coils or liquid embolic agents are delivered inside the aneurysm itself, to endoluminal therapies with standalone stents known as *flow-diverting stents* (FDS). These stents promote aneurysm occlusion by modifying intrinsic aneurysm properties such as wall shear stress, redirecting blood flow away from the aneurysm. The end result is facilitation of endothelial growth within the stent struts, repairing of the vessel, and, ultimately, permanent exclusion of the aneurysm. This chapter analyses how these variables are modified in vitro, discusses computational methods used both clinically and experimentally to analyze hemodynamic changes, and reviews the current challenges that remain with this technology.

Keywords: cerebral aneurysm, computational fluid dynamics, flow-diverting stent, hemodynamic modifications

20.1 Introduction

Hemodynamic changes are known to play an important role in the etiology, growth, and rupture of cerebral aneurysms. The higher incidence of cerebral aneurysms in (1) patients with aortic coarctation, (2) vessels proximal to a stenosis, (3) feeding arteries of arteriovenous malformations, and (4) contralateral side of an occluded internal carotid artery are prime examples of the impact of altered fluid dynamics. However, the precise cause of cerebral aneurysm formation is still unknown. Complex interactions between the vessel wall and hemodynamic forces are believed to contribute to the process.[1] Endovascular techniques allow modification of hemodynamic variables leading to a powerful means of therapy toward promoting thrombosis and eventual aneurysmal occlusion.

During the past two decades, coil embolization has been the most popular endovascular treatment for cerebral aneurysm repair. Recently, the endovascular treatment paradigm has shifted from intrasaccular therapies (where coils or liquid embolic agents are delivered into the aneurysm sac) to endoluminal therapies (where standalone stents are deployed along the parent vessel, across the aneurysm neck). Standalone stents, called *flow-diverting stents* (FDSs), change the flow between the aneurysm and parent vessel promoting stagnation. The stagnant flow within the aneurysm sac promotes gradual thrombosis which ultimately will occlude the aneurysm. Over time, endothelial growth within stent struts facilitates reconstruction of the parent vessels, ultimately resulting in permanent exclusion of the aneurysm from circulation. This chapter examines the impact of FDSs on cerebral aneurysm hemodynamics and the different methodologies used to analyze these changes.

20.2 In Vitro Techniques

Various in vitro techniques have demonstrated the effects of FDSs on cerebral aneurysm hemodynamics.[2,3,4] One of the main advantages of in vitro techniques over in vivo techniques is the repeatability of the experimental process with different devices and configurations, vascular models, and flow conditions. Furthermore, idealized cerebral aneurysm models can be employed to investigate the effects of factors, such as aneurysm geometry and stent configuration, under controlled conditions to provide a fundamental understanding of the impact of different factors on treatment success. In general, in vitro experimentation involves (1) reconstructing or designing the computational aneurysm geometry, (2) translating the computational model to a physical model, (3) connecting the physical model to a flow loop with a blood analog as a circulating fluid, (4) measuring fluid flow through the model using techniques such as optical imaging, and (5) deploying FDS into the physical model to measure the effects of treatment on cerebral aneurysm flow.

Particle image velocimetry (PIV) is a popular flow visualization and analysis technique often used in cerebral aneurysm research.[2,5,6,7] One of the methods for constructing the physical aneurysm model used for experimentation is the lost-core manufacturing technique (▶ Fig. 20.1). The optically clear model is connected to a flow loop for experimentation. The solution is seeded with reflecting particles that are illuminated by a laser, and then imaged by one or more cameras. Hemodynamic information, such as flow velocity, is calculated based on particle movement between subsequent images. Detailed information about PIV can be found in the study of Adrian and Westerweel.[8] The experimental process can be repeated to investigate the effects of different FDS on cerebral aneurysm hemodynamics (▶ Fig. 20.2).

20.3 Computational Techniques

Advances in computational modeling and simulation techniques have facilitated the use of computational fluid dynamics (CFD) in cerebral aneurysm research, which may be the most popular technique for investigating the effects of endovascular treatment on cerebral aneurysm hemodynamics. CFD models blood flow by solving the Navier-Stokes equations (governing equations of fluid flow), consisting of continuity and momentum equations, using numerical methods and algorithms. The Navier-Stokes equations for an incompressible fluid can be written as follows:

$$\nabla \bullet \vec{v} = 0, \tag{20.1}$$

$$\frac{\partial \vec{v}}{\partial t} + \vec{v} \bullet \nabla \vec{v} = -\frac{1}{\rho} \nabla P + v \nabla^2 \vec{v} + \vec{g}, \tag{20.2}$$

where $\vec{v}$, ρ, P, and v are the fluid velocity, density, pressure, and kinematic viscosity, respectively, and $\vec{g}$ is the gravitational force

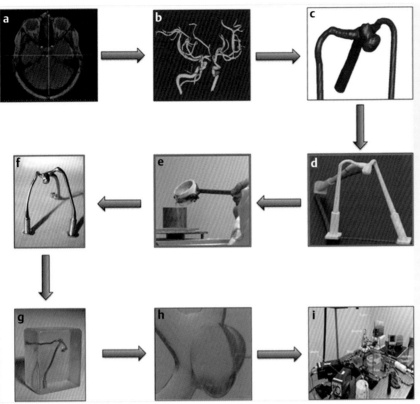

Fig. 20.1 Constructing the physical model for particle image velocimetry (PIV) experimentation. **(a)** Medical image acquisition, **(b)** geometry segmentation and reconstruction, **(c)** computational model, **(d)** 3D wax model, **(e)** translation of the wax model to metal model, **(f)** polished metal model, **(g)** metal model encapsulated in clear urethane, **(h)** lost-core aneurysm model, **(i)** PIV experimentation. (Reproduced with permission from Nair.[39])

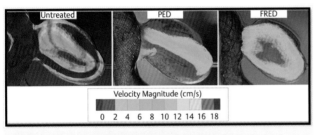

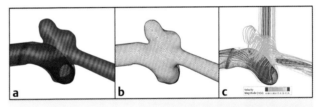

Fig. 20.3 (a) 3D computational model, **(b)** meshed geometry, and **(c)** stream traces obtained after computational fluid dynamic simulation.

Fig. 20.2 Velocity vector plots (left) before treatment and after treatment with the (middle) Pipeline Embolization Device (PED) and a Flow Redirection Endoluminal Device (FRED, right).

acting on the fluid. One of the main advantages of CFD over in vivo and/or in vitro techniques is the flexibility to investigate large patient populations without the tedious and expensive process of physical model construction. CFD also allows virtual treatment with endovascular devices, and has the potential to be used as a treatment-planning tool. However, various assumptions have to be made to simplify the complexity of modeling blood flow. Blood is often modeled as an incompressible and Newtonian fluid, and the vessel walls are assumed to be rigid. There are techniques that can be used to overcome this, but at the cost of computational time.

Flow analysis using CFD usually entails (1) construction of the three-dimensional (3D) computational model; (2) discretization of the computational model into mesh elements; (3) applying suitable boundary conditions to the inflow(s), outflow(s), and vessel walls; and (4) simulation of blood flow (▶ Fig. 20.3).

20.4 Effects of Flow-Diverting Stents on Hemodynamics

One of the main factors that plays an important role in the success of FDSs is the stent porosity.[9] Specifically, a correlation exists between aneurysm occlusion rates and stent porosity.[10] Porosity is defined as the ratio of the metal-free surface area to the total (equivalent to the preoperative condition). Therefore, reducing the porosity of an FDS would improve the likelihood of flow reduction and diversion. This would in turn lead to increased stagnation within the aneurysm sac promoting thrombosis, and ultimately aneurysm occlusion. However, stent porosities less than 65% can occlude neighboring perforating vessels, thereby compromising cerebral perfusion.[11] Higher metal coverage (i.e., lower porosity) has also been found to cause in-stent stenosis, secondary to intimal hyperplasia.[12]

Furthermore, low porosity stents can lack the flexibility needed to navigate through cerebral vasculature. Another important consideration during the deployment of an FDS is that aneurysms often occur in the greater curvature of curved vessels. Deploying an FDS in such geometries would "open up" the stent pores at the aneurysm neck, increasing the porosity at the ostium. Fortunately, emerging technologies in CFD and modeling have enabled assessment of treatment effectiveness prior to clinical deployment of FDSs, such as effects of the stent on (1) flow diversion, (2) neighboring vasculature, and (3) parent vessel morphology, as well as the impact of different stent deployment strategies, including the use of multiple telescoping stents.

Quantitative hemodynamic responses include intra-aneurysmal velocities, aneurysmal inflow, intra-aneurysmal pressure, wall shear stress (WSS) and WSS gradients, vorticity, and turnover time. Qualitative responses include flow complexity and impingement zones. The remainder of this subsection details the effects of FDSs on hemodynamics.

20.4.1 Intra-aneurysmal Velocity and Aneurysmal Inflow

The amount of blood crossing the aneurysm neck per second, or aneurysmal inflow, and velocities inside the aneurysm can serve as indicators for FDS treatment effectiveness. In general, FDSs have proven to be superior to other stents in terms of reducing aneurysmal flow velocities, correlating with favorable clinical outcomes.[10,13,14,15] Intra-aneurysmal flow velocities in an untreated cerebral aneurysm are sometimes up to 70% of the parent vessel velocity at the end of systole.[9] Various clinical trials, along with experimental and computational studies, have demonstrated the effectiveness of a FDS in cerebral aneurysm treatment. In a PIV-based study, previously conducted by our group, reductions in aneurysmal velocities were observed when comparing the effects of cerebral aneurysm hemodynamics after treatment with the Pipeline Embolization Device (PED) and the Flow Redirection Endoluminal Device (FRED). Intra-aneurysmal velocity reductions of more than 55 and 65% were observed after treatment with PED and FRED, respectively, under steady and pulsatile flow conditions (▶ Fig. 20.4). In another CFD-based study, Kulcsár et al analyzed eight patients with para-ophthalmic aneurysms treated with SILK flow diversion (not available in the United States).[16] Velocity reductions of 44% were observed after virtually treating the aneurysm with this device. Roszelle et al have also compared the effects of PED with those of telescoping high porosity stents showing that PED treatment was associated with the greatest reductions in intra-aneurysmal flow.[2]

20.4.2 Intra-aneurysmal Pressure

Intra-aneurysmal pressure is the outward force applied by blood on the aneurysmal wall. The effects of FDSs on intra-aneurysmal pressure remain a topic of controversy. Furthermore, pressure changes within an aneurysm following stent placement have been found to be insignificant compared with physiologic blood pressure.[17,18,19,20] A study by Larrabide et al demonstrated that FDSs do not alter intra-aneurysmal pressure.

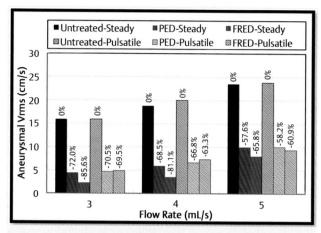

Fig. 20.4 Intra-aneurysmal flow velocities in a patient-specific sidewall aneurysm model measured using particle image velocimetry. The black, red, and blue boxes correspond to untreated, Pipeline Embolization Device (PED), and Flow Redirection Endoluminal Device (FRED) cases, respectively. The solid and patterned boxes correspond to steady and pulsatile inflow conditions, respectively.

Their results suggested that regardless of the size and shape of the aneurysm, flow diversion affected only the dynamic pressure (i.e., <3% of the pulse pressure, or <2 mm Hg).[18] However, in a retrospective CFD study by Cebral et al that investigated pre- and posttreatment conditions following treatment of three ruptured and four successfully treated aneurysms (seven aneurysms in total), increased intra-aneurysmal pressure was observed in the three ruptured cases following treatment with FDS.[17] They suggested that the increase in posttreatment pressure could possibly be due to the proximal parent vessel stenosis (observed in two of three ruptured cases), or due to an initial decrease in local aneurysmal flow, followed by cerebral autoregulation working to maintain perfusion pressure, resulting in an increase in intra-aneurysmal pressure. In another study by Schneiders et al, experimental hemodynamic measurements using a dual-sensor guidewire (corroborated with computational studies) suggested that flow diversion did not protect aneurysms from stresses induced by pressure changes.[21] The authors argued that these continued stresses could contribute to aneurysm rupture at a later phase. Thus, alterations in intra-aneurysmal pressure after treatment with FDSs have been proposed as a contributor to late rupture.

CFD may also have the potential to be used as an important tool for preprocedural analysis to identify potentially dangerous cases after simulation of patient-specific CFD models. These studies could assist the interventionalist in considering other deployment options, such as using embolic coils to optimize the posttreatment hemodynamic environment.

20.4.3 Wall Shear Stress and Wall Shear Stress Gradient

Wall shear stress is defined as the tangential force produced by blood flowing past the endothelial surface.[22,23] Like in the case of intra-aneurysmal pressure, whether high or low WSS is detrimental to an aneurysm remains a topic of debate. While increased WSS levels have been associated with aneurysm initiation by triggering the remodeling of the blood vessel wall, low levels of WSS weaken the integrity of the vessel wall, causing aneurysm growth and eventual rupture.[24,25] Microscopically, high WSS leads to fragmentation of the internal elastic lamina, resulting in outward destructive remodeling in an effort to decrease WSS, and low WSS triggers inflammatory and atherosclerotic changes.[22,26] Meng et al proposed a bimodal theory identifying both low and high WSS as factors in aneurysm rupture.[27] Specifically, low WSS and high oscillatory shear index induce an inflammatory cell-mediated response, which can be associated with atherosclerotic aneurysm phenotypes. High WSS combined with a positive WSS gradient triggers a mural-cell–mediated response which can also be associated with bleb-like aneurysm growth and rupture.

Additionally, stent placement is known to reduce WSS. A study by Levitt et al demonstrated a decrease in WSS and WSS gradients following virtual stent placement.[28] Meng et al used an in vitro dye model and CFD to analyze the impact of Wallstent placement to vessel curvature.[29] Stent placement resulted in decreases of 61, 96, 98, and 56% in saccular aneurysms with parent vessels of increasing curvature from sidewall (0 mm) to 0.03 mm, 0.07 mm, and 0.11 mm, respectively.

20.4.4 Vorticity

In vitro experiments and CFD simulations have demonstrated a well-defined vortical structure near the proximal neck of a sidewall aneurysm during early systole.[30] An unsteady three-dimensional vortex forms in early systole and propagates toward the distal neck during diastole, with vortex dissipation at the end of diastole.[30] Vortex formation links flow pulsatility and aneurysm formation and growth.[31,32] Using a digital PIV system, Cantón et al compared vorticity and shear stress fields following deployment of one to three Neuroform stents.[33] The authors measured a consistent decrease in vorticity with the addition of each subsequent stent. Specifically, the decrease in magnitude of vorticity after the first stent was significant, while the addition of the second and third stents led to less significant reductions. Regardless, the study demonstrated flow diversion to decrease vorticity that could lead to aneurysm growth and rupture. A study by Meng et al demonstrated that reduction in vorticity also depended on the geometry of the parent vessel, in addition to stent placement.[29]

20.4.5 Turnover Time

Turnover time is defined as the ratio of aneurysm volume to the inflow rate at the neck plane, and can be described as the time taken by blood to enter and exit an aneurysm. Deployment of a FDS results in contrast stagnation within the aneurysm. Virchow's triad suggests that stasis of blood favors thrombosis. Xiang et al investigated three complex aneurysms using CFD.[34] The results indicated that the aneurysm with the greatest reduction in inflow and greatest increase in turnover time occluded within 3 months. Turnover time is also affected by the geometry of the parent vessel, particularly vessel curvature, where small vessel curvatures were found to correlate with higher turnover times. A study by Kim et al demonstrated that two different stents (i.e., the Tristar and Wallstent) were ineffective at

curvatures of 0.07 mm or greater.[35] Tremmel et al also analyzed turnover time using Enterprise and Vision stents.[20] In this study, a single stented aneurysm model did not significantly change turnover time. However, double and triple stenting increased turnover time by factors of 1.1 to 1.2 and 1.27 to 1.28 times, respectively. The stasis index is another metric similar to turnover time. It is calculated as the half-peak width of the time–intensity curve, or the duration of time a dye remains in the region of interest. Meng et al reported that the best results and greatest stasis index occurred in sidewall aneurysms with parent vessels of low curvature.[29] Similar calculations were performed by Struffert et al demonstrating that, in an elastase-induced aneurysm following placement of a Neuroform stent or PED, the maximum opacification was increased.[36] Furthermore, this effect was most prominent in the PED group, indicating that the PED had the greatest intra-aneurysmal stasis efficacy.

20.5 Qualitative Hemodynamic Responses

Flow patterns are known to play a role in cerebral aneurysm rupture.[37] In a retrospective study investigating 210 patient-specific cerebral aneurysm models using CFD, 83% of the aneurysms that ruptured were associated with concentrated inflow jets, small impingement regions, and complex flow patterns, while the aneurysms with simple flow patterns were found less likely to rupture.[25] Simple flow patterns involve one inflow jet and a single vortex structure, while complex patterns involve several inflow jets and multiple intra-aneurysmal vortices. Complex flow patterns are also associated with inflammatory cell infiltration, typically found in the walls of ruptured aneurysms.[38] While a FDS may not entirely disrupt a vortex, a single stent can dampen flow complexity considerably.[20]

20.6 Conclusion

With the increasing prevalence of flow diversion in the treatment of cerebral aneurysms, there is a distinct need for a better understanding of the hemodynamic effects flow diversion has on aneurysms and its relationship with future occlusion. As more information is gathered, practitioners will hopefully be able to better utilize this new tool, while engineers continue to improve on its design. Ultimately, the hope is to provide better patient care through a more complete understanding of this treatment modality.

References

[1] Lasheras JC. The biomechanics of arterial aneurysms. Annu Rev Fluid Mech. 2007; 39(1):293–319
[2] Roszelle BN, Gonzalez LF, Babiker MH, Ryan J, Albuquerque FC, Frakes DH. Flow diverter effect on cerebral aneurysm hemodynamics: an in vitro comparison of telescoping stents and the Pipeline. Neuroradiology. 2013; 55 (6):751–758
[3] Roszelle BN, Babiker MH, Hafner W, Gonzalez LF, Albuquerque FC, Frakes DH. In vitro and in silico study of intracranial stent treatments for cerebral aneurysms: effects on perforating vessel flows. J Neurointerv Surg. 2013; 5(4):354–360

[4] Dorn F, Niedermeyer F, Balasso A, Liepsch D, Liebig T. The effect of stents on intra-aneurysmal hemodynamics: in vitro evaluation of a pulsatile sidewall aneurysm using laser Doppler anemometry. Neuroradiology. 2011; 53 (4):267–272

[5] Lieber BB, Livescu V, Hopkins LN, Wakhloo AK. Particle image velocimetry assessment of stent design influence on intra-aneurysmal flow. Ann Biomed Eng. 2002; 30(6):768–777

[6] Ford MD, Nikolov HN, Milner JS, et al. PIV-measured versus CFD-predicted flow dynamics in anatomically realistic cerebral aneurysm models. J Biomech Eng. 2008; 130(2):021015

[7] Bouillot P, Brina O, Ouared R, Lovblad KO, Farhat M, Pereira VM. Particle imaging velocimetry evaluation of intracranial stents in sidewall aneurysm: hemodynamic transition related to the stent design. PLoS One. 2014; 9(12): e113762

[8] Adrian RJ, Westerweel J. Particle Image Velocimetry. Cambridge University Press; 2011

[9] Tang A, Chan H, Tsang A, et al. The effects of stent porosity on the endovascular treatment of intracranial aneurysms located near a bifurcation. J Biomed Sci Eng. 2013; 6:812–822

[10] Darsaut TE, Bing F, Salazkin I, Gevry G, Raymond J. Flow diverters can occlude aneurysms and preserve arterial branches: a new experimental model. AJNR Am J Neuroradiol. 2012; 33(10):2004–2009

[11] Trager AL, Sadasivan C, Lieber BB. Comparison of the in vitro hemodynamic performance of new flow diverters for bypass of brain aneurysms. J Biomech Eng. 2012; 134(8):084505–084505

[12] Tominaga R, Harasaki H, Sutton C, Emoto H, Kambic H, Hollman J. Effects of stent design and serum cholesterol level on the restenosis rate in atherosclerotic rabbits. Am Heart J. 1993; 126(5):1049–1058

[13] Chong W, Zhang Y, Qian Y, Lai L, Parker G, Mitchell K. Computational hemodynamics analysis of intracranial aneurysms treated with flow diverters: correlation with clinical outcomes. AJNR Am J Neuroradiol. 2014; 35(1):136–142

[14] Kojima M, Irie K, Fukuda T, Arai F, Hirose Y, Negoro M. The study of flow diversion effects on aneurysm using multiple enterprise stents and two flow diverters. Asian J Neurosurg. 2012; 7(4):159–165

[15] Ouared R, Larrabide I, Brina O, et al. Computational fluid dynamics analysis of flow reduction induced by flow-diverting stents in intracranial aneurysms: a patient-unspecific hemodynamics change perspective. J Neurointerv Surg. 2016:pii: neurintsurg-2015–012154. [Epub ahead of print]

[16] Kulcsár Z, Augsburger L, Reymond P, et al. Flow diversion treatment: intra-aneurismal blood flow velocity and WSS reduction are parameters to predict aneurysm thrombosis. Acta Neurochir (Wien). 2012; 154(10):1827–1834

[17] Cebral JR, Mut F, Raschi M, et al. Aneurysm rupture following treatment with flow-diverting stents: computational hemodynamics analysis of treatment. AJNR Am J Neuroradiol. 2011; 32(1):27–33

[18] Larrabide I, Aguilar ML, Morales HG, et al. Intra-aneurysmal pressure and flow changes induced by flow diverters: relation to aneurysm size and shape. AJNR Am J Neuroradiol. 2013; 34(4):816–822

[19] Shobayashi Y, Tateshima S, Kakizaki R, Sudo R, Tanishita K, Viñuela F. Intra-aneurysmal hemodynamic alterations by a self-expandable intracranial stent and flow diversion stent: high intra-aneurysmal pressure remains regardless of flow velocity reduction. J Neurointerv Surg. 2013; 5 Suppl 3:iii38–iii42

[20] Tremmel M, Xiang J, Natarajan SK, et al. Alteration of intra-aneurysmal hemodynamics for flow diversion using enterprise and vision stents. World Neurosurg. 2010; 74(2–3):306–315

[21] Schneiders JJ, Vanbavel E, Majoie CB, Ferns SP, van den Berg R. A flow-diverting stent is not a pressure-diverting stent. AJNR Am J Neuroradiol. 2013; 34 (1):E1–E4

[22] Hashimoto T, Meng H, Young WL. Intracranial aneurysms: links among inflammation, hemodynamics and vascular remodeling. Neurol Res. 2006; 28 (4):372–380

[23] Jou L-D, Lee DH, Morsi H, Mawad ME. Wall shear stress on ruptured and unruptured intracranial aneurysms at the internal carotid artery. AJNR Am J Neuroradiol. 2008; 29(9):1761–1767

[24] Shojima M, Oshima M, Takagi K, et al. Magnitude and role of wall shear stress on cerebral aneurysm: computational fluid dynamic study of 20 middle cerebral artery aneurysms. Stroke. 2004; 35(11):2500–2505

[25] Cebral JR, Mut F, Weir J, Putman CM. Association of hemodynamic characteristics and cerebral aneurysm rupture. AJNR Am J Neuroradiol. 2011; 32 (2):264–270

[26] Masuda H, Zhuang YJ, Singh TM, et al. Adaptive remodeling of internal elastic lamina and endothelial lining during flow-induced arterial enlargement. Arterioscler Thromb Vasc Biol. 1999; 19(10):2298–2307

[27] Meng H, Tutino VM, Xiang J, Siddiqui A. High WSS or low WSS? Complex interactions of hemodynamics with intracranial aneurysm initiation, growth, and rupture: toward a unifying hypothesis. AJNR Am J Neuroradiol. 2014; 35 (7):1254–1262

[28] Levitt MR, McGah PM, Aliseda A, et al. Cerebral aneurysms treated with flow-diverting stents: computational models with intravascular blood flow measurements. AJNR Am J Neuroradiol. 2014; 35(1):143–148

[29] Meng H, Wang Z, Kim M, Ecker RD, Hopkins LN. Saccular aneurysms on straight and curved vessels are subject to different hemodynamics: implications of intravascular stenting. AJNR Am J Neuroradiol. 2006; 27 (9):1861–1865

[30] Le TB, Troolin DR, Amatya D, Longmire EK, Sotiropoulos F. Vortex phenomena in sidewall aneurysm hemodynamics: experiment and numerical simulation. Ann Biomed Eng. 2013; 41(10):2157–2170

[31] Aenis M, Stancampiano AP, Wakhloo AK, Lieber BB. Modeling of flow in a straight stented and nonstented side wall aneurysm model. J Biomech Eng. 1997; 119(2):206–212

[32] Lieber BB, Stancampiano AP, Wakhloo AK. Alteration of hemodynamics in aneurysm models by stenting: influence of stent porosity. Ann Biomed Eng. 1997; 25(3):460–469

[33] Cantón G, Levy DI, Lasheras JC, Nelson PK. Flow changes caused by the sequential placement of stents across the neck of sidewall cerebral aneurysms. J Neurosurg. 2005; 103(5):891–902

[34] Xiang J, Damiano RJ, Lin N, et al. High-fidelity virtual stenting: modeling of flow diverter deployment for hemodynamic characterization of complex intracranial aneurysms. J Neurosurg. 2015; 123(4):832–840

[35] Kim M, Taulbee DB, Tremmel M, Meng H. Comparison of two stents in modifying cerebral aneurysm hemodynamics. Ann Biomed Eng. 2008; 36 (5):726–741

[36] Struffert T, Ott S, Kowarschik M, et al. Measurement of quantifiable parameters by time-density curves in the elastase-induced aneurysm model: first results in the comparison of a flow diverter and a conventional aneurysm stent. Eur Radiol. 2013; 23(2):521–527

[37] Cebral JR, Castro MA, Burgess JE, Pergolizzi RS, Sheridan MJ, Putman CM. Characterization of cerebral aneurysms for assessing risk of rupture by using patient-specific computational hemodynamics models. AJNR Am J Neuroradiol. 2005; 26(10):2550–2559

[38] Chiu J-J, Chen CN, Lee PL, et al. Analysis of the effect of disturbed flow on monocytic adhesion to endothelial cells. J Biomech. 2003; 36(12):1883–1895

[39] Nair P. Characterization of the Effects of Cerebral Aneurysm Geometry on Hemodynamics and Endovascular Treatment Outcomes. Arizona State University; 2016

21 FUTURE DEVELOPMENTS AND RESEARCH

ADAM S. ARTHUR, CHRISTOPHER NICKELE, and BRANDON BURNSED

Abstract

Novel flow diversion therapies on the horizon are an evolving brainstorm of multifaceted strategies to modify the treatment of cerebrovascular pathologies, generating new therapeutic options for the endovascular community. Favorable experiences within the peripheral world prompted biomechanical advances to facilitate the navigation of the tortuous cervicocerebral vasculature for device delivery. Limited off-label application of covered stents within the cerebrovasculature has shown reduced recanalization rates, creating opportunities for an innovative design tailored to treat specific pathologies.[1,2] Polymer coatings may be applied to cover the bare metal of stents, providing corrosion resistance and increased hydrophilicity among other favorable characteristics. Methods of coating and polymer selection are highly scrutinized variables in current research models targeted to promote neoepithelialization, while combating intimal hyperplasia and thrombogenicity.[3,4,5] Clinical demand to create a flow diversion model averse to thrombotic events, while averting the side effects of dual-antiplatelet therapy required for current models, has driven experimental designs that could potentially preclude the use of antiplatelet therapy.[6] Transitioning to state-of-the-art surface modifications, bioengineers are able to link polymers in a more favorable profile, and electropolish the flow diverter alloys improving their biocompatibility. Concerns of permanent metal constructs piloted the development of bioresorbable vascular scaffolds. Currently being evaluated in the cardiovascular trials, biodegradable vascular stents may have their place in cerebrovascular therapies.[7,8,9] Ultimately, today's flow diverters will be supplanted by a more-modern generation that promotes rapid vascular regenesis while providing bioresorbable capabilities with a low thrombogenic profile.

Keywords: bioresorbable stent, coated stent, covered stent, flow diverter

21.1 Introduction

Novel flow diversion therapies on the horizon are an evolving brainstorm of multifaceted strategies to modify the treatment of cerebrovascular pathologies, generating new therapeutic options for the endovascular community. Modifications of flow diversion are currently being tested in some cardiovascular trials with elegant, bioresorbable stent scaffoldings.[8,9] Additionally, stent coating alternatives and their method of application to the stent construct, techniques for corrosion prevention, enhanced lubricious coatings for improved delivery, and coating/surface modifications for reduced thrombogenesis are just a small example of current areas of study in the laboratory for improved in vivo tolerability.

21.2 Bioresorbable Stents

Interests in long-term effects of adverse complications associated with permanent metal stents have opened doors to investigation of bioresorbable scaffolds. Vascular tissue bioengineers have worked with multiple substrates, including decellularized constructs, natural polymers, and synthetic polymers. Neovessel generation with epithelialization across the extracellular matrix construct, while preserving mechanical strength of the native vessel, is one hurdle faced when considering in vivo applications.[10] Concern for small-vessel patency continues to be evaluated with experimental research progressing to the achievement of an engineered tissue model of a vascular scaffold suitable for smaller diameter vessels.

21.2.1 Decellularized Vascular Scaffolds

Laboratory animal models of decellularized vascular scaffolds have shown mixed results with reduced biodegradation rates and biocompatibility issues. The decellularization process can be performed in several different ways (chemical/detergent-based, mechanical abrasion, enzymatic catabolism, etc.), but the ultimate goal of the process is to maintain the extracellular matrix while reducing the immunogenicity of the scaffold. Studies have also attempted adding extracellular matrix components or endothelial progenitor cells to vascular scaffolds to promote rapid endothelialization, that is, human saphenous endothelial cells on a decellularized porcine aorta and hybridization of a polymer scaffold with human allogenic smooth muscle cells.[10] However, none of these models have been utilized in human cerebrovascular trials.

21.2.2 Polymer Vascular Scaffolds

Nondegradable Polymers

Expanded Teflon, ePTFE, and Dacron, polyethylene terephthalate (PET), have been used as vascular conduits for decades. The patency rate of ePTFE is more favorable due to its electronegative luminal surface, although the patency rate reduces as it is applied to vessels with smaller diameters.[10] While both ePTFE and PET alone have shown poor vascular regenesis, autologous endothelial cells have been harvested and applied with fibrin glue to luminal surfaces of ePTFE grafts with similar long-term patency results as autologous vein grafts.[11]

Natural Polymers

While naturally occurring extracellular membrane components have been investigated due to their biocompatibility, the biodegradation profile and mechanical properties of these components may raise some concern. Collagen as a vascular scaffold has several limitations. Its production is expensive and its mechanical properties may not withstand arterial loads. Furthermore, catabolism of collagen results in thrombogenic amino acids.[10] However, elastin has shown favor due its endothelial progenitor cell recruitment while abating hyperplasia.[12] Fibrin, which can be isolated from a patient's blood sample for autologous application, may demonstrate increased immunocompatability.[10] These, and other natural polymers, can be blended with synthetic polymers for a tailored scaffold amenable to restoration of the vessel wall.

Synthetic Polymers

Biodegradable vascular scaffolds have the mechanical profile suitable for the smaller diameter vessels commonly encountered in neurointerventional procedures. Fabricating a synthetic scaffold gives the tissue engineer the opportunity to alter the degradation process and mechanical properties of the substrate. Additionally, synthetic polymers have gained favor within the vascular tissue engineering field due to the revival of electrospinning. This process allows a micro- to nanoscale topographical arrangement of the extracellular matrix components and a large surface to volume ratio for attaching pharmaceuticals, natural polymers, proteins, nucleic acids, etc.[12] Although many synthetic polymers exist, the favorable degradation of a few polymers to the end-products of the Krebs cycle shows more favorable biodegradation profiles. A bioresorbable poly(L-lactide) semicrystalline polymer (PLLA) scaffolding with a poly(DL-lactide) coating (Absorb bioresorbable vascular scaffold, Abbott Vascular) is currently being evaluated in the ABSORB trials. The Absorb everolimus-eluting bioresorbable vascular scaffold was recently found to be within the prespecified range of noninferiority when compared to a cobalt-chromium, everolimus-eluting stent at the 1-year analysis for target-lesion failure.[9] Further long-term analysis is ongoing with the ABSORB IV trial.

21.3 Improved Delivery

Access burdens for distal pathologies within the cerebrovasculature brought bioengineers back to the drawing board to design devices that could manage the tortuosity and narrow lumens of vessels in need of repair. Not only has stent design technology improved, but the catheters and delivery apparatus used to deploy and capture the device at the targeted flow diversion site have also been modernized. As experience is gained with the current generation of flow diversion devices, collaborative efforts are once again creating the next delivery system on the horizon.

21.3.1 Lubricious Coatings

There is a shift toward enhanced lubricious coatings on catheters to maintain a reduced level of friction against the lumen wall of the vessel. Lower water droplet contact angles on the polymer surface are used to quantify the hydrophilicity of the coating membranes, while the amount and degree of friction are considered for the erosion of the polymer surface.[13] These advances, however, may not be without risk. Recently, postmortem analysis of three patients with lethal intraparenchymal hemorrhages after Pipeline Embolization Device treatment, revealed polyvinylpyrrolidone (PVP) deposition within the lumen of distal vessels in the region of the hemorrhage. The polymer compound identified in the specimen showed a similar spectroscopic absorption band profile as the PVP coating on the diagnostic and guide catheters.[14] Additionally, in vitro models comparing friction behavior in commercially available polymer Biogel coatings versus a coating of a biodegradable, natural polysaccharide with fatty acids has shown comparable results.[13]

Based on these studies, future changes in the lubricious coating of catheters may improve the safety and biocompatible profile of delivery systems.

21.3.2 Stent Technology Modifications

Navigating the tortuous anatomy to approach a cerebrovascular aneurysm requires a superelastic alloy that permits longitudinal flexibility for navigation, all the while maintaining shape memory for radial tension when deployed. The tendencies of device foreshortening or migration which can affect the optimal construct porosity upon deployment must also be considered. Braided stent designs have proven successful in the flow diversion model to mitigate the trade-off of reduced flexibility versus increased porosity. Shape memory alloys are frequently used for the braiding process due to their favorable radial tension features upon deployment. The braiding angle of the shape memory alloy wires determines the longitudinal flexibility as evidenced by increased stiffness at angles greater than 45 degrees for both 16- and 32-wire constructs.[15] Longitudinal flexibility can also be modified by altering longitudinal waves in a flow diverter braid, provoking creative flow diverter designs.[16] Thus, it is imperative to find a balance between flexibility, porosity, and radial tension to design a successful flow diverter.

21.4 Reduced Thrombogenesis

Thromboembolic phenomena are an unwelcome consequence in the setting of flow diversion. Bioengineering modifications to combat thrombogenic responses to endothelial damage require similar coating mechanisms as previously described. Multiple other attempts at reduction of thrombogenesis have been described in the literature with new techniques constantly evolving. As an example, innovative surface modifications have been developed to reduce thrombogenesis on the new generation of flow diverters.

Electropolishing of implanted vascular constructs has gained favor since the turn of the century. This process, applied to nitinol, has shown improved reduction of fibrin and thrombus deposition when compared to stainless steel in the absence of dual-antiplatelet therapy.[6] Modern adhesive techniques include chemical covalent bonding of surface phospholipids or glycosaminoglycans to improve biocompatibility and thwart thrombotic cascades. Covalent bonding appears to provide a thumbprint with a lower profile on the diverter surface when compared to alternative coating methods. This has been applied to the new Pipeline Flex with Shield Technology (Medtronic, Irvine, CA).[17] Phosphorylcholine, a phospholipid recognized on the surface of erythrocytes and many other cells, is covalently bonded to the surface of the Pipeline Flex diverter, reducing platelet adherence and thrombosis.[17] Heparin, a glycosaminoglycan with a significant negative charge density, has been used in a similar process to preserve patency in bypass circuits.

21.5 Conclusion

The continued excitement in research in device and delivery technology will hopefully lead to improved patient outcomes.

Ultimately, the prospect of a bioresorbable, flow diverting, vascular scaffold that provides rapid neoepithelialization and vascular regenesis with minimal thrombogenetic complications seems feasible in the future. With further experimentation and clinical trials, the new era of endovascular treatment of cerebrovascular pathology may lead to a tailoring of endovascular therapies targeted to the specific patient.

References

[1] Tan HQ, Li MH, Zhang PL, et al. Reconstructive endovascular treatment of intracranial aneurysms with the Willis covered stent: medium-term clinical and angiographic follow-up. J Neurosurg. 2011; 114(4):1014–1020

[2] Zhu YQ, Li MH, Lin F, et al. Frequency and predictors of endoleaks and long-term patency after covered stent placement for the treatment of intracranial aneurysms: a prospective, non-randomised multicentre experience. Eur Radiol. 2013; 23(1):287–297

[3] Parkinson RJ, Demers CP, Adel JG, et al. Use of heparin-coated stents in neurovascular interventional procedures: preliminary experience with 10 patients. Neurosurgery. 2006; 59(4):812–821, discussion 821

[4] Komatsu R, Ueda M, Naruko T, Kojima A, Becker AE. Neointimal tissue response at sites of coronary stenting in humans: macroscopic, histological, and immunohistochemical analyses. Circulation. 1998; 98(3):224–233

[5] Jamshidi P, Mahmoody K, Erne P. Covered stents: a review. Int J Cardiol. 2008; 130(3):310–318

[6] Thierry B, Merhi Y, Bilodeau L, Trépanier C, Tabrizian M. Nitinol versus stainless steel stents: acute thrombogenicity study in an ex vivo porcine model. Biomaterials. 2002; 23(14):2997–3005

[7] Mauri L, Kereiakes DJ, Yeh RW, et al. DAPT Study Investigators. Twelve or 30 months of dual antiplatelet therapy after drug-eluting stents. N Engl J Med. 2014; 371(23):2155–2166

[8] Ormiston JA, Serruys PW, Onuma Y, et al. First serial assessment at 6 months and 2 years of the second generation of absorb everolimus-eluting bioresorbable vascular scaffold: a multi-imaging modality study. Circ Cardiovasc Interv. 2012; 5(5):620–632

[9] Ellis SG, Kereiakes DJ, Metzger DC, et al. ABSORB III Investigators. Everolimus-eluting bioresorbable scaffolds for coronary artery disease. N Engl J Med. 2015; 373(20):1905–1915

[10] Thottappillil N, Nair PD. Scaffolds in vascular regeneration: current status. Vasc Health Risk Manag. 2015; 11:79–91

[11] Deutsch M, Meinhart J, Zilla P, et al. Long-term experience in autologous in vitro endothelialization of infrainguinal ePTFE grafts. J Vasc Surg. 2009; 49(2):352–362, discussion 362

[12] Sill TJ, von Recum HA. Electrospinning: applications in drug delivery and tissue engineering. Biomaterials. 2008; 29(13):1989–2006

[13] Niemczyk A, El Fray M, Franklin SE. Friction behaviour of hydrophilic lubricious coatings for medical device applications. Tribol Int. 2015; 89:54–61

[14] Hu YC, Deshmukh VR, Albuquerque FC, et al. Histopathological assessment of fatal ipsilateral intraparenchymal hemorrhages after the treatment of supraclinoid aneurysms with the Pipeline Embolization Device. J Neurosurg. 2014; 120(2):365–374

[15] Kim JH, Kang TJ, Yu WR. Mechanical modeling of self-expandable stent fabricated using braiding technology. J Biomech. 2008; 41(15):3202–3212

[16] Ma J, You Z, Peach T, Byrne J, Rizkallah RR. A new flow diverter stent for direct treatment of intracranial aneurysm. J Biomech. 2015; 48(16):4206–4213

[17] Girdhar G, Li J, Kostousov L, Wainwright J, Chandler WL. In-vitro thrombogenicity assessment of flow diversion and aneurysm bridging devices. J Thromb Thrombolysis. 2015; 40(4):37–443

Index